STRETCHING THE LIMITS

Lee Torrey

STRETCHING THE LIMITS

Breakthroughs In Sports Science That Create Superathletes

DODD, MEAD & COMPANY

NEW YORK

To the South Street Stars
for incredible half-time entertainment

Published by Dodd, Mead & Company, Inc.
79 Madison Avenue, New York, N.Y. 10016
Distributed in Canada by
McClelland and Stewart Limited, Toronto
Manufactured in the United States of America
Designed by Tom Mellers

First Edition

Library of Congress Cataloging-in-Publication Data

Torrey, Lee.
Stretching the limits.

Bibliography: p.
Includes index.
1. Sports—Physiological aspects. 2. Athletes—
Physiology. 3. Sporting goods. I. Title.
RC1235.T67 1985   796'.01'5   85-15866
ISBN 0-396-08585-7

CONTENTS

v

CONTENTS

LIST OF FIGURES

ACKNOWLEDGMENTS

Art: Arti Torrance with Grover Freedman.

Research: Gail E. Santarelli.

Research assistants: Paulo Albuquerque, Ann Monteith.

Editorial assistants: Jackie Jordan, Patrick Lions.

Sources: The following people granted interviews or supplied materials to the author or his staff: A. Terry Bahill, University of Arizona; Arthur M. Bernhang, Stony Brook Medical Center; Howard Brody, University of Pennsylvania; George A. Brooks, University of California, Berkeley; Peter Cavanagh, Pennsylvania State University; Kenneth C. Clark, director of sports medicine at the Olympic Training Center (OTC), Colorado Springs; Charles A. Czeisler, Harvard Medical School; Charles J. Dillman, director of the biomechanics lab, OTC; Byron Donzis, American Pneumatics Company, Houston; Herbert Fensterheim, Cornell University; Nancy Greer, University of Massachusetts; Voight R. Hodgson, Wayne State University; Tzu C. Huang, University of Wisconsin; Ernst Jokl, University of Kentucky; Aladar Kogler, Columbia University; Daniel Landers, Arizona State University; Rick McKinney, Arizona State University; Richard C. Nelson, Pennsylvania State University; Stephen Reid, Northwestern University; Elizabeth Roberts, University of Wisconsin; Steve Sagedahl, University of Minnesota; Ron Stratton, Childrens Medical Center, Tulsa; Richard M. Suinn, Colorado State University; Peter VanHandle, director of the physiology lab, OTC.

Special contributors: The following gave support and advice and many provided valuable information: Tom Cunningham; Leslie D'Angelo; Scott DeGarmo; Jerry Gross, my editor at Dodd, Mead; Ken Halpern; Ron Kaplan, *South Street Star;* Philip Katz, First Capital Press; Harold D. Kemp, Sports Equipment, Inc; Ronald F. Lochocki, Kistler Corporation; René Long; Michael Marten,

Science Photo Library; George Quinn, for insights about the sedentary life; Jim Reed, Transkinetics Telemetry Systems; the staff of J. C. Dobbs; Full-Year Shuen; my agent Nat Sobel; Peter G. Stide, Nike, Inc; Stanley Torrey; John Trux.

STRETCHING THE LIMITS

INTRODUCTION

In sports as in biology, new phenomena will arise unexpect-
edly, shatter our perception of what is normal, and con-
stantly surprise us about the ability of the human body to
adapt and excel.
                              —Ernst Jokl
                              University of Kentucky physiologist

In the late 1940s it was commonly believed that running a
mile in less than four minutes was beyond human capability.
It was an insuperable physiological barrier, an absolute limit to
human performance.

A few people, however, felt this athletic miracle might just
be possible and sat down to calculate the theoretical conditions under which such a race might occur. This embryonic
group of sports scientists included a physician, a physiologist,
a psychologist, a few trainers, and a meteorologist.

After much consultation the experts concluded the event
would happen in Scandinavia, where it was thought that higher
levels of ozone would give the new athletic hero an extra lift, a
theory still in dispute. They said the wind would be still, the
temperature moderate, the race would be held on a dry track
to the cheers of a large, ecstatic crowd, and most important,
the athlete would exercise cautious pacing, slowly increasing
his speed, lap after grueling lap.

In 1954, Roger Bannister ran right over those predictions on
a wet cinder track in a chilly 15-mph wind before only a handful of restrained spectators in Oxford, England—running suc-
cessively *slower* laps on his way to the tape.

Despite the embarrassing miscalculation, this early collaboration of experts was a sign of dramatic changes in the scientific study of sports. The end of World War II allowed scientists to resume freewheeling inquiry into the nature of man
and the world. The reopening of national borders was paralleled by the renewed exchange of scientific information on an

international level. Research once classified now circulated freely. The result was a spectacular information explosion in all fields of endeavor.

Borrowing extensively from this wealth of information outside their own discipline, biologists began to draw a new portrait of the athlete: performance could no longer be defined or predicted solely by the internal functions of respiration and locomotion. External factors such as the design of stadiums, the weather, the number of spectators and their level of enthusiasm, the physical properties of sports equipment, even the time of day all had potential impacts—for better or worse—on how far, fast, or high the body would soar.

The end of the war, along with improvements in communication and transportation, brought more athletes to competition than at any other point in history. By 1960, advances in training techniques and equipment design, coupled with the burgeoning number of new athletes, led to what the popular press described as a "performance revolution." The turnover of athletic records soon acquired a rhythmic transience, prompting British middle-distance runner Sebastian Coe to observe that "world records are only borrowed." As records remained in flux, the limits of human performance defied definition. No one could pinpoint the absolute limits in any sport—and those who dared guess would soon be as embarrassed as those who confidently predicted that the mile could not be run in under four minutes.

Bannister's 3:59.4 mile is run routinely today, and it's not uncommon to witness a race in which the last-place finisher comes in at 3:55. In fact, New Zealand Olympian John Walker and U.S. mile record holder Steve Scott have both run the sub-four-minute mile 100 times.

Over 1,500 years ago, the original marathon was run by a single Greek messenger. Today, a million Americans can run the 26 miles, and as many as 100,000 do so competitively every year.

The implication is not just that elite athletes are bettering each other year after year, but that the general level of fitness and performance for *all* athletes has risen at a commensurable pace. Indeed, an argument can be made that the health and fitness of the human population as a whole improves at the rate at which champions set new records.

2

INTRODUCTION

At every distance, races are now being run at average speeds that are from 4 to 10 percent faster than in Bannister's day. But even more dramatic than the increase in speed is the increase in endurance. Top runners can now go up to twice as far at a given average speed as they did in the 1950s. The 10,000-meter run is now being covered at an average speed of just over 13.5 mph, the same average speed that was used to set the record at 5,000 meters in 1957. This constitutes a 100 percent increase in endurance at this speed—a remarkable achievement reflecting a doubling of the efficiency at which the human body can move.

Improvements in running performance are the easiest to quantify due to the large number of events of varying speeds and distances, but progress on the track has been matched in almost every other major sport. Proficiency in golf is measured by a player's stroke average for 18 holes, and the lowest in twenty years was set in 1980 by Lee Trevino's 69.7. In ice hockey, Wayne Gretzky eclipsed the eleven-year-old goal-scoring record by 21 percent in 1982 with 92 goals in one season. In football, Walter Payton broke Jim Brown's 12,312-yard career-rushing total in 1984, a record that stood unchallenged for nineteen years. The list is endless.

What makes these improvements possible? To what extent can science and technology be credited?

A few years ago, Gideon Ariel, a biomechanist who works with U.S. Olympians and has introduced computer technology to many sports, looked into these questions with an interesting experiment comparing the performance of past and present track stars. He began by analyzing the track films and race times of Olympic sprinter Jim Hines, who set a world record of 9.95 seconds for the 100-meter sprint in 1968, and then did the same for Jesse Owens, who clocked 10.3 seconds for the same distance in the 1936 Olympics. The data on both athletes were fed into a computer loaded with a special program that could simulate an imaginary 100-meter race under contemporary conditions. Ariel ran the program, pitting Hines against Owens— and they both broke the tape at the same instant, matching the current world record. Owens gained almost a half second over his 1936 time because, according to the computer analysis, fifty years ago he didn't have sprinters' starting blocks and the tracks didn't have the favorable rebounding characteristics of modern track surfaces. In other words, even without the benefits of modern training, if Jesse Owens were alive and in his prime today he'd perform better simply because of advances in sports technology.

High technology began to invade sports during the 1970s, and today its influence is pervasive. No athletic endeavor has been untouched by miniaturized electronics or advanced materials engineering. The simple stopwatches and barometers of Bannister's day have evolved into a sophisticated realm of wind tunnels, high-speed video, computer graphics, strain gauges, oscilloscopes, and treadmills equipped with sensors to monitor the respiration, heart rate, muscle activity, and metabolism of an athlete. Complex predictions of an individual's time to exhaustion and a multivariable analysis of the efficiency of his limb motions are commonplace.

Outside the sports lab, athletes can be wired with remote telemetry systems to monitor any physiological function under actual field conditions. Lightweight protective equipment made from a wide range of new shock-absorbing materials is reducing injuries in contact sports. Athletic shoes and even the fabrics used in playing uniforms are designed by computers, which balance such factors as durability against heat retention.

It often seems that world-class amateur and professional athletes are getting the same kind of high-tech attention once reserved for astronauts. In fact, one of the motivating forces behind this development was a "sputnik effect" in amateur sports. At the end of the 1976 Olympics, the Russians went home with more gold than any other country, and East Germany didn't trail far behind in second place. This fact underscored the complaints lodged for years by U.S. athletes that competitors from the Soviet Union and East Europe were enjoying an unfair advantage because of their advanced sports technology. Not to be outdone, the U.S. Olympic Committee put together a multimillion-dollar sports science program of their own in 1981, and the knowledge from their research has trickled down to every type of athletic activity.

Performance has been affected by new technology in two ways. First, more is accomplished in an event due to direct energy contributions from the equipment itself. In pole vaulting,

4

the additional lift of the new fiberglass pole increased world records by 9 inches in the year it was introduced—a gain that had taken twenty years to accomplish with aluminum and bamboo poles. The introduction of the aluminum baseball bat has had a similar effect on the national pastime. These metal weapons launch a baseball about 4 mph faster than wooden bats, a difference that corresponds to a 10 percent increase in the distance the ball travels. Since the aluminum bat would ultimately destroy the sacred batting averages of the immortals enshrined in the Hall of Fame, it was outlawed by major league clubs, but it is used widely by university and amateur teams and was sanctioned by the International Olympic Committee for use in the 1984 Games in Los Angeles.

The second contribution of the new technology is as an adjunct to training. The ability to make multiple observations of an athlete in practice, and simultaneously process and display the information, provides that athlete with a quick, objective tool to attain his training goals. Trial and error have been virtually eliminated from training. A video camera, for example, can record a player kicking a football, its electronic signal digitized—converted into numbers a computer can digest—and a computer-generated "stick man" will appear on the monitor along with the usual video image. If the kicker had an inefficient motion, that problem could be isolated on the screen in about the time it takes the ball to reach the goalposts. Accessories such as pressure platforms, which measure shifts in body weight, can be used in tandem with video analysis to provide even more information. Add electromyleograph (EMG) sensors to the kicker's legs and the storm of electrochemical activity inside his muscles can also be measured and integrated into his performance profile. All this information can be stored on tape and used later to review progress, help bust slumps, or teach other would-be punters.

The major advantage of portable, high-speed training equipment is that it provides *instant* feedback, which is essential in acquiring motor skills. In the wake of any physical activity, sense organs in the muscles transmit information to the brain, subjectively perceived as how the movement "feels." Known as the proprioceptive trace, this sensation is weak and usually fades within 30 seconds. If an athlete can obtain feedback on his actions before the feeling dissipates, studies have shown a motor skill can be learned faster and the ability to recall it is greatly enhanced.

In many respects, technological changes in sports have had a more profound effect on beginners and athletes of intermediate skill than on world-class professionals. The oversize Prince tennis racket, with its larger face and "sweet spot," is more forgiving than conventional rackets if the ball is hit off center—a common mistake of novices—whereas John McEnroe or Jimmy Connors will probably fare just as well with any style of racket. Computer analysis of a baseball lineup can provide a rookie manager with information he may lack from experience, but Billy Martin was known to come up with baseball strategies seconds before the Yankee's computer terminal. The net effect is that sports invested with a high level of technology are more accessible to nonathletes, novices, and challengers. Greater accessibility attracts more public interest and new players, increasing the size of the talent pool from which more and better champions should emerge.

Despite the visibility of the new sports technology, the principle force behind the sustained improvement in athletic performance comes from new forms of training.

When analysts note that athletes can now run twice as far at the same speed as their counterparts thirty years ago, the degree of improvement is far greater than that wrought by technology alone. Something has happened inside the human body that is unrelated to external improvements in the design of running shoes or the elasticity of track surfaces. If we could go back in time some thirty years and subject runners to the training techniques used today, chances are they too could go twice as far at the same speed, even if they were still to run on cinder tracks in canvas sneakers.

The essence of all training is to induce an adaptive change in the body. Stress a muscle hard enough and its fibers will swell in size; progressively increase the stress, and they will grow even larger—the most common effect of strength training. Push a distance runner until he runs out of breath, and adaptations begin to arise in the heart, lungs, and circulation—functional alterations that occur only as a result of endurance training. In this sense, an athlete is literally reshaping himself for his sport, sculpting microscopic changes in millions of cells, which will yield macroscopic changes in the structure and function of his body.

Because adaptations mirror the stress that provokes them, they are said to be "training specific." An outfielder who wants to make it with a major league ball club, but hasn't enough punch in his bat, must do more than simply increase the size and strength of the muscles in his torso and arms; he has to strengthen them with exercises that come as close as possible to simulating the swinging of a baseball bat. Huge muscles are useless to a would-be slugger if they don't contract fast and forcefully, in a coordinated sequence, moving the arms along the specific range of motion used in batting.

Adaptation is never limited to building bigger hearts or biceps. For every adaptation, there is a ripple effect that pervades every physiological system remotely associated with the tissues being stressed. Body builder Lou Ferrigno is unquestionably stronger than tennis star John McEnroe, but McEnroe has a stronger service, backhand, and forehand than Ferrigno, and it's much more than technique. Through constant use, the adaptations in McEnroe's arms provide him not with bulkier muscles, but with muscles that contract faster and more forcefully than the body builder's in motions involved in wielding a racket.

The modern realization of the precise specificity of adaptive changes in an athlete has led to a revolution in training techniques and technology. The fashionable practice of carbohydrate depletion and loading to enhance endurance in events such as the marathon is based on an adaptation inside muscles that are starving for fuel. When an athlete eats a very low-carbohydrate diet while maintaining a high level of exercise, his active muscles begin to manufacture extra enzymes that cause an increase in the storage of glycogen, a basic fuel of muscle contraction. Then, if he reverses the process by stuffing himself with complex carbohydrates, which are broken down and overstocked in the muscles by the increased enzyme activity, he can time it just right so his muscles are maximally loaded with fuel to provide him with more energy on the day of the race.

It seems that for every conceivable contingency there is an

adaptive response, and sports scientists are constantly looking for new ways to fool the body into using these adaptations by creating spurious emergencies. It is well known, for example, that when alpine climbers ascend above 10,000 feet, the shortage of oxygen in the air stimulates an increased production of red blood cells, which carry oxygen from the lungs to tissues. Researchers are now searching for the most effective method of eliciting this response to high altitudes with the hope of giving endurance athletes more oxygen-carrying capacity and thus better performance at sea level. At a laboratory at Harvard Medical School, athletes are kept awake for 24 to 48 hours while exercising. Physicians take regular samples of their blood and saliva, and analyze them for changes—on the order of billionths of a gram—in the levels of key hormones. This research, funded in part by the U.S. Olympic Committee, is the stuff breakthroughs are made of. The goal is to assess the body's adaptations to changes in time zones, daily cycles, and sleep to see if they can be manipulated to the athlete's advantage. The name of this field, chronobiology, may sound like science fiction, but to those involved in this work, "time stressing" may become a practical tool in future training programs.

Of course, some discoveries and innovations have been abused, and sports scientists are often blamed, although they are seldom responsible for an athlete's ultimate use of their work. Blood doping received widespread publicity after it was disclosed that seven members of the U.S. Olympic cycling team—including four medalists—had received extra blood through transfusions during the 1984 Games. This practice was unheard of before 1975, when Swedish physiologist Bjorn Ekblom announced that tests of the procedure gave athletes a 25 percent increase in endurance, due to the greater number of red blood cells to carry oxygen. Ekblom has recently disassociated himself from the controversy, saying that his discovery was the result of basic research, and that no one can foresee how some individuals might use freely available information to cheat.

Many athletes appear to be all too willing to try anything to gain an edge over the competition. It's no secret that professional football players take amphetamines to increase strength and aggression, or that major league baseball players have hollowed out their bats to hit balls faster and farther. Less known

8

and more dangerous is the surreptitious testing of substances by a very small number of ambitious amateur athletes. One physician reported that three weight lifters had injected a dangerous mix of hormones because they had *heard* that the procedure was effective for adding bulk to domestic cattle.

Despite the media coverage of the abuses and controversy associated with a few discoveries, the benefits from the sports lab greatly exceed the detriments. In sports medicine alone, countless lives and injuries have been spared because researchers have taken an active role in investigating the effectiveness of safety equipment and making recommendations to further protect the athlete's body from the punishing collisions that occur in football, ice hockey, and boxing.

Indeed, the willingness of athletes "to try anything" has actually led to phenomenal gains in the health and well-being of the general population. From one perspective, the athlete can be seen as someone who has donated himself to be an experimental prototype, a biological test pilot, stretching the known limits and tolerances of the human anatomy and physiology, ostensibly for his own personal gain, but ultimately the products of his endeavor are shared by all. In recent years, exercise physiologists have discovered that some of the training programs used by endurance athletes can be adapted for use by anyone to *reverse the effects of aging*—a breathtaking idea. Research with scuba divers has led to a form of medical therapy known as hyperbaric oxygenation, where oxygen is administered to patients at pressures many times higher than occur at sea level, a procedure that has been found effective for treating infections in burn patients and has been used experimentally for victims of cancer or strokes.

Sports psychology has made similar advances, transforming the aggression that surfaces naturally in many contact sports—as it does with the general population—into a purposeful and constructive energy source to enhance performance. The techniques pioneered by athletes to acquire a perfect state of relaxation and concentration under pressure have wide application outside the sports arena.

The collaboration of science and sports has also helped alter social perceptions about race, sex, and age. Fifty years ago, Jesse Owens, like many other black and minority athletes, struggled to the top solely on the basis of his courage and God-given talents, and finally dismayed Hitler during the Berlin Olympics when he won three gold medals, proving that Aryans were not the world's superior race. Today, research has accelerated the acceptance and integration of almost every segment of the population into sports, by clearly and objectively demonstrating the essential biological equality of all people. As recently as the 1970s, women and children were deemed to be unsuited for vigorous physical exercise: the thought of training a six-month-old infant to swim was as shocking as a woman daring to enter the Boston Marathon. That has all changed. By the turn of the century, some analysts expect women to equal or even surpass men's records in several sports. Adolescents are seen in many sports beating players ten or fifteen years older, and wheelchairs are a common sight in many marathons.

All the advances seen on and off the field are not the result of breakthroughs in any particular branch of science as much as the result of the integration of over a dozen disciplines under the loose heading of sports science. In some cases, researchers, who traditionally have little to do with athletics, make substantial contributions to athletic performance. Mechanical engineers, architects, and physicists can be found visiting the modern sports lab, working next to physiologists, physicians, and psychologists. In fact, at present there are no degrees to be earned or jobs to be filled under the specific heading of sports science. The term may be something of a misnomer, but it remains useful to explore how separate sciences pool their resources in the service of sports. In the future, it's entirely possible that the scientific investigation and management of athletes may revert to more familiar hands. According to Irving Dardik, director of sports medicine for the U.S. Olympic Committee, "Athletics is science in action and one day all coaches will be scientists."

The purpose of this book is to give athletes and nonathletes, scientists and nonscientists, an overview of how these diverse disciplines fit together to shape the present and future state of sports. Instead of organizing the material under the traditional headings, such as biomechanics or sports medicine, the contribution of each field is presented in relation to some of the most popular sports in North America. For those who wish to pursue the progress in only one field of research, there is an index and a bibliography, and cross-references appear throughout the text.

Each chapter has been designed to look at various aspects of sports science through the performance of particular athletes, such as the physiology involved in a touchdown run by John Riggins, the explosive physics of Arnold Palmer's full-shot swing, and the graceful biomechanics behind Wayne Gretzky's skating and shooting skills. The idea is to build a cumulative profile of "championship material" in *human* as well as scientific terms.

If there is a real danger in applying science to sports, it's not in the occasional discovery of techniques like blood doping, but rather in the possibility of digitizing the flair, beauty, and guts of athletes like the "stick men" on a computer screen. To preserve the vitality of sports, it's absolutely essential that we don't allow the scientific quantification of athletes to obscure their qualities as human beings. An overly mechanical, manipulative approach to sports will only backfire: performance will decline, and such abuses as blood doping will seem like innocence itself. But there's a better reason not to dehumanize the athlete: the roots of sports extend back beyond the dawn of civilization. It's a social activity as old and universal as religion, and perhaps much more fundamental to our existence than science.

Human beings are a playful species. Whether on the field, on the bleachers, or at home watching a game on television, we derive a great deal of joy and amusement from sports. It's more than the competitive spirit of an event that attracts us. It's the sheer amazement and wonder we feel when we see the human body twisting and contorting itself beyond what anyone thought possible the day before. In the modern arena, advances in training and technology have created much of that magic, and an appreciation of the science behind a champion's performance can only enhance our enjoyment of his triumph.

We should always remember, however, that the triumph is entirely of his own making.

ONE

FOOTBALL

Rushing on the Computerized Gridiron

An athletic spectacle occurred on January 30, 1983, that smashed records, electrified millions of fans across America, and gave the Washington Redskins their first world championship in forty years.

In the Rose Bowl, set like a jewel at the foot of the mountains in Pasadena, California, John Riggins ran with the ball 38 times, gained 166 yards, and in the longest touchdown run from the line of scrimmage in Super Bowl history, rolled through the Miami defenders like a locomotive, covering the 43 yards to the end zone in just under 6 seconds.

The pivotal play that put the Redskins in front of Miami for the first time in the game and settled Super Bowl XVII occurred in the fourth quarter. Redskins quarterback Joe Theismann had a drive going until he tried to throw a deep downfield pass, which was intercepted. When the Skins got the ball back, 11:43 remained on the clock. They rushed three times for a gain of over 9 yards and on the fourth down at the Miami 43-yard line with inches to go, the Dolphins called a time out.

When they returned to the field, the entire Miami squad assembled in a virtual goal-line defense, with ten players close to the line of scrimmage, forming a wall to deprive Washington of the first down (see *Fig. 1.1*). Only cornerback Don McNeal had any substantial depth behind the wall, allowing him to maneuver against anyone breaking through for a pass. But everyone in the stadium, and everyone watching at home, expected a

FIGURE 1.1

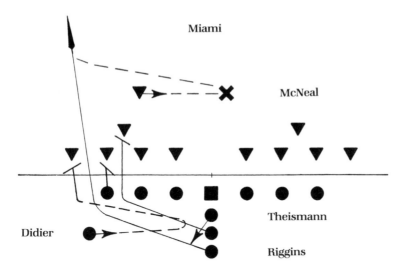

Miami

McNeal

Theismann

Didier

Riggins

"It's just a basic short-yardage play." That's how fullback John Riggins described the Redskins' rushing pattern called the 70-Chip—which turned out to be the longest touchdown run from the line of scrimmage in Super Bowl history.

Crowded along their own 43-yard line in a fourth down, inches-to-go situation, Miami's defense was designed to deprive Washington of a first down. Only cornerback Don McNeal had any distance behind the wall of Dolphins. He might have been able to contain Riggins, except that he shifted toward the center of the field as he followed Redskins receiver Clint Didier's zoom fake, slipping on the turf during the about-face.

Meanwhile Riggins took the ball from quarterback Joe Thiesmann, broke through the Dolphins defenders being blocked by his linemen, and by the time McNeal was on him, the burly fullback had only to shove off the tackle and sprint to the end zone.

Washington won the game, 27–17.

handoff to Riggins, who had now gained over 100 yards in the game.

Theismann didn't disappoint them. He took the snap and placed it in the hands of his 235-pound fullback, who charged to the left, looking for a hole in the Miami defense. A split second earlier, Redskins receiver Clint Didier dashed from the left end of the line toward the center and then abruptly turned around and retraced his steps, a maneuver the Redskins called a "zoom fake." The effect was to make Miami's McNeal follow Didier toward the center, drawing the only man deep behind the Dolphin defense away from the area Riggins intended to penetrate.

The zoom fake worked better than anticipated: McNeal slipped on the turf as he attempted to keep up with Didier's about-face. Riggins rushed between two Miami defenders being blocked by his offensive linemen, the incredible Hogs, and by the time McNeal was on him, Riggins had the momentum. With hardly a break in his stride, he brushed off the tackle and began pounding the turf.

In the next few seconds, within 16 strides, he'd be in the end zone. In these short moments, his heart beat only 10 times, but 434 muscles were saturated with over 1,000 milliliters of blood, fueling over 4 billion microscopic muscle fiber contractions. Countless nerve cells were telegraphing chemical messages at the speed of 300 feet per second from the brain to the spinal cord to every extremity and back again. Hormones were mobilized. Metabolism increased and body temperature was elevated. Trillions of molecules were dissolving and recombining to produce more than 7,000 watts of power.

Of course, the burly fullback was aware of only one thing. Eleven angry men from Miami were in pursuit, keen to mash him into the earth if he gave them a chance. And he didn't. Dolphin safety Glenn Blackwood came the closest to Riggins before he scored—almost 15 yards.

Riggins, like every other athlete and spectator, takes the internal flurry of biological activity for granted. It's impossible for the human mind to comprehend the sheer number of chemical transactions taking place during exercise or rest, and certainly there's no way to directly control them. As long as everything is working smoothly and painlessly, people seldom think about their bodies. Yet the shuffle of microscopic particles inside the human body is where sports science acquires the fundamental knowledge so essential to understanding and improving performance on the field.

Increasing the speed of a running back, the momentum of a lineman, or the agility of a receiver requires cunning manipulation of body chemistry. Stressing key muscle fibers stimulates the intricate assembly of specific chains of molecules, a phenomenally complicated process known to players simply as "more strength" or "bulking up." In training sessions, certain leg muscles can be forced to contract faster than they ever could on their own, modifying the electrical properties of a network of nerve cells to pass a billionth of a gram of the right chemical to each other, fractions of a millisecond faster. As a result, the rate of muscle contraction is set higher, providing greater speed on the field.

An athletic trainer may not fit the image of a gentlemanly scientist, but he most definitely is a chemist.

STRENGTH TRAINING FOR THE RUSH

Whereas the quarterback tends to be glorified as the modern star of the game, it's the running back who is the classic hero of football. The roots of this sport stretch back to 1823, when an English soccer player named William Ellis, frustrated because he was unable to get a good foot on the ball, picked it up and ran to the goal. His impulsive act at Rugby College gave birth to the sport of the same name. In the 1860s, Americans mixed soccer and rugby, added a few innovations of their own, and created football. For the next four decades the sport remained a rushing game, the ball carrier its star. Forward passing wasn't legal until the 1930s, when several rule changes opened the game up to pass plays and strategies, which today are profusely exploited by quarterbacks. In recent history, only the Chicago Bears and the Los Angeles Rams have accrued more rushing than passing yardage.

Making the legs of a running back move more powerfully and quickly has always been a central feature of football training. Running flat out or blasting through the defense with sheer power, dodging, darting, leaping like a gymnast—these have been the hallmarks of every great running back from Bronko Nagurski, Jim Brown, Larry Csonka to O. J. Simpson and Walter Payton. Those who followed Riggins's eleven-year history in the National Football League (NFL) saw him practice and compete in sprints; but they also knew he had the potential to become one of the great running backs.

After the Super Bowl victory over Miami, Redskins general manager Bobby Beathart recalled watching Riggins compete in a professional 40-yard dash back in the 1970s when he was playing with the New York Jets. He ran against Larry Brunson of the Denver Broncos and Cliff Branch of the Oakland Raiders, two of the fastest men in the NFL, and shot-putter Brian Oldfield. Riggins was wearing suspenders, black socks, and striped Olympic Speedo swim trunks. Although he didn't look like a serious contender, he beat Oldfield by a lot and wasn't far behind Branch and Brunson. His time was 4.6 seconds. Not bad, considering the world record at that time for the 100 meters (109 yards) was 9.9 seconds.

Curious about how Riggins trained to obtain this kind of speed, Beathart later watched him at the Redskins' training camp. After he'd finished his morning workout, Riggins would strip down to shorts and track shoes and run quarter-mile intervals. He'd run one, then jog one, and run the next even faster. "I started timing him," said Beathart. "He was running 10 quarters in under 75 seconds each, an incredible pace."

As football has evolved, so has the science of rushing. Players may still push themselves with quarter-mile runs, but today they can choose from a wide selection of more effective techniques.

For the first hundred years of the game, training consisted primarily of general conditioning, ball handling, running patterns, sprint drills and the inevitable laps around the field. The legs of "galloping ghost" Red Grange or Bronko Nagurski, who used to plow the hard Minnesota soil *without a horse*, were considered a natural endowment, a God-given talent that could not be significantly enhanced. "Tampering" with these skills was liable to backfire, especially when coaches, who may have known the game inside out, knew very little about the effects of training on the human body. This may seem unbelievable today, with NFL clubs spending millions of dollars on high-tech gadgets to improve strength, speed, agility, flexibility, and balance, but in 1970 most professional teams did not even have simple weight-lifting programs.

"Back in the 1960s and '70s, there was an attitude that guys who lifted weights all the time were a little bit strange," says Stan Jones, defensive line coach of the Denver Broncos. "There are still some coaches around the league with a bias against weight lifters, but they are a dwindling breed."

Running backs and receivers in particular were advised against weight lifting because coaches mistakenly thought it made a player tight. If a body was tight, speed was diminished. This notion was gradually dispelled by two observations. First, Olympic sprinters had been using weight lifting for many years and continued to set new world records; second, players who had greater muscle mass had consistently fewer injuries and thus longer careers—which really drove the point home in terms of the longevity of their salaries and contracts.

Today, progressive coaches believe the key to improving explosive power in a pair of legs is to use carefully designed training cycles, consisting of weight lifting; flexibility exercises, such as passive stretching; speed training; and a form of ballistic exercise known as *plyometrics*, building leg muscles through repetitive long jumps, triple jumps, and hurdle hops.

Plyometric exercises strengthen the muscle responsible for an athlete's vertical jumping ability, which is linked to his explosive acceleration as a sprinter. These exercises work by suddenly loading a muscle and forcing it to stretch before it can contract and elicit movement. The simplest example is jumping backward from an elevated box onto the ground, rapidly absorbing the load as the legs struggle to rebound back to the box again.

In a twelve-week test of the effectiveness of adding plyometrics to conventional training at the University of Maryland, football players shaved an average of 30 seconds off their 1.5 mile run, 2 seconds off a 30-yard cone sprint (which tests the ability and speed at which players can change direction), and increased the maximum weight they could lift in a parallel squat by 16 pounds.

Trainers refer to the *overload principle* when they devise strategies to apply sufficient stress to specific muscles to produce greater strength and speed. In sprint training, muscles respond to overloads in two ways: they undergo *hypertrophy*, or grow larger, and they recruit more of their constituent muscle fibers to contract together. In the locker room, the new guy who's slow and uncoordinated is often ridiculed because of deficiencies in his motor skills. But his condition is not terminal: proper training will eventually induce the thousands of individual fibers in each muscle to pull together at about the same time, making each physical motion faster, stronger, and surer. Many players think of strength training only in terms of hypertrophy, equating increases in girth with increases in performance; but for rushing it's just as important to maximize muscle fiber recruitment, and then increase the rate at which they can contract in unison. To accomplish this, sprint training must stress muscles in a manner that mirrors the exact rhythm and forces used in rushing. (The physiology and new technology of general strength training is covered in Chapter 5.)

As a child, the brilliant Finnish runner Paavo Nurmi developed a natural method of speed training: he ran while hanging onto the slow-moving trains of his native land, which pulled him along faster than he could run under his own power. This is a classic example of a stress overload that enhances muscle recruitment. Modern coaches have adopted this method of *sprint towing*, initially hauling their athletes behind cars at speeds faster than they could attain unassisted.

According to George B. Dintiman, an exercise scientist at Virginia Commonwealth University, towing is the most practical and effective means of increasing sprint speed in use today. At Dintiman's summer speed camps, football players have knocked up to 0.6 second off the 40-yard dash after tow training, but he doesn't haul them behind cars. Using a stationary machine called a Sprintmaster, a runner grabs the handles of a 95-yard rope and pulls it behind him while jogging until the line is fully played out. The athlete then begins sprinting toward the machine at his top speed as the motor reels in the line until it's taut. Using a joystick, the coach can accelerate the rope, initially about 0.3 second faster than the athlete's best time for the 40-yard dash. Improvements are such that a 5.1-second player can be realistically converted to a 4.8-second player, a critical difference for aspiring pro linebackers and fullbacks who must beat the 5-second barrier for the 40 to avoid preseason cuts.

While some sports scientists continue to find ways to enhance the size and recruitment patterns of existing muscle fibers, others are working on methods to grow *new* muscle fibers, something once thought impossible. In fact, most physiologists still believe that athletes cannot grow more muscle fibers, because the number of fibers per muscle is thought to be fixed at birth by genetic factors—the obvious growth of muscles is attributed only to hypertrophy. The philosophy that accompanies this outlook is that would-be champions had better pick the right parents. New evidence suggests that this depressing idea may not be true, at least for certain areas of human anatomy and physiology, but it will take a good deal of research and explanation to uproot the old philosophy and clear the way for new training strategies that might exploit this discovery.

At present, sprint training is designed specifically to develop only one type of muscle fiber, called *fast twitch*. Not only do these fibers look different from any other type of muscle cell— they are the "white meat"—they have a very distinctive way of contracting. Fast-twitch fibers are recruited for rapid and explosive movements because they contract very forcefully and very quickly, usually shrinking down to their smallest size within 40 milliseconds. This prodigious production of power, however, causes them to fatigue quickly.

In all skeletal muscles, these fibers are complemented with *slow-twitch* fibers, which have a lower tension capacity, contract at the relatively sluggish time of 100 to 120 milliseconds, but are fatigue resistant. A marathon runner relies on his slow-twitch fibers to keep him going for over two hours of exertion, contracting faithfully throughout the 26-mile race. A player like Riggins, however, is only interested in covering the 40 yards to the end zone as fast and as powerfully as possible. He relies on his fast-twitch fibers to get him there before somebody gets him.

Both types of fibers are individual threadlike cells, millionths of an inch in diameter, but up to several inches in length. Both can contract by as much as 50 percent of their resting length and can exert a tension of about 100 pounds per square inch of cross-sectional area. This is why the thicker the fiber, the more force it can exert, the payoff for the painful training that causes hypertrophy.

The traditional belief that each individual is born with a fixed number and ratio of fast- and slow-twitch fibers is based on research done with *muscle core biopsies*. During this procedure, an area of an athlete's leg or arm is numbed with local anaesthetic and a needle is plunged into the tissue, extracting a small sample for microscopic analysis. Over the years it's been found that the muscles of successful sprinters have a high ratio of fast- to slow-twitch fibers, and successful endurance athletes, such as marathoners, have a high ratio of slow- to fast-twitch fibers. These core biopsies have been conducted on hundreds of elite athletes, and no one doubts their veracity. The question, however, is whether the biopsies show the *exact* ratio the athlete was born with, or did training affect this ratio? Since successive samples have never been taken from a champion's infancy, childhood, adolescence, right through his adult training years, there's no way of knowing how the use of a muscle may have affected its number of specialized fibers. The belief in the constancy of fiber content throughout life is based on the older biological premise that muscle cells, like nerve cells, cannot divide and multiply.

William J. Gonyea, a physiologist at the University of Texas Health Sciences Center in Dallas, recently challenged this whole line of reasoning when he reported a staggering *20 percent increase* in the number of muscle fibers in response to strength training. Gonyea suggests this increase can be attributed to a longitudinal division of a muscle fiber—producing a new muscle cell of the same fiber type—a phenomenon that had never been reliably reported before. If true, this means an athlete can increase the number as well as the size of the muscle fibers he needs to excel in his chosen sport; he need not have been a "born sprinter" to become a successful running back. Although this work is controversial, other scientists have since reported similar findings in animals.

Before every contender who's been told he hasn't had the right stuff since birth can sign up for a radical training program based on Gonyea's discovery, a considerable amount of further research is needed. So are some answers. Why hasn't this been observed before? Even without looking at muscle biopsies, why hasn't traditional training been able to accomplish this kind of miraculous transformation in terms of performance out in the field? No one knows. But despite the problems, this type of pioneering research is always exciting because, if nothing else, it stimulates new ideas and provokes further inquiry with the hope of finding ways to enhance performance.

Until Gonyea's findings are confirmed there is only one established method to help a player compensate for an innate shortage of fast-twitch fibers. This capitalizes on the same physiological principle—the specificity of adaptation—used in sprint towing, where speed can be increased by stressing the muscles in *exactly* the same way an athlete wants them to work out on the playing field.

Research has shown that, regardless of the ratio of muscle fibers, selective training can increase the functional capacity of either type. For receivers, running backs, and track sprinters, studies have found that high-intensity, low-repetition strength training of the leg muscles causes selective hypertrophy of the fast-twitch fibers, but produces no significant change in slow-twitch fibers.[1] The implication is that the right form of strength training can transform a player with a high ratio of slow-twitch fibers and gradually build his fast-twitch fibers to the point that he can compete with the "born sprinter."

But watch out: studies have revealed that selective hypertrophy will not occur if the same muscle is also involved in the opposite form of endurance training. For a sprinter developing his fast-twitch fibers to increase speed, this means his efforts will be wasted if he engages in distance running within a day or two, because this form of exercise will stimulate his slow-twitch fibers. No one understands why this happens, but one theory proposes that the nervous system cancels out one motor-recruitment program to accommodate the other; another explanation is that muscles are incapable of supplying building materials to both types of fibers simultaneously. Although there are problems with both of these theories, the point should be well taken that *any* kind of training is not necessarily better than no training at all—some forms of exercise can be absolutely detrimental to the athlete specializing in a particular event.

In the present highly competitive environment of amateur and professional sports, the corollary of this is that serious athletes can no longer afford to haphazardly indulge in just any kind of training in the mistaken hope of improving performance. A shot-putter who does push-ups because this form of calisthenics stimulates the same muscles in approximately the same way he uses them in his event is likely to place second to the shot-putter who stresses those same muscles in *exactly* the way he wants them to perform. As training becomes more sophisticated and more precise, competitors are less likely to succeed if they base their training on guesswork, sports lore, or common sense.

It's interesting, in this regard, to recall Bobby Beathart's anecdote about Riggins's personal training program: here is an explosive runner doing 10 quarter-mile intervals and jogging in between. Whereas a single quarter mile in 75 seconds will primarily stimulate fast-twitch fibers, the successive runs and jogs also affect slow-twitch fibers. A modern trainer might have considered one study, which found that athletes who simultaneously engage in both strength and endurance training acquire 20 percent less strength than athletes who engage in strength training alone. The findings of this study may not have any application to Riggins, who is an exceptional player, but just *imagine* this fullback with leg strength that is 20 percent or even 10 percent stronger, and you get the idea.[2]

FOOTBALL BY COMPUTER

For running backs and receivers, leg strength is only part of the formula. Biomechanics, the study of human motion in terms of mechanical engineering, can produce optimal pacing for any player by adjusting his gait to the position he plays, tinkering with factors such as his stride length and stride frequency. Studies have found that every athletic endeavor involving some form of sprinting imposes its own special gait requirements on its players. The gait used by track sprinters, for example, is not the best for rushers, and the stride of a fullback should not be used by a wide receiver.

In 1963, Bob Hayes set a record of 9.1 seconds for the 100-yard dash, covering the distance between the 60- and 75-yard marks in an astonishing 1.1 second (or 27.89 mph)—generally considered the highest instantaneous speed ever attained. When Hayes became a receiver for the Dallas Cowboys, however, he said he had to relearn how to sprint. Prolonged, all-out blasts are seldom required in football, because players must alter their speed and direction when running a pattern to avoid or confuse potential defenders. A player's ability to change speed and direction depends on his ability to rapidly exert large forces against the ground, in any direction, at the instant it's required, without causing an injury.

The gait of a runner in any sport is analyzed by the distance he covers in each stride, which is his *stride length*, and the number of strides he takes in a given time, which is his *stride frequency*. His speed is the product of stride length multiplied by stride frequency. Because of the simple and universal nature of this relationship across all sports, the treadmill has become an essential piece of equipment in the sports laboratory. Not only can it be used to adjust stride length and frequency to obtain maximum speed for any event, it can be used to measure oxygen consumption, energy expenditure, heart activity, and other factors, comparing them to a runner's gait to assess efficiency. If identical twins have the same heart and lung capacity, and both are equally trained, but one consistently uses more oxygen during a run equal to his brother's, it's a clear signal to the biomechanist that he's developed an inefficient motion in his gait that's burning more oxygen and fuel, and that can be corrected by adjusting his gait.

In football, the biomechanic analysis of wide receivers suggests that acceleration is faster and safer when a foreshortened gait is used—a shorter stride length with a higher stride frequency. The validity of these lab tests, which were conducted on treadmills, was assessed against performance in the field using high-speed films of top NFL receivers and examining them frame by frame. The films confirmed that the best players did use this quick-step gait to rapidly accelerate and decelerate, a movement similar to the mincing footwork seen in ballet dancers anticipating a jump—which is exactly what a receiver is about to do when he slows and rises to catch a pass above any nearby defenders. Long gaits, by contrast, give slower acceleration and put greater stress on the hamstring when decelerating and stopping, which often leads to a painful pull at high speeds, landing the player on the bench.

The same film studies also discovered that wide receivers run best in an almost upright position, which facilitates the foreshortened gait, whereas a halfback performs best with a forward tilt or angle to his body, with a significantly longer gait. As a result, the halfback has his center of gravity in front of his waist, which is ideal for collisions, but disadvantageous for sudden cuts and stops *(see Fig. 1.2).*

Biomechanics obtains this type of information by breaking the human body down into separate mechanical parts, examining muscles, bones, and ligaments as if they were pistons, levers, and pulleys. The same laws of physics that apply to suspension bridges and automobiles also apply to the human body. Bone fractures from constant overuse can now be predicted in terms once reserved for stress fractures in the wings of aircraft due to metal fatigue. The elasticity of red blood cells as they change shape snorkeling through capillaries with microscopic diameters are discussed in the same language used to describe the sway of skyscrapers in a gale-force wind.

The tremendous number-crunching ability of the computer has made it as indispensable to biomechanics as the pencil and slide rule once was to mechanical engineering. In fact, twenty hours of slide-rule work can now be performed in one minute on most computers. By hand, it would take weeks or months to compose a comprehensive profile of an athlete due to the sheer number of variables. Oxygen consumption, heart rate, and energy expenditure, for example, are all known to be interrelated, the smallest change in one factor affecting all the others. In competitive sports, the drop of only a few milliliters of oxygen per minute per kilogram of body weight can mean the bronze instead of the gold medal in amateur sports, and can make or break a $100,000 contract for a professional. By saving an athlete those precious few milliliters of oxygen, computer-assisted biomechanic analysis is affecting performance in almost every sport.

A rusher who is looking for extra speed can go to a biomechanics laboratory, now at most major universities and contractually linked with many amateur and professional clubs. At such a lab the technicians first measure all the major landmarks on the athlete's body, particularly the bones attached to major joints. Dots or grids are painted onto key landmarks on the legs, which helps to track precise limb movements captured on film. The player is then put on a treadmill and run at various speeds approximating those he might use in the field, while three high-speed 16-mm cameras (200 to 6,000 frames/second) or high-speed video cameras record the pat-

FIGURE 1.2

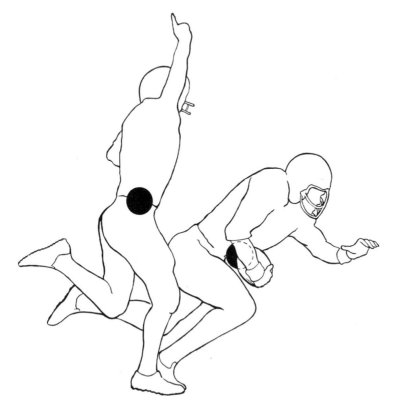

A player's gait affects his center of gravity. Film studies of top NFL receivers found that a foreshortened, quick-step gait is used for rapid starts and stops without causing a hamstring pull, as the center of gravity is above their feet. The longer gait of the halfback, by comparison, results in his center of gravity being in front of his waist, which is ideal for collisions. Note how the center of gravity in the halfback coincides with the position of the ball, so that if he is tackled, he is more likely to roll around the ball as he falls, rather than fumbling.

terns of motion in his limbs. The films are then digitized, or translated into numerical data a computer can use to plot the motions of the limb landmarks. If information is added to the computer on the athlete's physical dimensions, precise calculation can be made about the amount of work being performed by each limb in each phase of the gait; this, in turn, provides

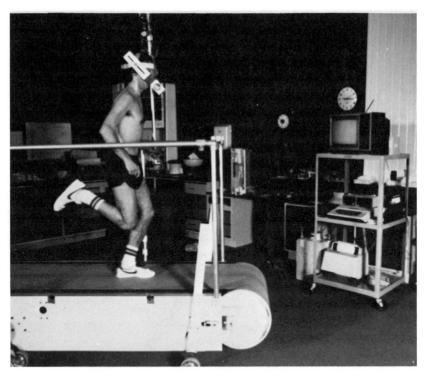

Treadmills have become essential equipment in all major sports labs. They can be used to test aerobic capacity and biomechanical efficiency. Here the oxygen demands of a runner are being studied. (Photo by Dennis Waters/Oak Street Studio, Exeter, NH. Courtesy of Nike, Inc.)

the biomechanist with an analysis of the power being generated by various muscle groups.

In the end, recommendations can be made to adjust gait, body angle, and other facets of running technique to improve acceleration and deceleration, and to avoid injuries. Suggestions can also be made about increasing strength in certain muscles if, say, the height of knee lift of one leg is significantly different from that of the opposite leg.

Computer-assisted film analysis is also used to assess player activity out on the field. In track events, it's been found that sprinters accelerate to 90 percent of their maximum speed in 2 seconds, and 99 percent of their maximum in 4 seconds. In football, however, some plays can be over in 4 seconds. As split seconds are so important in sprint starts from the line of scrimmage or from the takeoff positions in the backfield, considerable attention has been given to the question of the ideal body angle, distance of leg separation, and stance for different players to adopt.

At the line of scrimmage, will a player take off faster if his feet are parallel or staggered? Studies suggest that the staggered position is superior due to the fact that the sum of the forces exerted by both legs rises as the distances between the feet increases, but this applies only up to a maximum separation of about 28 to 36 inches.

Five separate investigations comparing takeoff speed from the line of scrimmage in the 2-, 3-, and 4-point stance (number of limbs in contact with the ground) discovered that the 4-point stance held definite advantages for the straight line charge, the 3-point stance best for sprinting away over 7 to 8 yards, and the 2-point stance quickest for darting over 3.3 yards.

Another consideration is the distribution of body weight in any stance. Research has found that reaction time to the snap signal decreased significantly as the amount of weight a player put on his hands in the 3- and 4-point stances increased. One study discovered that the time it took players to travel one yard forward was fastest when only 5 percent of the body weight was supported by the hand on the ground.

In the future, this kind of information can be poured into a computer during preseason training, the variables processed in relation to new play patterns being introduced by the offensive coach, and the optimal stance can be obtained for any man in a given position for a particular play. If, for example, a player needed to charge 8 yards forward in the first leg of a pattern, he might shave a half second off his time by using a 26-inch staggered 3-point stance with only 5 percent of his body weight on his hand.

Is a half of a second too trivial to worry about? Ask the player in the trenches who's within spitting distance of defensive end Lyle Alzado, the six-three 270-pound Raiders roughneck who thinks face ripping is a finesse move.

At present, computers are revolutionizing both offensive and defensive strategies for coaches who are willing to learn how to use the keyboard to obtain an edge over their rivals.

Miami Dolphins coach Don Shula has never been hesitant to experiment with new ideas and technology, especially when it comes to settling old scores. In 1984, still smarting from their Super Bowl loss to the Redskins, Shula and his staff dedicated a large portion of their preseason training to smothering rushers like Riggins while simultaneously opening the skies with spectacular passes by quarterback Dan Marino.

In their first game after summer training, the Dolphins' twenty-two-year-old quarterback broke records in three of the four categories in the NFL rating system when he led Miami to a 35–17 victory over Washington. Marino completed 21 of 28 passes for a total of 311 yards. Five of the passes resulted in touchdowns, and he had no interceptions in the entire game. The Elias Sports Bureau in New York, which handles all league statistics, gave him a 150.4 ranking—158 is the perfect ranking in the Elias system for quarterbacks.

The Dolphins' defense also contained the run. In preseason exhibition, no team rushed for 100 yards against them and in the contest against the Redskins they held Riggins to 98 yards, despite his 15 carries—a standard of performance that bought Miami the 1984 division championship.

Although it's impossible to discount Shula's cunning, the pinpoint precision of Marino's arm, or the tenacity of the Dolphins' defensive line, some credit must be given the microchips on the Miami bench—a computer system called Sportspac. This system was invented in 1968 by Burt Gilner, a self-styled football nut who, at the time, was working with a small software company near Tampa Bay, Florida. When the city became the home of the Buccaneers, they also acquired a new coach, John McKay, who came from Gilner's alma mater, the University of Southern California. Gilner approached McKay and introduced him to a computer system that would handle the complexities of the player payroll. The system was such a success that it was expanded to cover ticketing and mailing lists, then player statistics, which proved helpful when it came time for the drafts. In fact, the data base became broad enough that Gilner could ask it for such things as the names of all eligible wide receivers who were free agents, who could run the 40 in under 4.8 seconds, and who stood between six feet and six-four. Naturally, it wasn't long before he was working with the coaching staff designing plays. Today, Sportspac, or a similar system, is used by almost every NFL team.

The San Diego Chargers have used Sportspac to analyze the defensive weaknesses of opposing teams to design new offensive plays. One of these is the 372-F shoot-pump (see Fig. 1.3). This play, when it was first designed in 1983, called for tight end Kellen Winslow to charge downfield about 8 yards and cut outside as fullback John Cappelletti blasted through to the same area to attract coverage from the opponents' strong safety. Meanwhile, quarterback Dan Fouts fakes a pass to immobilize the linebacker covering Winslow, who suddenly runs upfield to the area left vacant by the strong safety and receives the pass. When the play works, Winslow should score a touchdown, or at least buy a lot of yardage.

The Chargers' 372-F shoot-pump evolved as a result of preparation for a game against the Kansas City Chiefs, when the coaching staff noticed that between the 20-yard line and the end zone the Chiefs' defensive formation was the same 70 percent of the time. Knowing this, pinpointing the holes to penetrate, mapping out the safest zones for a reception, planning the decoys, and then selecting the best players for the job led to the play's creation.

The software is now so advanced that a coach can study over fifty variables in any individual play. Based on information like this, Bill Walsh, coach of the San Francisco Forty-niners, often scripts the first twenty plays of a game before he walks onto the field. After each play, advanced systems can produce a breakdown of cumulative statistics only minutes after the action has stopped. In fact, after the half-time gun, the first half of a game, play by play, can be dissected and in the printer for distribution before the players reach the locker room. Gilner has estimated that football computers are increasing a coach's productivity by up to 25 percent, relieving him of a lot of dreary paper work and giving him a tool with which to be more creative.

According to Ed Hughes, offensive coordinator coach of the Chicago Bears, when computers first entered football many coaches wondered whether the microchip might take their jobs, but "now I know coaches who make up their entire game plan with computers and don't even look at the game films."

FIGURE 1.3

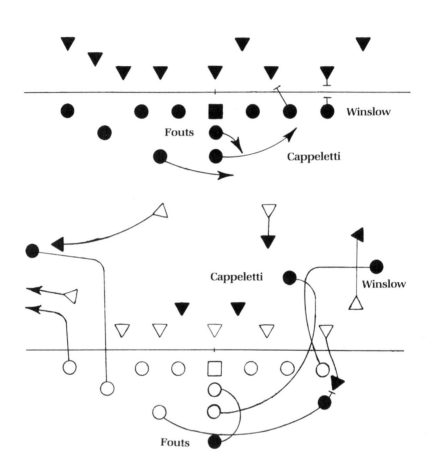

COLLISIONS AND INJURIES

Recall for a moment the Redskins' zoom fake, used so successfully to get John Riggins through the Miami defense in Super Bowl XVII. What if Miami's Don McNeal had not been fooled by Didier's maneuver *(see Fig. 1.1),* or what if he hadn't slipped on the turf? A head-on collision with Riggins might have occurred, but who would have been pushed to the ground?

Although Riggins weighed 235 pounds and McNeal only 192,

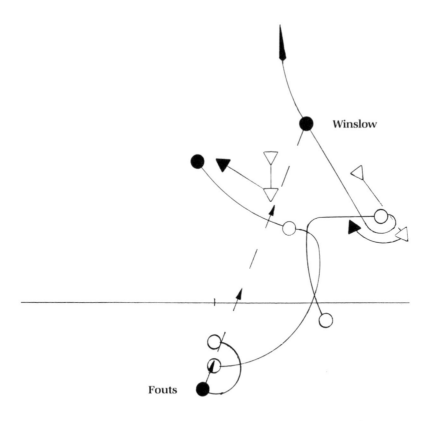

Winslow

Fouts

Football by computer. The San Diego Chargers designed a play similar to the one above, called the 372-F shoot-pump, in preparation for a game against the Kansas City Chiefs when a computer analysis of the Chiefs' defense found that their formation was the same 70 percent of the time when Kansas City was between the 20-yard line and the end zone.

For the first seconds after the snap (top left) it appears as if quarterback Dan Fouts is going to hand the ball to one of his running backs (as Theismann did in Fig. 1.1). Tight end Kellen Winslow, who will eventually receive the pass, appears only to be blocking to create a hole for the rush. Winslow suddenly slips through, charges downfield for 8 yards as fullback John Cappelletti follows his tail, slanting inside, drawing coverage from the Chiefs' safety (bottom left), who would otherwise be in a position to stop Winslow. Fouts fakes a pass to Winslow, causing the Chiefs' linebacker, who's been following Winslow, to charge forward. At that moment, Winslow does a button-hook and runs downfield to receive the real pass (above).

the outcome of their impact cannot be anticipated by weight alone: momentum is everything. As Riggins's initial rush was slowed by squeezing through the line, his speed when he came in contact with McNeal might have been 20 feet/second. McNeal, in the open, would have had longer to accelerate and could have been moving at 25 feet/second. In which case, on impact the burly Riggins would have been stopped and shoved into reverse at the rate of 4 inches/second, not enough to bowl him over, but enough to trot him around until help arrived or the whistle blew.[3]

In the actual game, Riggins had greater momentum and McNeal landed on the turf. As the Miami cornerback later recalled, "I wanted to make him bounce outside, but I never did get my arms all the way around him. He was like a train."

Vince Lombardi, the much loved, hated, and quoted coach of the Green Bay Packers, once said, "Football isn't a contact sport, it's a collision sport. Dancing is a contact sport." A recent study at Stanford University dramatized Lombardi's words: when two professional football players collide at top speed, head on, they release enough energy to move a 30-ton object a distance of 1 inch. With impacts of this magnitude it is surprising that the injury rate in football, which ranks highest among all contact sports, is not even higher.

Surveys have found that injuries are highest among high school teams, with about 72 reported per 100 players. University teams have a lower rate, and NFL players have 51 injuries per 100 players. Since 1931, an average of 19 fatalities per year have been reported in the United States from football played at all levels. (See Figs. 1.4 and 1.5 for injury rates for different player positions and for different areas of the body.)

One of the most tragic injuries in recent years occurred on August 12, 1978, when the New England Patriots were in Oakland to play an exhibition game against the Raiders. Near the end of the second quarter, five-year veteran wide receiver Darryl Stingley ran downfield for 8 yards, then slanted toward the center at a 45-degree angle ready for a reception. Patriot quarterback Steve Grogan gave him a pass that was just inches too high, despite Stingley's ball-hawk leap into the air. As he returned to the ground, he was struck by the Raiders' free safety,

FIGURE 1.4
Injury Rates by Body Area

Body Area	1969–72 Study	1976–79 Study
Head and neck	13%	8%
Shoulder	8%	13%
Elbow	2%	3%
Wrist	2%	3%
Hand and fingers	8%	12%
Chest and ribs	3%	3%
Back	5%	5%
Hip	3%	2%
Knee	20%	22%
Ankle	15%	11%
Foot and toes	3%	4%

Do rule changes reduce injuries? The most dramatic change in the rate of injuries per body area over a seven-year period has been a reduction of head and neck injuries and a proportional increase in shoulder injuries. This may be explained by the 1976 NCAA rules banning head blocks, putting the burden on the shoulder. The rise in hand injuries is more difficult to explain, but is likely due to the same reason, as hands and shoulders are now more often the first areas of the body to make contact in a block or tackle.

The 1969–72 study, by Blyth and Mueller (1974), reported on 4,278 high school football injuries in North Carolina. The 1976–79 study, by Culpepper and Niemann (1983), reported on 1,877 high school players in Alabama. The lag time between the surveys and the publication of the data accounts for the absence of more recent injury statistics. (See bibliography.)

210-pound Jack Tatum, who connected with Stingley at the base of his skull.

In his book *Happy to Be Alive*, Stingley recalled, "I hit the ground with a thud and tried to get up, as I had so many times before, but I couldn't move. I felt like I was the cornerstone of a high-rise building, as if an elephant had planted his foot on my chest." Today, the former receiver is the Patriots' executive director of personnel, although he remains a quadriplegic, paralyzed from the neck down.

Stingley's injury, the result of a legal tackle, posed a chal-

FIGURE 1.5
Injury Rates by Player Position*

Player Position	Percentage of Injuries
Running back	21%
Linebacker	11%
Defensive back	10%
Defensive tackle	10%
Defensive end	9%
Guard	7%
Defensive guard	6%
Quarterback	6%
Tackle	5%
Tight end	4%
Wide receiver	3%

*Source: Blyth and Mueller (1974). (See bibliography.)

lenge for sports scientists: they needed to test the adequacy of protective equipment to absorb the force of any kind of collision likely to be encountered on the playing field. As soon as they started to look for published research on protective equipment, they discovered that a lot of the equipment on the market had been developed on a trial-and-error basis, with little objective laboratory evaluation. In fact, as recently as 1983, a survey of the scientific literature by Robert W. Norman, a kinesiologist at the University of Waterloo in Ontario, found that no work has as yet been submitted to refereed journals on the arm pads or shoulder pads in football, despite the large numbers of injuries to these areas of the body (see Fig. 1.4). Studies on other types of football equipment have been extremely limited and have begun to appear only within the last ten years.

In his survey, Norman concluded that "biomechanic assessments of protective equipment should be required of manufacturers before the product reaches the marketplace and not emerge as a reaction to injury problems which occur after the equipment has been purchased."

Today, safety standards for football helmets are set by an independent committee of scientists, and all new models are evaluated for their ability to absorb and deflect impact forces. The results are published with the hope that consumers will shun helmets found to be unsafe and that the consequent market forces will prevail upon manufacturers to produce truly protective equipment.[4]

The evaluations are conducted by mounting the helmet on a "headform" and dropping the dummy head-first onto an anvil or striking it with an impactor. The headform, helmet, and striking surface are usually loaded with instruments and the impacts are recorded on high-speed film. Impact velocities are typically between 15 and 25 feet/second, which corresponds to running speeds on the field, but are below the resultant velocity of a head-on collision between two players who are each running at 15 to 25 feet/second.

Since the invention of the plastic helmet in 1939 by Gerry Morgan of the John T. Riddle Company in Chicago, external injuries to the head have been dramatically reduced, particularly lacerations, tooth loss, nose fractures, and ear detachments. Internal head injuries persist, but at a lower rate; they are due to the traumatic beating of the brain as it bounces around and against the interior of the skull when the head is violently moved (graphically shown in *Fig. 4.1*). These internal injuries are studied in terms of the acceleration—the rate at which velocity increases over time—of the head, and are measured in meters or feet/second squared. Another unit of acceleration is the "G," short for the acceleration imposed on everything on the earth's surface by the planet's gravitational field, where 1 G equals an acceleration of 32 feet/second squared. Air force test pilots blackout if their jet fighters expose them to 8 or 9 G's, whereas the brain of a player hit in a football game while wearing a helmet can be as high as 100 or even 200 G's—and it's this kind of force that causes concussions and brain damage.

Because wired mannequins cannot simulate the complexity of the collisions and resultant forces that occur for an active player in a real game, Stephen E. Reid, a sports physician at Northwestern University Medical School, invented a system to wire a player to measure accelerations to his head in a live environment. He mounted accelerometers on the suspension lining of an experimental helmet at three locations; these instruments are sealed transducers that pick up the energy of acceleration, but are not sensitive to the movement of the helmet liner or to normal head motion. Strain gauges, which measure impact forces, were mounted on the shoulder pads. The effects on the brain itself were detected with electroencephalograph (EEG) wires attached to the player's scalp; these surface probes are sensitive enough to detect the storm of electrical activity in the brain through the skull. All these sensors were then connected to an "impact telemetry system," which coded, amplified, and transmitted the signals over an FM radio frequency to a receiver Reid set up on the sideline.

During one Northwestern University football season, Reid tested his system on a middle linebacker, who participated in 418 plays in seven Big Ten Conference games. These games were also recorded on film, so the signals from the wired player could be correlated with collisions on the field. In the course of these seven games, the linebacker received 169 head impacts, with peak acceleration ranging between 40 and 230 G's, each impact transmitting these awesome forces within 20 to 420 milliseconds.

There is considerable disagreement among safety experts about the exact tolerance threshold of the human brain to acceleration, although the general consensus is that concussions and other forms of brain injury begin to occur with impacts between 110 and 200 G's lasting less than 70 to 400 milliseconds. For Reid's linebacker, there were 15 impacts in this high-intensity range, one of which clearly registered as a concussion on the EEG.

In assessing injury in relation to acceleration, the duration of the blow is a critical measure of its intensity. The importance of time in acceleration is well known, at least intuitively, to anyone who has ridden in an automobile. If a car's velocity increases from 0 to 60 mph in 30 seconds, the passenger's body is noticeably pushed back against the seat. But if the velocity increases from 0 to 60 over 5 minutes, the acceleration is hardly perceptible. In equivalent terms, the brain of Reid's linebacker was accelerated at *hundreds* of miles per hour within *thousandths* of a second.

Of course the brain is spared from the full force of these collisions by the helmet, which lengthens the time of acceleration by absorbing the blows through the compression and deformation of several layers of material. Helmets of the 1980s are made of a tough outer shell composed of a shiny surface layer of polycarbonate, a layer of aluminum lined with vinyl foam,

36

and a layer of styrene plastic. Inside, there are a variety of suspension systems holding the hard shell away from the player's head. Some are padded liners, others are plastic pods filled with antifreeze or pure alcohol. Recently, liners have been made of many mini-airbags that expand to snugly fit the head once inflated with an ordinary bicycle pump inserted into an intake valve inside the helmet's earhole.

Generally, successive generations of safety equipment have decreased injury rates, but sometimes a particular piece of equipment, designed with the best intentions, can actually cause more injuries of a totally unexpected nature.

In the mid-1970s, a few sports physicians noted that the rate of head and neck injuries was increasing; in fact, the majority of football deaths resulted from head and neck injuries. This realization sparked studies to investigate the cause of the problem, and before long blocking and tackling techniques came under close scrutiny. Using a rapid series of X-ray films (4 to 6 frames/second) and transposing them onto 16-mm motion picture frames, a technique known as *cineradiography*, physicians examined the motions of the head and neck of volunteers who wore helmets in laboratory simulations of typical football collisions. The X-ray films clearly showed that blocking with the head, using the helmet as a battering ram, caused the neck to bend violently backward and forward (hyperflexion and hyperextension), effectively breaking the vertebrae.

These findings were supplemented by a 1976 survey by the National Alliance Football Rules Committee, which found that 38 percent of the coaches questioned said they taught blockers to make initial contact with their heads. This technique of "butt blocking" or "spearing" arose with the advent of the plastic, hardshell helmets, first used by the U.S. Military Academy football team in 1944. To their credit, football officials acted quickly and outlawed butt blocking in 1976, and the rate of head and neck injury fell *(see Fig. 1.4)*.

A similar irony applies to the face guard or mask on a modern football helmet. Initially introduced to reduce injuries to the eyes, nose, and mouth, the face mask was also implicated in the rise of head and neck injuries. Cineradiographic analysis found a lever effect was imposed on the head and neck when a projecting face mask, especially a single bar mask, was caught

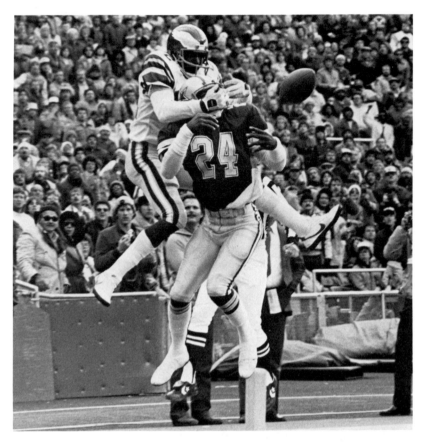

It is illegal to touch or tackle a player's face mask. Here a Philadelphia Eagle free safety is not attempting to harm the Dallas receiver, only to block his vision, but if the face mask is even touched, the referee could call a 15-yard penalty. The extreme sensitivity about face-mask violations stems from studies in the mid-1970s that found any pressure applied to the mask acts like a lever, snapping the neck. This play was called on pass interference. (Courtesy of Philip Katz/First Capital Press.)

on the ground or by another player. This finding led to the ban of face tackling and face mask violations.

Although injuries to the trunk and ribs are much rarer than those to the head and major joints, a tremendous advance in upper-body protection occurred when Houston sports designer Byron Donzis developed the "flak jacket." Introduced in

1978 to protect the broken ribs of Oilers quarterback Dan Pastorini, the jacket is made of layers of urethane-coated nylon, which are heat sealed to take the shape of several cylinders once inflated with air. The cylinders are interconnected with fabric valves, which stay open during normal body movement to allow the shape of the jacket to conform to that of the body. Upon impact, the sudden increase of air pressure within the jacket closes the valves, stiffening the cylinders to absorb the blow.

Over the past five years, the Donzis flak jacket has been widely used by players throughout the NFL—but only to protect existing injuries, not to prevent them. This limited use of the flak jacket prompted some researchers to wonder if the equipment was really effective.

Thomas E. Cain, an orthopedic surgeon at Baylor College of Medicine and a consultant to the Houston Oilers, decided to evaluate Donzis's invention, but instead of fitting a mannequin with strain gauges and accelerometers, he opted to fit a flak jacket on a live human subject, then take a baseball bat and hit the jacket as hard as possible—all done scientifically, of course.

Cain used high-speed films (500 frames/second) to calculate the force of impact of the bat being struck against a rib cage area of 4.5 square inches. Normally, the bat would break a few ribs, but the volunteer subjects of this test reported no discomfort. Cain's study illustrates the usefulness of high-speed films in analyzing a wide range of phenomena in sports. Because the film moves through the camera at a uniform speed, he was able to measure the distance the bat traveled in each frame (0.002 inches/second), calculate the acceleration of the bat in feet per second, obtain impact force as the product of the bat's mass and acceleration, and finally divide impact force by the square inches of impact area to determine the force per square inch.

The result: the flak jacket deflected an incredible 587 pounds per square inch. To inflict this kind of force in a game, a player would have to run down the field at *60 miles per hour*, leap up, and strike his opponent with the heel of his boot.

Donzis, inspired with the success of his flak jacket, went back to the drawing board to make similar protective equipment for thighs and shoulders. He worked with Oilers running back Earl Campbell to design a uniform jersey with a teflon fabric that would help Campbell glance off, rather than stick to, opposing players or the turf. He is now refining an inertial-reel knee brace that will lock the knee in a safe position if a runner makes too sudden a cut or stop, or falls, shifting the pressure to the thigh.

A vocal advocate of safety equipment in contact sports, Donzis says, "I don't think any sport is so violent that equipment can't eliminate most injuries." And to prove his point he has designs for hockey, soccer, and lacrosse, but he insists there's one piece of equipment he'll never manufacture—a protective cup.

"I personally test everything before it goes out the door and I'll be damned if I'll stand there and let someone take a swipe at me with a baseball bat."[5]

TWO

BASKETBALL

Courting Coordination

In 1962, Wilt Chamberlain owned a Harlem nightclub, a Los Angeles apartment project, and a boy's camp. He spoke four languages, played guitar and bass fiddle, had cut three folk music records, and on March 2, he broke five National Basketball Association individual scoring records. In the best game of his fourteen-year NBA career, Chamberlain scored the most field goals (36), most foul goals (28), most points in one quarter (31), most points in one half (59), and most points in one game (100), to lead the Philadelphia Warriors to a 169–147 victory over the New York Knickerbockers. The combined score of 316 was an NBA record as well.

In Hershey Stadium, before a crowd of only 4,124 spectators, Wilt started the game as he finished it, exploiting every weakness in the Knicks' defense, shooting at every opportunity. His opponent at center was the six-ten Darrell Imhoff, who was the strongest defensive player on the New York bench, but he couldn't keep up with Wilt's performance: Imhoff committed four fouls in the first quarter trying to prevent the seven-one Philadelphia star from scoring. In the second quarter, Knicks coach Eddie Donovan replaced Imhoff with Cleveland Buckner, who was quicker on his feet, but much shorter. Unaffected by the substitution, Chamberlain continued his scoring spree, especially with quick lay-ups and dunks, and made thirteen out of fourteen baskets from the foul line.

During the half-time break, Philadelphia coach Frank Mc-Guire, perhaps intuitively sensing what his center was about to

41

accomplish, told his team to give the ball to Wilt. And Knicks coach Donovan was thinking exactly the same thing. He told his players, "There's no way he's gonna get a hundred against us." The Knicks were going to do anything to avoid being the victims of a historic rout.

In the third quarter, Chamberlain scored ten of sixteen shots and eight for eight at the free-throw line. The public address announcer kept the fans alerted to Chamberlain's point total and they started to respond by yelling, "Give it to Wilt, give it to Wilt." Imhoff came back onto the court in the last quarter, but committed two more fouls against Chamberlain and was forced to sit out the game.

With 89 points and five minutes left in the game, the stadium was in a frenzy. For over two minutes Chamberlain didn't score and the Knicks were eating up time with every possession, hogging the ball. With less than three minutes left, Wilt scored with two short-range jumpers and a few free throws to bring his total to 96 points. Then, with a minute remaining, Wilt took a pass under the hoop and dunked it for 98.

He stole the next pass, dribbled it down the foul line, leapt for a jump shot, and missed. Pandemonium broke out in the stands. The Knicks took the ball and missed. The Warriors took control and fed the ball to Chamberlain, who shot and missed, grabbed the rebound, went up, and missed again. The Tribe still got the rebound, waited for Chamberlain to clear from the pack, then charge inside, and they fed him the ball—which he stuffed through the hoop with both hands, with only 46 seconds left on the clock. The stadium erupted, fans pouring onto the court to congratulate the greatest player in basketball history.

Fans can be a fickle lot. It's tempting to wonder, when Chamberlain missed those baskets near the end of the game, generating such tension, how many Philly fanatics asked each other, *"How could he have missed that shot?"*

Passing a basketball 9.71 inches in diameter through an 18-inch rim mounted 10 feet above the floor seems to be such an easy task that some players have actually been booed if they missed half of their shots. Compared to other sports, the scoring average of a basketball player per game is relatively high. Most baseball players seldom hit the ball more than a third of the time at the plate. In fact, basketball game scores have been so high in recent years, with some shooting percentages up almost 50 percent since 1948, that officials have considered raising the height of the net to 12 feet to increase the excitement of the game.[1]

Yet behind the apparent simplicity of a basketball shot there is a mind-boggling interaction between nerves and muscles. Suppose for a moment that the NBA awarded you with a lucrative contract to build a motorized, mechanical basketball launcher, which could be moved around the court by remote control, parked in any location, and programmed to shoot a perfect swish. The mechanical engineering of such a contraption would be fairly simple. The difficulty would come in designing a computer program coupled to an optical range-finder that could measure the horizontal and vertical distances to the basket and calculate the angle, force, and speed with which the ball should be launched—from any position on the court.

Fortunately, in 1981, Peter Brancazio, a physicist at City University of New York, published the equations necessary for such a program (see Fig. 2.1) and they could be incorporated into the software by a competent programmer.

However, if the NBA contract called for the mechanical player to make shots while it was moving like a human player, jogging down the court at fifteen feet/second, you'd run up against a serious obstacle. If the machine was parked in a stationary position, such as the free-throw line, there would be plenty of time for the on-board computer to make the necessary optical measurements and integrate them with Brancazio's equations, then adjust its launch mechanism and release the ball. But today's computers and machines do not work fast enough to simulate a basketball player shooting on the trot, in spite of the lightning speed of contemporary data processors and servos. When the contract was lost, you could at least take heart from the fact that no one else would be able to make the NBA's mechanical player.[2]

The mundane process of eye-hand coordination still has no rival. A player running down the court, who unexpectedly has a basketball enter his peripheral vision, unconsciously makes countless calculations and motor commands that lock his eyes onto the ball for at least 60 milliseconds *before he even knows he's looking at the ball.*

FIGURE 2.1
Effects of Distance to Basket on Launch Angle, Speed, and Force*

Distance to Basket (feet)	Minimum Launch Angle (degrees)	Optimal Launch Angle (degrees)	Minimum Launch Speed (feet/second)	Average Launch Force (pounds)
10	45.6	50.7	19.82	3.93
15	41.6	48.8	23.49	5.52
20	39.4	47.9	26.68	7.12
25	38.0	47.3	29.53	8.72

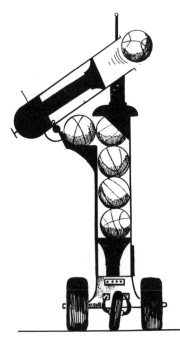

To program a 6-foot mechanical basketball launcher with a fixed point of release 8 feet above the floor, thirteen equations must be performed; the results for four distances are given in the columns above. The numbers will be different for every change in horizontal and vertical distance from the basket. Of course, the situation is actually more complex: lateral angle (left to right) and air resistance calculations must also be considered to achieve a swish.

*Source: Brancazio (1981). (See bibliography.)

The automatic response to a moving object sensed—but not yet seen—by peripheral vision is a very predictable and orderly series of events. First, a very fast eye movement, called a *saccade*, signals the muscles of the eyes to contract just enough to move the most sensitive part of the retina, or *fovea*, onto the ball, a process that takes about 40 to 50 milliseconds. Although the conscious brain does not realize it, the visual image of an object during a saccade is effectively blacked out during the eye movement, and it can take an additional 10 to 20 milliseconds after the eye movement has stopped to obtain a conscious visual image. After a delay of another 20 to 40 milliseconds, the head itself begins to turn in the same direction. As the eyes have independently moved first, and much faster than the head, a rapid series of adjustments must be made to coordinate the dual movement of eye and head muscles. If there was no compensatory movement, the eyes would overshoot the ball as the head turned.

At three separate locations in the brain, the angular distance between the line of sight and the moving basketball must be compared and recalculated, millisecond by millisecond, with the position of the rotating head. This is done through a network of nerves that control *vestibulo-occular tracking*, taking signals from a kind of biological accelerometer in the vestibule of the inner ear, and calculating how much the head has moved since the last signal, comparing that information to the ongoing movement of the eyes—then making the required alterations in the rate and force of contraction in selected fast-twitch muscle fibers in the eye and head.

If the ball is also moving at an angle away from or toward the player, depth perception must simultaneously be controlled to keep the ball in focus. Motion in depth is perceived by comparing the minute differences in the visual signals fed to the brain by the two separate eyes, and comparing the stereoscopic image with past memory images of how large or small a ball should appear as it approaches or recedes.

For the player moving down the court at 15 feet/second, this *entire series* of neural calculations and muscle contractions involved in controlling *only* eye and head coordination is performed at least ten times in the space it takes the player to make a single stride forward. The process is updated and recalculated over a billion times in the course of a game.

If we consider the infinitely more complex process that occurs during a fast break, where the player runs down the court at top speed, receives a pass, and hooks the ball into the hoop on the trot, it becomes apparent why the NBA's moving mechanical basketball player is beyond the present state of technology.

From a coach's point of view, this awesome phenomenon may have a practical side. Although there's no way to integrate Brancazio's equations into the conscious actions of a basketball player to assure accurate shots—because the conscious mind works far too slowly and too linearly to handle the rapid simultaneous calculations—contemporary sports psychologists have found methods to program the brain to improve shooting performance. The programming secret is something of a paradox: teach a player to mentally visualize a shot or imagine a perfect play before it's executed, but once the body goes into action, teach him how to stop thinking entirely. In fact, give him methods to shut down the analytic areas of his brain.

SHUTTING DOWN THE BRAIN

Long before scientists began probing the brain with a view to enhancing performance, Bob Cousey intuitively grasped some of the psychological requirements of consistent shooting. In 1963, after retiring from the Boston Celtics, Cousy took over as head coach at Boston College, and during his six-year tenure, he built a nationally ranked team with a record of 177 wins and 38 losses. Among the many elements of his winning formula, he taught players to condition themselves to eliminate distracting thoughts and feelings when they were playing, especially when they were about to shoot.

Cousey once observed that "the seemingly superhuman coolness some players have under pressure is nothing more than a kind of *practiced absentmindedness* regarding everything but the immediate task." He believed that a successful player at the free-throw line possessed a "trancelike consciousness" when sighting the basket.

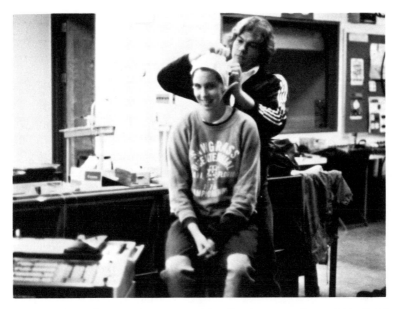

Daniel Landers at the University of Arizona and Brad Hatfield at the University of Maryland pioneered the investigation of brain activity in athletes by initially wiring elite marksmen. Here an EEG helmet is being placed on a subject. The helmet, as light and pliable as a swimming cap, holds the sensitive EEG leads in place on the subject's scalp. (Courtesy of Daniel Landers and Brad Hatfield.)

Assuming Cousey's statement is an accurate psychological observation, what exactly is going on inside the player's brain to produce such trancelike behavior?

Since the mid-1970s, brain researchers have gathered evidence that different types of skills are directed by either the left or right hemisphere of the brain. In a right-handed person, verbal, mathematical, and strategic functions are processed in the left hemisphere; nonverbal, artistic, and spatial functions occur in the right hemisphere. For a left-handed person, the opposite hemispheres process these functions.

One of the most intriguing suggestions to emerge from this discovery is that complex perceptual and motor processes, such as those involved in sports, preferentially engage the right hemisphere and sometimes result in an altered state of consciousness, in which the perception of time or pain is modified.

47

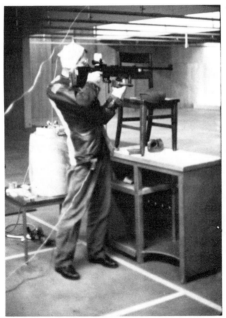

The marksman in action at the rifle range, EEG helmet on, data flowing from his brain to the recording machines. Landers and Hatfield discovered that when the athlete is setting up the shot, the left brain is very active, but when he begins to focus and calculate the spatial distances, the left brain tends to shut down. (Courtesy of Daniel Landers and Brad Hatfield.)

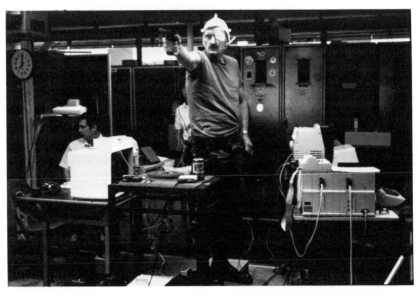

The marksman at the range with EEG helmet on, leads running into the recorder at his side. Sensitive to the storm of electrical activity inside the brain, the EEG leads pick up signals measured in millivolts. Landers and other investigators went on from these landmark experiments and discovered that archers and basketball players also shut down the left brain when shooting. (Courtesy of Daniel Landers and Brad Hatfield.)

Curious about the implications of this idea, Charles Rebert, an experimental neurologist at SRI International, a think tank in California, placed electroencephalograph (EEG) electrodes on the heads of fourteen volunteers and had them play several games of Pong, a video tennis game. He found that all the players had a flurry of electrical activity in the right hemisphere while playing TV tennis—and these bursts of energy occurred while the players were automatically calculating angles, velocities, and points of intersection in space and time.

In the past few years, Daniel Landers, an exercise scientist at Arizona State University, has conducted similar EEG studies with rifle shooters and Olympic archers to see if this phenomenon might have any practical value for coaches. Like Rebert, he has found that brain activity diminishes in the left hemisphere when the marksmen begin to concentrate on the target.

"We think this happen for several reasons," says Landers. "Spatial-positioning tasks, involved in aiming and sighting, are known to be a right-brain specialty. Also, the automatic response is so quick and complex that the marksmen can't really think about it. It seems that if they do try to think about it, they clutter their performance. So, one practical application of this work may be that we can teach athletes how to shut down the left half of their brain at critical moments."

In EEG studies of basketball players at the free-throw line, Landers discovered that after they set up for the throw, if they concentrated intensely on the basket for about seven seconds, during this period the left brain would turn off and the right brain would take over. Landers is quick to caution that more work is needed to establish that performance improves for any player with this technique, but he is certain that the good shooters he studied possessed the ability to shut down their left brain.

Rick McKinney, one of the Olympic archers who worked with Landers, believes he has some idea of what the EEG recordings of his own shot are showing. "At first I found it puzzling to learn that I was turning off the analytic areas of my brain, but after I began looking into the studies of left and right brain functions and compared the EEG findings to what I am doing subjectively when I shoot, it all made sense. If I just 'go with the flow' of the shot, I perform well, but if I start thinking about what

49

I'm doing while I'm aiming, I don't do as well. It's as if I momentarily step out of my normal consciousness and something else takes over."

In light of these recent EEG studies, it is interesting that coaches like Bob Cousy have always taught their players psychological conditioning techniques—usually a combination of concentration, relaxation, and confidence—to remove all thoughts and distractions while shooting. Today, using the new EEG findings as clues to the neurological activity behind a perfect swish, psychological conditioning techniques are being shaped to produce dramatic improvements out on the court.

About the time Bob Cousy retired as coach at Boston College, Richard Suinn, a psychologist at Colorado State University, was giving therapy to an intelligent doctoral candidate who had twice failed his oral examinations, although he had maintained a 3.64 grade point average. Suinn assumed that his patient's oral performance was being blocked by emotional obstacles, which he attempted to remove with a technique he called Visuo-Motor Behavior Rehearsal (VMBR). With this technique the patient tenses all his muscles, then relaxes and imagines the entire task he wishes to improve. The process is repeated many times; anxiety and other emotional obstacles are eliminated because, in the imaginary task, failure is impossible. After this student had finished his VMBR sessions with Suinn, he glided through his oral exams with remarkable ease. In fact, his college adviser was startled by the deftness and originality of the student's answers and commented to Suinn, "It's just not his style!" This prompted Suinn to suspect that an unexpected effect of VMBR produced new behavioral styles that *were not rehearsed in therapy.*

Suinn reasoned that if VMBR facilitated the spontaneous emergence of new adaptive behaviors, as well as removed psychological obstacles, then the technique might be useful for normal individuals, such as athletes. As it happened, the ski coach at Colorado State approached Suinn at this time and asked him if he could help manage some of the routine competitive tensions experienced by his team. Suinn gladly accepted the assignment, and in his VMBR sessions with the college skiers he made another observation. During deep relaxation, the skiers told Suinn that the mental imagery became very rich: the athletes began to imagine the course in vivid color, could feel the cold temperature, hear the sounds of their skis on the snow, and feel their muscles move as they raced downhill. Some of the skiers could actually imagine they were racing in slow motion and began to detect some of the errors they had been making, which in an actual run would have happened too fast to notice. Ironically, Suinn's experiment was so successful that the coach used only the VMBR skiers in competition, excluding those from a matched control group of skiers who had not had VMBR, making it impossible to quantitatively measure the difference in performance between the two groups in actual races. The results did, however, reinforce Suinn's theory that VMBR was more than a therapeutic tool; it could dramatically enhance performance.

Though the VMBR sessions proved to be successful for the ski team, Suinn continued to look for hard experimental evidence to show that his technique did more than build confidence and soothe anxieties. To do this, he connected electromyograph (EMG) leads to the leg muscles of an Alpine ski racer and subjected him to VMBR sessions in which he verbally described an imaginary downhill race, moment by moment. When Suinn compared the tapes of the session to the EMG recordings, he found that the electrical activity in the muscles mirrored every bump and turn in the imaginary course—even though the muscles were apparently relaxed. These invisible muscle contractions were the first piece of physical evidence that Suinn's method of behavior rehearsal occurred not only in the imagination of an athlete, but that the entire nervous system—right down to the motor units that excite muscle fibers—was rehearsing and practicing for the real event.

According to Suinn, analytic thinking is a left-brain activity and the visualization behind VMBR is a right-brain activity.

"When athletes get into an event, the left brain is active when they are setting up strategies, but the right brain takes over just prior to executing certain motor activities. With VMBR, we may have a practical tool to program various parts of the mind and body for sports activities, even though the athlete doesn't move a muscle," says Suinn.

Herbert Fensterheim, a psychologist at Cornell University Medical Center who has worked with several U.S. Olympians, tried Suinn's technique to see if it could be used to improve the percentage of successful foul shots. He studied eight college basketball teams, using the first half of the season without VMBR as a control period, and the second half of the season experimenting with VMBR with the players. According to Fensterheim, "With VMBR the overall performance improved 6 percent, which is not only statistically significant, but the coaches figured it was worth about eight games a year."

The key to this process is that whatever happens in mental imagery appears to carry over to real-life situations.

Says Fensterheim, "William James, the writer, used to say 'You learn to ice skate in the summer and to swim in the winter.' And what he was referring to was the mental rehearsal phenomenon, systematically learning and improving a skill with your brain, not with your muscles. Of course, you still have to get into a real game for feedback and fine tuning, but it seems certain that mental rehearsal accelerates the learning process."

THE PHYSICS OF SLUMP BUSTING

Despite the widespread myth of beginner's luck, someone who has never shot a basketball cannot stand at the free-throw line and make a long series of consecutive baskets. The most advanced methods of visualization and psychological conditioning can only fine tune an acquired skill, not create one.

Shooting skills have traditionally been acquired through trial and error at an early age, and by the time a player reaches the varsity level, most coaches concentrate on techniques of ball handling and play strategies, but they won't tamper with a player's shooting skill. As in other sports, coaches are saddled with the dogma that a good shooter is born, not made; it's a natural talent that some people have, and it can't be improved, aside from minor tips on position and timing. And even if it could be improved, coaches have had no *objective* criteria with which to suggest changes.

The reluctance to tamper with an acquired skill stems from the conservative and protective attitudes we have toward our *kinesthetic memory*. Kinesthesia is the perception of muscular movement, tension, and coordination, also known as muscle sense. Kinesthetic memory is that internal program of coordinated muscular contractions that has worked so well in the past, against which we unconsciously compare present movements to perform successfully—without it every action would be based on trial and error. In those sports where there is no instant feedback on performance, like a long drive in golf, a player will say his swing "felt good" long before the ball has reached its intended target. Here, the golfer has compared his present performance to his kinesthetic memory and feels confident about the outcome of his shot.

In basketball, there are now objective standards for either learning or refining shooting skills, if players and coaches can overcome their resistance to tampering with "natural talent." Our mechanical basketball player, which was not equipped with any form of kinesthetic memory, used precise physical equations to compute the angles and forces required for every shot. Of course, these formulas were not concocted for imaginary robots. Peter Brancazio published them in the hope of lending a scientific basis to the art of shooting.

Brancazio began by examining an attribute of all the best shooters, the "soft shot," where the ball arrives at the basket with the minimum amount of speed necessary to go in. If a shot does not result in a swish, the slow speed will help make it "lucky"—as it hits the rim or backboard, its kinetic energy will be exhausted on impact, making it more likely to drop into the basket rather than bounce away. Brancazio found that there are two ways, one old and one new, for any player to develop a soft shot: impart backspin to the ball and shoot with what he termed the *minimum-force angle.*

If a basketball is shot with no spin, when it hits a surface a fraction of its forward motion is translated into angular momentum, or a forward spin. If the ball is shot with forward spin (that is, the ball is spinning in the same direction it's moving), when it hits there's a decrease in its original spin, but an increase in the speed at which it bounces off the backboard or rim. Backspin minimizes the unpredictable rebound effect: after impact, there is a decrease in both spin and speed. These basic laws of motion apply to every game where there is a round ball and a flat surface—soccer, tennis or squash, for example.

The importance of developing backspin can be seen in comparing two different shooting styles at the foul line. The free throw is a critical and often decisive element in any game; one study found that about 25 percent of all victories were the result of free throws. Given the importance of this shot, there has been considerable debate about the best shooting style—overhand push shot versus underhand loop shot. Statistics published in three separate studies between 1950 and 1964 all show that the highest percentage of successful free throws were made with the underhand shot. In fact, it was once recommended as the only shot from the foul line. Yet, in recent years, Golden State Warriors' Rick Barry has been the only NBA player to use this style. He retired in 1980 but still holds the highest career free-throw percentage of any professional player: 89 percent.

An analysis of the physics of the two styles reveals that they both have advantages and disadvantages regarding angles and velocities, which appears to make both shots about equal. The slower entry velocity of the underhand makes it a softer shot, but the larger entry angle of the overhand makes it "see" a bigger rim area.[3] Why, if the two styles are about the same, does the underhand shot produce more baskets? After torturing the problem, Brancazio concluded that the major advantage of the underhand shot is that it is naturally thrown with a larger amount of backspin.

Despite the statistics and the physical analysis, modern players all shun the underhand shot because, they say, it conflicts with their overhand shot, used so effectively in field goals. Many players feel that learning a second shooting style will ruin their game. Yet Rick Barry mastered both styles, and had a higher career field goal percentage with the overhand shot than did such greats as Bill Bradley, Bob Cousey, Dave DeBusschere, and John Havlicek.

Since the distance of any shot directly influences the launch speed required to get the ball to the basket, the softness of a shot, regardless of spin, is going to decrease with distance. A lay-up requires much less speed than, say, a 15-foot jump shot. Since the speed and angle of launch required for a successful shot are interdependent, as demonstrated in the programming of the mechanical ball launcher, the distance of a shot influences the launch angle. Juggling these factors, Brancazio began his search for the minimum-force launch angle—the ideal compromise between angle and speed.

At one extreme is the rainbow shot, the high arc with the largest entry angle. To attain an entry angle of 87 degrees from the court (a 90-degree entry angle is a practical impossibility unless you're standing on a step ladder) the ball must be released with a speed of 65 feet/second (44 mph)—a feat beyond the ability of any known athlete using an orthodox shot. Even if the ball could be released at this speed, it would rise to a height of over 70 feet above the court, considerably higher than most arena ceilings.

At the other extreme is the flat shot, a line drive that requires the least amount of launch speed. A very tall player, releasing the ball over his head, can actually be shooting above the 10-foot rim, but even if he could look directly at the basket and throw the ball at the minimum entry angle of 33 degrees, there would be absolutely no margin for error; the ball must land in the dead center of the basket or it will bounce off the rim.

Between the two extremes lies the optimal launch angle and optimal launch speed—for a machine. For humans, there is the minimum-force angle. "Force" is the key here because it can be sensed and adjusted, whereas angle and speed are abstract concepts that are difficult to integrate into a player's technique. In any type of basketball shot, the final forces are imparted to the ball through the fingertips, where split-second adjustments in trajectory are made. In any activity, control of a movement decreases as muscle tension increases. In shooting, this means that the more force you apply to the ball, the less control you have of it as it leaves your fingers—hence larger errors in launch angle. For any position on the court, Brancazio has found a minimum-force angle at which the ball can be launched; this shot incorporates the old factors of high entry angle and low entry velocity with the minimum amount of force required to achieve both.

For a busy, pressured NBA player or coach this may all sound interesting, but is there any way to learn or teach shooting at the minimum-force angle? According to Brancazio, pure shooters *can* be made—it is possible to develop and improve one's ability to shoot a basketball accurately by taking a scientific approach to basketball shooting.

To find the minimum-force angle a player can practice

shooting the same shot at different launch angles, subjectively feeling the difference in the amount of force required to score; the purpose is to find the most effortless movement. At 15 feet, a 5-degree change in the launch angle corresponds to a 1-ounce change in launch force, which to sensitive basketball hands feels like a ton—a sensation with which a player can relate. Players should also notice where the ball sits in the air at the peak of its trajectory, in relation, say, to the top of the backboard or a row of bleachers, and compare this observation to the most effortless shot. A more objective method involves suspending strings or other markers from the ceiling at the peak trajectories for minimum-force shots.

To test his theoretical calculations against reality, Brancazio filmed college players considered to be good shooters—assuming that they had found the minimum-force angle by instinct—and analyzed their shots in slow motion through a film-editing machine. The trajectory of each shot was traced out on a plastic sheet that covered the viewer, and the launch angle was thus calculated. Brancazio found that most of the best shooters were, in fact, using the minimum-force angle.

But even the best players have occasional slumps, and Brancazio suggests that intentionally altering the launch angle and feeling for the effortless shot is a sure guide for slump busting.

Considering the importance of the minimum-force shot, an enterprising inventor might think about designing and testing a device that could measure the best launch angle for each player using tight beams of light, similar to those used in intruder alarm systems. When a player launched the ball at the correct trajectory, the light beams would be broken, and a small computer would assess the shot and provide the player with feedback, using a buzzer or bell.

This type of innovation is not as far off as some might imagine. In baseball and golf, work is now being conducted on a 3-D hologram-laser system, which athletes will use to practice their skills. The most significant use of these futuristic machines, however, may prove to be slump busting.

The old adage "practice is just practice" refers to the fact that repeating a flawed technique or motor skill won't necessarily correct the error—it may actually reinforce it. But if an athlete can obtain objective feedback about his performance, he then has external information, often more reliable than that provided by a coach or fellow player, against which he can compare the internal kinesthetic sensations of his movements.

Of course the introduction of high-tech slump-busting machines is possible only because sports scientists, like Brancazio, take the first step toward unraveling the complex physics behind phenomena like the simple swish.

IS "OXYGEN DEBT" A MYTH?

The fifth game of the 1984 NBA play-offs between the Los Angeles Lakers and the Boston Celtics was held at Boston Garden, an ancient arena that had no air conditioning. In the third quarter, as the temperature on the boards approached 100 degrees Fahrenheit, Kareem Abdul-Jabbar, the thirty-seven-year-old Lakers center, was pulled off the floor, apparently exhausted. The television cameras zoomed in on his face as a trainer gave him an oxygen mask, which he used again several times during the game.

The use of supplemental oxygen before exercise to give athletes a boost and after exercise to hasten recovery was first introduced by the Japanese at the 1932 Olympics in Los Angeles. The technique is still thought to be effective and is used in many sports as a sideline aid, particularly in football. The use of oxygen seems to make such good sense that its efficacy has seldom been challenged. In recent years, however, new information about endurance, fatigue, exhaustion, and recovery has raised interesting questions about oxygen therapy. Did Kareem Abdul-Jabbar really benefit or were the effects wholly imaginary?

As a player sits on the bench waiting for a game to begin, all the energy he needs comes from a fundamental chemical process occurring inside his muscle cells: carbohydrates, fats, and proteins are taken from the blood and combined with oxygen to manufacture ATP (adenosine triphosphate), the principal chemical that fuels muscle contraction. This is known as *aerobic* metabolism. Once the game has started and the player begins intensive exercise, his body cannot always supply enough oxygen to keep up with the demands of ATP production, and his muscles go into a short-term overdrive, or *anaerobic* metabolism. Here, carbohydrates and other substances stored in the muscles are broken down to make ATP without using oxygen.

The primary drawback to anaerobic energy production is that waste products begin to accumulate in the blood and they exert negative effects on the body's metabolism, a phenomenon associated with fatigue. In response to this stress, there is an increase in heart rate, blood pressure, and breathing to provide more oxygen for the muscles. In this way aerobic metabolism takes over again, and the wastes from the anaerobic phase are cleared from the blood as the fresh supply of oxygen is used to convert them back to carbohydrates.

Unlike football, where players exert a maximum energy output for the seconds that it takes to complete a play, basketball requires that a player pace himself. Because the game requires almost constant exertion, he must maintain a balance between his oxygen supply and oxygen demand to prevent fatigue caused by anaerobic metabolism. In football, a running back can theoretically hold his breath all the way to the end zone: the explosive bursts of energy are provided by anaerobic metabolism and the time between the plays allows his body to recover so he can exert a maximum effort play after play. If a basketball player exerted a continuous maximum effort he would have to be carried from the floor after the first few minutes of the opening quarter.

Everyone has his own upper limit of how much oxygen can be supplied to muscles during exercise. This maximum volume of oxygen that can be consumed by the body is called VO_2max, and is measured as milliliters of oxygen consumed per minute, per kilogram of body weight. Studies of trained basketball players have found that on the average they consume 35 milliliters of oxygen per minute of exercise per kilogram of weight. Kareem Abdul-Jabbar, who weighs 232 pounds (105 kilograms), consumes about 3.6 liters of oxygen every minute during a game—but that is not his VO_2max. It has been estimated that trained basketball players function at about 50 percent of their VO_2max. In Kareem Abdul-Jabbar's case this would mean that at maximum exertion he would consume no more than 70 milliliters of oxygen per kilogram per minute or 7.2 liters (7.6 quarts) of oxygen per minute.

An individual's VO_2max can be increased by 20 percent or more through endurance training (see Chapter 9). The more an athlete can increase the maximum amount of oxygen he can extract from the air and transport to his tissues, the less he will depend on anaerobic metabolism, and thus go farther and faster out on the court without fatigue. In this sense, VO_2max is an important measure of an individual's physical fitness (see Fig. 2.2).

Fatigue from exercise is caused by several different factors. An insufficient supply of oxygen, nutrients, and ATP, coupled with an accumulation of anaerobic waste products, will bring even the best-trained athlete to the threshold of fatigue. Those who push themselves beyond this point feel as if they are "running out of breath," the subjective experience of reaching an uncomfortable level of anaerobic waste products in the blood. Further exertion sometimes produces a "second wind," a sensation most physiologists once considered wholly imaginary. Evidence now suggests that a sudden decrease in the neural stimulation of the diaphragm as measured by EMG, allows the lungs to take in more air with less effort, which is accompanied by a sense of relief. But whether or not a player experiences a second wind, prolonged exertion using his anaerobic reserves will lead from fatigue to exhaustion until he collapses.

In the 1920s, physiologists theorized that when exercise involved anaerobic metabolism, the body developed an "oxygen deficit." The principal cause of this deficit was believed to be *lactic acid,* an anaerobic waste product, the same chemical that makes old milk taste sour. After exercise, the deficit was repaid with interest. The extra oxygen consumed as an athlete gulped for air following exertion was thought to support the combustion of a fraction of the lactic acid, providing the energy required to convert the remainder back to the ready-to-use sugar, glycogen. In this way, the extra oxygen consumed after exercise was thought to be a yardstick of the amount of anaerobic metabolism involved in exertion.

When athletes are placed on treadmills, scientists have found that their VO_2 increases in proportion to the intensity of exercise, but the level of lactic acid in the blood remains unchanged until exercise brings oxygen consumption up to or beyond 60 percent VO_2max—and then it rises dramatically. The

FIGURE 2.2

Comparison of Maximum Oxygen Uptake in Male Athletes in Eight Sports

Sport	Age	Height (feet and inches)	Weight (pounds)	VO_2max (milliliters per kilogram per minute)
Baseball	21	6'1"	182	48
Basketball	25	6'2"	185	55
Football	20	6'1"	211	51
Ice hockey	26	6'	189	53
Marathon	26	5'11"	141	77
Soccer	26	5'10"	167	58
Tennis	32	6'	169	50
Weight lifting	25	5'8"	178	40

One of the most accurate measurements of physical fitness, maximal oxygen consumption, or VO_2max, is the amount of oxygen an individual can extract from the air and deliver to his tissues. It is commonly measured as milliliters of oxygen delivered per kilogram (2.2 pounds) of body weight per minute, or ml/kg-min. VO_2max is primarily determined by the cardiovascular system, which adapts to endurance training by increasing blood volume, the number of red blood cells that carry oxygen, the size of selected arteries, and after prolonged training, increasing the size of the heart. As cardiovascular functions and VO_2max increase, so does the maximal sustained power output of an athlete.

The table above shows VO_2max values for male athletes, age twenty to thirty-two, in eight sports. The values are typical of the sports shown. Note the high VO_2max for the marathon runner, who must force his body over twenty-six miles, compared to the baseball player, who seldom runs more than a half mile in the course of a nine-inning game. (See Chapter 9 for more on the adaptations to endurance training.)

classic theory of oxygen debt contends that this takeoff point represents the *anaerobic threshold,* the point at which muscles have an insufficient supply of oxygen and anaerobic metabolism kicks in.

Recent research has shown that the sudden elevation of lactic acid may not mark the onset of anaerobic metabolism. In fact, there are several factors that do cause an increase in blood lactate and none of them has any direct connection with the anaerobic process.

First, as VO_2 increases, the blood in the body is automatically redistributed from lactate-removing to lactate-producing tissues. Second, hormones released during strenuous endurance training accelerate the rate at which glycogen is used up and lactate acid is produced. Third, as exercise intensity increases, the nervous system selectively recruits a greater number of fast-twitch muscle fibers, which are heavy users of glycogen and thus produce more lactic acid.

If blood lactate levels don't accurately reflect anaerobic metabolism, then the design and testing of athletes in endurance events like basketball may be flawed. In fact, some exercise physiologists select or reject athletes for training or competition on the basis of lactate levels in relation to exercise intensity.

The role of lactate and oxygen in exercise becomes clearer in light of findings deep inside muscles, where microscopic energy factories, called *mitochondria*, consume oxygen, break down carbohydrates and fats, and produce ATP. At the University of California, physiologist Kelvin J. Davies has discovered that endurance training causes a 100 percent increase in the number of mitochondria in muscles—and this doubling of energy factories was associated with a 400 percent increase in running endurance. VO_2max, however, increased by only 15 percent from the training.

This landmark finding led to the notion that endurance is determined by the muscles' capacity to use oxygen to burn fuels, whereas VO_2max is determined by the body's ability to transport oxygen from the lungs through the blood to the tissues. It is also interesting to note that these same studies found that strength training does not cause an increase in the mitochondrial content of muscles: bulk is no indication of endurance.

For reasons that remain unclear, mitochondria have an ability to consume much more oxygen than the blood can ever supply. This anomaly explains, in part, why *blood doping*, or induced erythrocythemia, is so effective in boosting endurance. This controversial process, reportedly used by seven U.S.

Olympic cyclists at the 1984 Los Angeles Games, involves taking up to a quart of an athlete's blood, or that of a matched donor, removing it for storage long before the event, and then reinfusing it to increase blood volume and the number of red blood cells that transport oxygen. One method separates, stores, and reinfuses only the red blood cells.

The first study that pointed to the potential for blood doping was conducted by physiologist Bjorn Ekblom at Stockholm's Institute of Gymnastics and Sports. He reported a 23 percent increase in exercise capacity in endurance events and a 9 percent increase in VO_2max following this procedure. Other studies have since found gains in endurance by as much as 37 percent and VO_2max by 26 percent. There are strict rules against blood doping set by the International Olympic Committee, but since the athlete uses his own or a matched type of blood, there are no reliable tests to detect the practice. Ekblom has recently said that a testing procedure to expose blood doping might be devised within a year.

To return to the original question posed in this chapter—whether supplemental oxygen was of any benefit to Kareem Abdul-Jabbar in Boston Garden—it is now possible to understand why the technique is mistakenly perceived to be advantageous.

When a player is pulled off the court for a rest, his breathing and heart rate remain high, even though exercise has ceased. In terms of the classic theory of oxygen debt, extra oxygen would seem to be needed to reconvert lactic acid to glycogen. Studies have shown, however, that *lactic acid does not cause oxygen debt.* Lactate serves to supply fuel to power the recovery process, but the combustion of lactic acid does not result in extra oxygen consumption. So why does the body work so hard after exercise—is there another reason why it needs more oxygen?

Physiologist George A. Brooks, of the University of California at Berkeley, believes he has the answer. He has proposed that the term "oxygen debt" be dropped from scientific vocabulary because it is misleading. He suggests the process be called *elevated postexercise oxygen consumption,* or EPOC. In his search for the causes of EPOC, Brooks looked at all the waste products of exercise and found that the major waste product is something so obvious it was apparently overlooked: heat. Unlike mechanical engines that use the heat of chemical reactions to move pistons and levers, the human body uses chemical reactions to directly make muscles contract. Heat is a by-product of biochemical locomotion, and if it accumulates in the body it can be deadly.

In tests of muscles in elevated temperatures, Brooks discovered that heat increases the rate at which mitochondria consume oxygen. Brooks explains that a mitochondrion can be likened to an automobile engine, which can run at full speed, take in oxygen, and burn fuel; but if the linkage in the drive train is faulty or inoperative, the wheels won't turn. During exercise, the elevated temperatures have the effect of disabling the drive-train gears in mitochondria; they are still consuming fuel and oxygen, but ATP production is diminished or halted until temperatures return to normal. Brooks's discovery corresponds to the work of other scientists. It is well known, for example, that basal or resting metabolism increases in humans during a fever by about 13 percent for every degree Celsius of increase in body temperature. Other studies have shown that EPOC volume rises with tissue temperatures.

In terms of the automobile analogy, giving supplemental oxygen to an athlete after exercise to speed recovery is like pumping extra oxygen into a car's carburetor to make it run, although the transmission was blown during a race. In fact, studies have been unable to detect any accelerated decrease in heart rate, blood pressure, or breathing with supplemental oxygen following exercise.

Breathing pure oxygen *before* exercise increases the amount of oxygen in the blood by 80 to 100 milliliters, and this has been associated with a 1 percent increase in maximal work capacity in exercise lasting less than two minutes. But because the extra oxygen in the blood dissipates so rapidly, oxygen before exercise is not practical. In the laboratory, oxygen taken *during* exercise has been shown to improve performance, but out on the basketball court any advantage would be more than offset by the weight of the tanks!

Athletes still swear they feel better after breathing sideline oxygen, and it may be that it does serve to clear their minds.

Perhaps the tanked gas is slightly cooler than the ambient air and it feels refreshing. A more likely explanation is that supplemental oxygen exerts a placebo effect, but most trainers would probably be reluctant to present this idea to someone with the stature of Kareem Abdul-Jabbar.

THREE

ICE HOCKEY

Fire on Ice

Referee Don Wicks was a busy man in the fourth game of the 1974 Stanley Cup play-offs. The Philadelphia Flyers and the Boston Bruins, two of the meanest teams in the National Hockey League (NHL), came roaring out of their dressing rooms and battled it out on the ice, devoting almost as much time spearing, hooking, high-sticking, and clubbing each other as chasing the puck.

As a result of the general mayhem, Wicks handed out twenty penalties in the opening period, which is ordinarily over within thirty minutes, but in this game took sixty-seven minutes to complete.

Of course the fans were not put off either by the fighting or the delay of game. Most were thrilled by the blood on the ice. One Flyers fan gleefully told author James Michener, who at first felt lucky to have tickets to the game, "How do you think we defeated New York last week? Our knuckle boys beat the living shit out of them and they were afraid to skate." Michener left the game appalled by the barbarity and went on a crusade against violence in sports in his book *Sports in America.*

For all its speed and flare, grace and beauty, ice hockey is a game rooted in violence. Even its most outspoken critics acknowledge that the fierce body contact and savage slashing of sticks is intrinsic to the sport. When sportswriters call for an end to "the senseless and unnecessary violence," their semantics logically accept a place for sensible and necessary violence. Indeed, psychologists who have studied hockey players distinguish between *instrumental aggression*, which is re-

65

quired to break through defensive formations, and *hostile aggression,* which is employed only to injure an opponent.

Purists rightly fear that the brawls might reduce hockey to the level of professional wrestling, but sports scientists hope to harness this form of natural, instrumental aggression to the players' advantage. By dissecting the chaos, pinpointing the source of violence, and redirecting the emotional power toward skating faster and scoring more goals, new training techniques can be developed that will be just as important as skating drills or practice shots on goal.

TAPPING VIOLENCE AS AN ENERGY SOURCE

The popular theories on hockey violence state that fights are provoked by players who are either psychologically deranged or victims of deprived economic backgrounds. This portrait of bloodthirsty goons, stereotyped as the notorious Hansen brothers in the film *Slap Shot,* is not typical of any player in the NHL today.

A study by Jean Poupart, a criminologist at the University of Montreal, has provided evidence that players are certainly tough and aggressive, but on their own, outside the context of the arena, they seldom if ever display the hostility seen so frequently on the ice. Almost all of the players interviewed confidentially by Poupart said they disliked the game's brutality, and most reported they were terrified when fights broke out on the ice. On the other hand, the players said they felt pressure from others to assume hostile roles—and once in those roles all the natural aggression of the game was freely expressed as overt hostility. In particular, they said they felt pressure from management to put on ever more spectacular performances, which they translated as ever more *violent* performances. Sound like a lot of rationalization?

Conn Smythe, owner of the Toronto Maple Leafs between 1927 and 1961, often quipped about hockey brawls and acknowledged their commercial value. He once said, "We've got to stamp out this sort of thing or people are going to keep on buying tickets." It's unlikely that any player on the Toronto bench hadn't memorized Smythe's maxim: "If you can't beat 'em in the alley, you can't beat 'em on the ice."

The practice of cashing in on violence has persisted since Smythe's heyday. Only two years ago, Paul Mulvey of the Los Angeles Kings was thrown off the team by coach Don Perry because he refused an order to jump off the bench and join a fight. Mulvey's defiance ruined his career. He was relegated to the minor leagues and it has been alleged he's blacklisted, if unofficially, as a clear signal to other players that they better fight if they want to play.

Players are also urged to violence by their fans. As in basketball, boisterous crowds in small arenas exert a powerful psychological effect. The home-court advantage adds to the effect; hockey teams display more aggression at home games. In fact, hockey fans cheer and applaud as much, and sometimes more, for fights as for goals.

A third source of hockey violence stems from the players' own peculiar code of honor. According to research conducted by Gordon W. Russell, a psychologist at the University of Lethbridge in Alberta, aggression in hockey tends to increase in intensity and frequency during the course of a game. From the first act of aggression, the tendency is for players to display more extreme forms of aggression. The escalation of violence, says Russell, stems from a "norm of reciprocity," which calls for aggrieved players to retaliate and settle unresolved insults and injuries.

In a survey of 160 professional and amateur hockey players in Canada, sociologist Kenneth Colburn, Jr., of Indiana University, discovered a distinctly chivalrous ritual in hockey fights. Although his players reported they disliked violence, they also felt obliged to retaliate for cheap shots, such as spearing with a stick from behind. These violations break the social code that binds competitors and teammates alike. Thus, in the eyes of these players, a fight is not violence, but is both a proper response and a deterrent to further infractions.

Colburn observed that the ritual fights on the ice have rules as clearly defined as those at a joust in Camelot. Just as the medieval knight would throw down the gauntlet, an aggrieved hockey player always drops his gloves and stick and assumes a fighting pose. In this way, both his opponents and other players are put on notice that a fight is about to begin. A player can skate away from a scuffle without a loss of honor, as long as his challenger has not dropped his gloves. Once the gloves are down, however, a player must respond by fighting or suffer the public disgrace of being a cowardly cheap shot who can strike with his stick from behind, but lacks the guts to fight face to face without the advantage of surprise.

Given that hockey players are inspired to play aggressive and often violent games, are there any positive benefits, other than at the box office?

In an archival study of hockey records over an eight-year period, John F. McCarthy, a psychologist at Fairfield University in Connecticut, found a significant relationship between high aggression and scoring. Those players rated high in aggression, using penalties and psychological tests as a guide, consistently scored more goals and had more shots on goal than those low in aggression. McCarthy found a similar, but less profound correlation between goal assists and aggression. "This finding suggests that not only is output high [in aggressive players], possibly because of generalized levels of motor output, but also the aggressive player is more efficient as well as effective," reports McCarthy.

These findings appear to corroborate conventional locker room wisdom that anger gets the adrenaline pumping, producing superhuman performances in which athletes go faster, farther, and hit harder. It also fits the prevailing view of contact sports as a constructive and healthy expression of aggression, which builds character, discipline, perseverance, and respect for authority. Certainly Vince Lombardi and Conn Smythe would agree. But from a scientific perspective, this philosophy is flawed, and if blindly embraced by coaches and players can impair performance.

Aggressive players may score more goals, but there is an aggression-hostility threshold that, once crossed, reduces a player's ability to concentrate on the motor skills required to perform successfully. NHL statistics, comparing penalties to goals, generally support McCarthy's study, but there are important exceptions: the Oilers' Wayne Gretzky and the Islanders' Mike Bossy, two top scorers in the NHL today, have the fewest penalty minutes of any of the top dozen scorers in the league.

Coaches, fans, and psychologists may quibble about the precise definitions of aggression and violence, but every player knows that once he has crossed his own aggression-hostility threshold, his performance will deteriorate.

"If you get so mad that you'd really rather injure an opponent or punch a referee, you're going to be off your game," says Thomas A. Tutko, a sports psychologist at San Jose University. "Coaches who exhort players to get mad at opponents are not enhancing performance. Anger, for most athletes, destroys concentration and gets them in trouble. While it's true that some players can channel the energy that anger generates to be more effective, most of them have never developed that capacity."

A perceptive coach who works closely with his players will know which individuals on the team can get angry without being hostile. Similarly, studying the temperaments of opposing players can provide clues about which individuals can be provoked. Tennis star John McEnroe, famous for his temper tantrums, often uses his anger to effectively distract his opponents. If a judge has made what McEnroe considers a bad call, he will interrupt play, rant and rave, and when he returns to the court, his opponent will often have lost his concentration and competitive edge.[1]

Is there any way to maximize player aggression without crossing the hostility threshold? When former Philadelphia Flyers coach Bob McCammon tried to reduce what he termed "dumb penalties" among his Broad Street Bullies, he found that fines did not reduce minutes in the penalty box. So, instead of taking their money, he took their playing time: players who drew petty penalties were benched. This reduced penalties, but also kept his best players out of the game.

Today, sport psychologists believe that concentration training and arousal control, not discipline, is the most effective way to harness aggression. One key lies in a player's own perception of grievances over time. In the studies of Russell and Colburn, the levels of aggression were observed to increase during the course of a game; other studies report that aggression increases in hockey players as they become older. It would seem that, to control aggression, a player must learn how to abort the effect of cumulative grievances.

Jeffrey H. Goldstein, a psychologist at Temple University in Philadelphia, who has studied sports violence for several years, believes that human beings possess a remarkable ability to transform an emotion, for example, mild personal insult into a great wrong—by rewriting history, effectively reinterpreting the past. For example, a player who feels wronged by an opponent during a game is capable of reinterpreting previous collisions, blocks, and other physical encounters—which had hitherto not been interpreted as personally offensive—as intentional attempts to injure, foul, slight, dishonor, or otherwise undermine his feelings of worth. A slight anger, says Goldstein, may thus become transformed into a great one, and it is this greater anger, fueled by a revision of past events, that is likely to be violently acted upon.

"If a player is sufficiently distracted from the task of revising history, the slight anger remains minor and, in fact, will dissipate with the passage of time," says Goldstein. "Sports that require complete attention and concentration may easily serve this distracting function, thereby preventing a negative emotion from becoming more intense."

Modern concentration training involves what sport psychologists call *stress management.* It's easy to tell a player to pay attention, to concentrate, but in the presence of stress—whether it's defined as physical wear and tear or psychological anxiety and tension—there is a physiological reaction. As the sympathetic nervous system speeds up in response to stress, the heart rate increases, palms sweat, and general metabolism goes into a higher gear. To prevent the physiological response to stress from causing psychological distractions, a player needs to learn how to relax, while still remaining alert and aggressive. Systematic imagery training, such as Visuo-Motor Behavior Research (see Chapter 2), deep muscle relaxation techniques, and biofeedback, have all been used effectively to minimize the effects of stress in U.S. Olympic athletes; but these techniques have never been broadly applied to professional hockey players.

Another factor in concentration training is *arousal control.* This refers to the ability to alter the intensity of behavior, from being very calm and relaxed to being extremely excited. The objective is to help the athlete find the optimal arousal level for the tasks required. Although this skill consists of both raising and lowering the level of arousal, the main objective is learning to lower arousal. In this respect, hockey coaches could learn from psychological training techniques used by world-class weight lifters. With these elite athletes, concentration is as important as muscle development. As part of their regular training, weight lifters pump iron while spectators intentionally taunt and jeer; the purpose is to teach the athlete to shut out all external distractions, no matter how provocative, and put all their concentration into lifting the weights.

"In the next few years, concentration training will become part and parcel with traditional physical training," predicts Goldstein. "Aggression can run high in sports like hockey as long as the player remains in control. Blind rage is not enough to score goals."

Ron Meyer, coach of the New England Patriots, who believes emotion is overrated in contact sports, recently remarked, "There was a lot of emotion at the Alamo, and nobody survived."

DO HOCKEY HELMETS REALLY WORK?

On a cold November night in 1959, Jacques Plante, goaltender for the Montreal Canadiens, crouched low on the ice of Madison Square Garden, squinting at the puck, which danced with the stick of Rangers right wing Andy Bathgate. About 25 feet from the goal mouth, Bathgate made a hard backhand shot that knuckled through the air, eluded Plante's glove, and smashed into his face.

The goalie toppled forward and lay on the ice. The game was stopped as concerned teammates surrounded Plante and frantically waved the Montreal trainer into the rink. Like Lazarus, Plante was soon back on his feet, but was escorted from the ice with a blood-soaked towel covering his face.

Down in the arena's medical room, Garden physician Kazuo Yanagisawa closed a jagged three-inch gash that ran from Plante's left nostril down to his lip with seven stitches. The thirty-year-old player knew from experience that the wound would leave another scar. After six seasons with the Canadiens, Plante had accumulated over 200 stitches, two broken cheekbones, had twice suffered a fractured skull, and had his nose busted four times.

Toe Blake, the Montreal coach, came down to the medical

room when the physician had finished his sewing and asked Plante how he felt.

"I'll go back in," Plante said, "if you let me wear the mask."

Having no other goalkeeper, Blake was forced to agree to let Plante wear a mask out on the ice, and his decision made history. No NHL goaltender had worn a mask in thirty years, not since Clint Benedict of the Montreal Maroons had worn one briefly to protect a badly broken nose. Everyone thought a mask would seriously reduce the breadth of vision required of a goaltender in the high-speed game of hockey. Besides, goalies were not supposed to fear injury, as they have always appeared immune to pain.

When Plante came back on the ice wearing a prototype fiber-glass mask he had experimented with during practice, the crowd was at first stunned into silence, then broke into howls of ridicule. After the arena settled down, the Canadiens won 3–1, with Plante making twenty-four saves while wearing the new protective equipment. After some hesitation, Blake let his goaltender wear the mask while his face healed and during this period became convinced that breadth of vision—and number of saves—was not impaired by the mask. Although Plante was called a coward for months, his record as a player for his insistence on wearing a mask ushered in a new era in hockey safety. Today, masks are not mandatory in professional hockey, but all goaltenders wear them. It can even be said that the mask has given players a wider variety of shots on goal, as the old rule "keep the puck down" no longer applies.

To say hockey is a hard-hitting contact sport is an understatement. Ten men skate at speeds of up to 30 mph on a stretch of ice that measures 200 by 85 feet—a rink that may seem large until you realize the players are bounded by immovable boards with little more than their noses to serve as bumpers. On razor-sharp skates, armed with 5-foot sticks, they slash at each other and a frozen rubber puck that can slice through the air at speeds up to 120 mph. The rink is like a bull ring . . . without a *burladero* to hide behind.

Despite the apparent lack and poor design of protective equipment, ice hockey has a surprisingly low injury rate compared to other contact sports, with the head and face being the most commonly injured part of the body.

Facial injuries account for 45 percent of all hockey injuries, most of which result from contact with the stick and puck. Injuries to the head and other parts of the body are a result of collisions between players and with the ice, boards or steel goalposts. Surveys have found that forwards are far more predisposed to injury than defense men, and the safest position on the ice is the goaltender.

A study of 174 NHL players conducted by Kent Wilson, an ear, nose, and throat specialist at the University of Minnesota Medical School, found that 93 percent of nongoalie players and 74 percent of goalies reported having sustained a facial injury during only one season. Over their careers, there was an average of fifteen facial lacerations per man, over one facial fracture each, with the nose being the most frequently broken bone, and a loss of about two teeth per man. Goaltenders had a significantly lower rate of lacerations and dental loss than nongoalies, which may be attributed to mask protection, although they had a higher rate of facial fractures.

Epidemiological studies of the type and rates of injury per player position provide important clues for sports physicians interested in preventive measures, but because the evidence is somewhat circumstantial it can also lead to faulty deductions. The goaltenders' injury rate is a case in point: survey data suggests that goalies have fewer facial injuries than any other players, but from this it cannot be concluded that current mask designs are necessarily safe or effective.

Plante's 1959 mask was made using a plaster cast of his face, and the mold was filled with fiberglass, which, once dried, fit snugly to the contours of his face. The mask undoubtedly served to quell Plante's fear of injury, but in fact would have offered very little protection had he been hit hard. Once the Plante face-molded mask became accepted by other goalies, similar contour designs quickly followed. Most were made of plastics about 5 millimeters (0.2 inch) thick, sometimes backed with thin rubber wedges of about the same thickness. As soon as they appeared on the market, the masks were advertised as capable of preventing lacerations and deflecting, distributing, and reducing impacts from pucks and sticks—although there was absolutely no published research to support these claims.

The first investigation of mask safety was conducted in 1973 by Robert Norman, a kinesiologist at the University of Waterloo in Ontario, Canada. Using techniques similar to those employed to evaluate football helmets (see Chapter 1), he developed a head model studded with strain gauges, which could be adjusted to support the mask at contact points on the player's face. He then struck the masks with a weighted puck suspended from a guide wire at various speeds. To no one's surprise he found that none of the face-molded masks could distribute the forces at velocities of about 70 feet/second. Subsequent to the publication of this research, some goalies adopted either cushioned face masks with wire grilles or clear plastic shields for eye protection. Manufacturers touted the new masks as providing protection for pucks traveling up to 100 feet/second; again, Norman and his skeptical colleagues tested the masks by propelling pucks from a shooting apparatus. Studying the effects with high-speed films, they found that eye or facial damage could be expected from pucks traveling over 85 feet/second.

Today, thanks largely to Norman's investigations, official skepticism of manufacturer's safety claims has led to the imposition of industry standards that are considered adequate. However, when the masks were worn with a helmet, the combined weight was over two pounds, which some players felt was too heavy. Moreover, the increased mass has been implicated in spinal cord injuries when the goalie was slammed to the ice. Nineteen cervical spine injuries were reported in the Province of Ontario over a period of two seasons with the heavy headgear worn, and one study of the helmet-mask factor advocated the use of restraining collars to reduce the chance of whiplash injuries.

A majority of professional players wear helmets today, some equipped with wire masks, but there remains a vocal minority who strongly object to headgear or being forced to wear any kind of protective equipment they think unnecessary. The fact is that head injuries are common in hockey, but seldom serious. Since 1903 there have been only three fatalities in professional hockey, two of which came from blows to the head. This death rate is lower than that of any other contact sport, as well as baseball.

The most recent fatality occurred in January 1968, when the

Minnesota North Stars played the Oakland Seals in the Metropolitan Sports Center in Bloomington, Minnesota. Four minutes into the game, Stars center Bill Masterton received a hard, but legal, body check from Seals right wing Ron Harris. Masterton bounced off another player, flew backward, cracking his bare head on the ice so hard that blood poured from his ears and nose. Reporters said they could hear the gruesome impact up in the press box. He fell so hard, in fact, that observers believe he may have been out before he hit the ice. Masterton never regained consciousness. Following this incident, the NHL allocated $5,000 for helmet research, which, critics charged, was merely a token response to blunt a public outcry.

Serious evaluation of hockey helmets did not begin until 1970. As in football or boxing (see Chapter 4), concussions and other forms of brain trauma are caused by either direct blows (linear acceleration) or oblique, twisting blows (rotational acceleration) to the head. Helmet research based its studies on the accepted fact that rotational acceleration produces a twisting motion of the skull around the brain, which, during the first few milliseconds of impact, remains stationary. As the skull moves around the outer surface of the brain, strains are imposed on the delicate tissues, often tearing the veins and capillaries, and inside the brain, severe traumatic hemorrhages can occur. Linear acceleration produces a squashing or compression of the brain tissue at the site of impact and an explosive expansion of tissue on the opposite side of impact (see Fig. 4.1). The extent of brain injury from either linear or rotational blows—and most injuries involve a little of both—depends on velocity of acceleration and duration of impact. At the same velocity, a few milliseconds can mean the difference between a headache and a concussion.

Knowing what impact velocities and impact times were capable of causing brain damage in linear and rotational blows to the head, René G. Therrien, a kinesiologist at the University of Sherbrooke in Canada, tested hockey helmets made in 1982 on dummy heads loaded with instruments. He found that impact velocities between 15 and 18 feet/second and impact times between 13 to 15 milliseconds produced accelerations that in a human head would be below acceptable injury thresholds for linear blows; but *all* rotational accelerations at these values turned out to be *above injury thresholds*. Remember, these are fairly modern helmets, which are manufactured to industry standards thought to be safe.

In real life, it's unlikely that the impact will be just linear. If you place a bowling ball on a flat, smooth surface and strike it with a hammer—no matter how hard you try to align the hammer with the center of the ball's mass—it will rotate away from the impact, either a little to the left or right. Therrien was equally convinced there must be rotational acceleration, even in an artificial situation using a dummy head. To document this effect he studied high-speed films (6,000 frames/second) of the impacts. These films showed that, at the onset of the collision, the outer layer of the helmet is deformed and flattened at the site of impact and simultaneously begins to rotate around the headform. After about 5 to 12 degrees of rotation, the helmet begins to regain its original shape and the dummy head begins to rotate—just as a human head would. There it was on film.

Therrien concluded that "the results presented clearly demonstrate that present day hockey helmets give a false illusion of protection against severe brain injury in oblique impacts . . . it is highly improbable that helmet design alone, even if it included some device producing a damping of the rotational motion, could bring high velocity impacts well below the tolerable thresholds for humans."

It should be noted that Therrien's impact velocity of 15 to 18 feet/second is below speeds that have actually been measured for hockey players who are *sliding* on the ice (up to 19 to 22 feet/second); in other words, if they are sliding on the ice they have already decelerated considerably. What if they were jammed into the boards or the steel goalposts at full skating speed? Or what if they were thrown to the hard ice?

In 1983, a teenage boy who was wearing a modern helmet, certified safe, suffered permanent brain damage when he hit the ice after being checked in a midget-league game in Spokane, Washington. The evidence convinced a jury that the player was wearing the helmet correctly, and he was awarded $3.5 million in damages, which the helmet manufacturer was forced to pay because the court found the company had not made a safe product. Therrien would not have been surprised.

In the rugged sport of ice hockey injuries have traditionally been shrugged off as an occupational hazard. In light of the low rate of fatality and serious injury in an aggressive, often violent sport, it would be a moot point to conclude that the masks and helmets are not safe, or that it is only by chance that the thigh protection in the poorly designed pants is in the right place at the right time as players crash into the boards, goalposts, or each other. If anything, it's ironic that some hardheaded, old-fashioned players are compelled to wear safety equipment that really doesn't seem to confer too much protection.

FEAR OF INJURY

No one will deny the tough nature of a professional hockey player, yet many of these men have confided to sports psychologists that they live with decidedly mixed feelings about violence and injury in the game. Studies of players' personality profiles have found that most fear fights, yet all see themselves as aggressive, capable men prepared to fight for honor, paychecks, and fan appreciation. This same ambivalence extends to their attitudes toward injury: no one wants to get hurt, but when it happens they are keen to get back on the ice as soon as possible, even if they have suffered a major laceration to the face or a broken nose. Defiance of pain is part of the game.

Considering the extent and number of injuries experienced by Jacques Plante, there can be no question about his courage. He did, however, once confess to a sportswriter that he had nightmares in the hospital while he recovered from those injuries. Some of these dreams were so vivid, he said, they were like movies in which "somebody takes a slap shot, but you don't see the puck until the last second; then it's a dark shadow coming at your face." Then, Plante said, he'd suddenly wake up in a cold sweat and find a nurse mopping his brow.

Rudy Pilous, coach of the Chicago Black Hawks, once recalled a play-off against the Canadiens when the game was stopped to clear debris thrown on the ice by the rowdy Chicago fans. As the referee was about to resume play, Pilous looked over at his goal and saw there was no one in the crease. A moment later, veteran goalie Glenn Hall came clomping up the stairs after using the team dressing room to throw up. Hall was never known as fainthearted. He had played 552 consecutive games, but he vomited before many of them.

Fear of injury is a big factor in most sports, including non-contact and individual sports. In particular, there is considerable anxiety about being struck in the face and the groin, even though the incidence of injury in the latter is very low. The severity of pain in a traumatized testicle, however, justifies what would otherwise be an irrational fear. The next time you are at a game and see a player catch a line drive in the groin and fall down, curling up into a fetal position, quickly look up and down your row of seats and see how many men have involuntarily clutched their own vulnerable area. A blow to the groin is like no other physical injury for males; not only is the pain incapacitating, it's accompanied by an emotional feeling of total helplessness, linked with the primal fear of castration and impotence.

Protective cups, made of plastic and rubber, offer limited protection. Many players won't wear them because they can be awkward, although no goalie in his right mind goes onto the ice without one. In 1981, Mike Liut, goaltender of the St. Louis Blues, caught a puck, estimated to be going about 70 to 100 mph, on his cup. When he reached the locker room he discovered the plastic had completely disintegrated as if a truck had run over it. At a nearby hospital, surgeons treated a testicular contusion and Liut was soon back in the crease, showing no shyness of the puck.

Behind the bravado, each player copes with his anxieties and fears in his own way. Some effectively deny their feelings, which are inevitably vented in some unconscious mode, such as nightmares. Others discharge the emotion with injury jokes, an aggressive playing style, binges, or pregame rituals and superstitions. Phil Esposito, throughout his eighteen-year career with the Boston Bruins and New York Rangers, prepared for every game with the same ritual. On the way to home games, he made sure he passed through the same toll booth he used before his last winning game. Once in the locker room, whether home or away, he put on his uniform in a precise sequence; underpants, pants, leggings, skates, and jersey. Once on the bench, he'd put a pack of gum next to him and put his gloves palms

78

up on either side of his stick. During the national anthem he'd say a Hail Mary, the Lord's Prayer, plus a prayer that his team played well and that no one would be hurt.

This kind of ritual is not rare among players and may continue for years unknown to anyone else on the team; indeed, the magical efficacy of superstitious ritual is perceived to be enhanced by privacy. On the other hand, entire teams may share certain superstitions. During the mid-1970s, the Philadelphia Flyers thought that Kate Smith's rendition of *"God Bless America"* brought them good luck, so they asked for the song to be played before critical games. During this period they won fifty-nine, lost nine and tied twice. Then the New York Rangers got hot (without team rituals) and began winning the Stanley Cup. The magic faded and the national anthem is now played before Flyers games.

Superstitious rituals, according to sports psychologists, are a way of reducing pregame fear and anxiety, directing and discharging emotions that might impair performance. As a form of structured behavior, rituals also help a player gain concentration. The net effect is to provide a sense of security about things they can't control.

The unspoken rationale of these rituals is that if the magic worked once, it'll work again. Studies have found that the greater the risk or adversity, the more superstition prevails. Of course, this is not confined only to hockey. In a survey of 137 intercollegiate athletes in several sports, psychologist Jane Gregory of Western Ontario University found that one-third of the athletes reported practicing superstitious pregame behavior, and half said they knew of others who had their own rituals with which to ward off bad luck.

Superstitions may seem irrational, but if they enhance performance, psychologists agree they should be given free expression. Certainly, the juxtaposition of contrary modes of behavior in ice hockey should come as no surprise. It's a game of contradictions: grace and brutality, players who prefer not to fight but have more brawls than any other team sport, the reluctance to adopt safety equipment despite the potential for serious injury.

Following the madness of the 1974 Stanley Cup play-offs,

Philadelphia Flyers owner Ed Snider summed up his feelings this way: "No other sport can make me irrational except hockey. And that's fine."

BIOMECHANICS OF SKATING AND SHOOTING

A living blur, barreling down the ice, Bobby Hull's missing front teeth gave his mouth a squarish, mechanical appearance like the intake vent of a small jet engine. He was once clocked at 28.3 mph skating with the puck and 29.7 mph without it—faster than Bob Hayes's all-time highest instantaneous speed for a human being on two legs. Hull could also slap a puck at 120 mph, or 35 mph faster than the average NHL player, or for that matter, faster than anyone who had ever played the game.

Hull's phenomenal speed was attributed to his strength. Years of chopping wood and other strenuous farm work gave him a physique like a bull. One Chicago newspaper said he was "a statue come alive from the Golden Age of Greece, incredibly handsome even without his front teeth." By contrast, Wayne Gretzky, the young record-smashing player with the Edmonton Oilers, has surpassed all of Hull's records except for his career totals, but he is thin and physically weak. One season he came in last on the team's strength tests.

Gretzky is a paradox. How can he hold so many NHL records and possess so little strength?

Today it has been established that a lack of strength in a hockey player can be compensated for with improvement in *technique*, although a strong player who also displays top form will be unbeatable in a race to the puck.

Hockey is characterized by *power skating*, which is distinct from speed skating or figure skating in that it involves rapid changes in velocity and direction. In some respects, the power skater is like the football rusher; but unlike sprinting, this style of skating has very slow acceleration, taking almost half the length of the rink to attain peak velocity. And by that time, a player often has to decelerate or even reverse direction, constantly recruiting his muscles for every maneuver.

From a stationary position, the power skater drives forward by digging the metal blade of his rear skate into the ice and pushing off. The power of the drive comes from the strength of

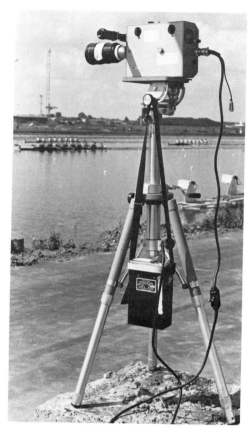

The Locam II high-speed 16-mm pin-registered motion picture camera can record athletic activities at frame speeds of up to 1,000 exposures per second. The lightweight, portable camera system is used by the biomechanics lab at the U.S. Olympic Training Center in Colorado Springs. Here the camera is set up to record the action in an eight-man crew race. The high-resolution films can be digitized and fed into a computer for analysis. (Courtesy of Redlake Corporation.)

the push, involving muscles in the hip and thigh. Traditionally, most power skaters fully extend their hip and knee with each stride, which then must be accelerated forward for the next stride, doing so with straight legs.

Charles J. Dillman, head of the U.S. Olympic Training Center's biomechanics lab in Colorado Springs, has recently discovered that the speed of hockey players can be significantly improved if the leg forces involved in a drive from a stationary position were applied from a flexed position. As over 75 percent of a player's acceleration occurs in the first 1.5 seconds— or within three strides after pushing off—Dillman found that by simply changing the drive technique to one with more flex in the knees, a player could increase his range of movement by 3 feet during the initial 2 seconds of acceleration—a critical difference in a race for the puck. Using three high-speed 16-mm cameras positioned around the rink to obtain a 3-D analysis, Dillman made his discovery after digitizing the films and feeding the data to computers. It soon became apparent that skaters who accelerated from a relatively upright, extended style lost speed because their skates literally *bounced* on the ice. By bending forward and flexing the knees, the forces that caused the bouncing were directed away from the skater in the opposite direction from which he was traveling.

A similar discovery was made by John F. Alexander, a kinesiologist at the University of Alberta: Technique may be more important than strength in shooting. His investigation began by measuring the speed and accuracy of the four basic hockey shots—the standing wrist shot, skating wrist shot, standing slap shot, and skating slap shot—using thirty players from four teams *(see Fig. 3.1)*.

The first surprise in this study was an inverse relationship between speed and accuracy: the skating wrist shot is the most accurate of all types of shot, although it is among the slowest. This has been confirmed by other scientists who found that the powerful slap shot, standing or skating, is 40 percent less accurate than the wrist shot.

But the really intriguing finding was a low correlation between grip strength and speed of shooting. In fact, *accuracy for all shots was unrelated to grip strength.* This was contrary to all expectations, as players have always been told to grip the stick firmly to increase accuracy as well as speed.

René Doré, a physicist at the École Polytechnique in Montreal, shed more light on this puzzle in an experiment in which he measured the force produced by a player's hands on the stick, placing strain gauges along the handle and blade. As his players skated, trailing an umbilical cord, the output signals from the strain gauges were amplified and recorded by an eight-channel oscilloscope in the penalty box. The puck velocity was measured with digital time counters, triggered and stopped by microphones that picked up the noise of the blade hitting the puck and the puck striking the target.

Using these methods, Doré compared wrist and slap shot velocities and found speeds that closely resembled those in Alexander's study. But he also found something unexpected.

First, the maximum force in the stick for *all* shots, located at the heel of the blade, was always about 22 pounds, except for

FIGURE 3.1
Mean Velocity and Accuracy of Four Types of Ice Hockey Shots by Two Teams*

Team	Wrist Shot				Slap Shot			
	Standing		Skating		Standing		Skating	
	Speed (mph)	Accuracy (30 max)	Speed (mph)	Accuracy (30 max)	Speed (mph)	Accuracy (30 max)	Speed (mph)	Accuracy (30 max)
Professional 11 players	63	20	79	20	75	19	86	21
University 6 players	54	18	76	19	60	15	76	18
Amateur 7 players	62	20	71	23	72	16	79	19

The skating slap shot is the fastest, and the standing wrist shot is the slowest for the teams studied by Alexander. The differences in shooting accuracy were not statistically significant by either shot type or team, although it appears that the skating wrist shot was the most accurate and the standing slap shot least accurate. Team averages have been rounded off to the nearest whole number and standard deviations omitted.

*Source: adapted from J. E. Alexander (1963), pp. 263–64. (See bibliography.)

the stationary slap shot in which, oddly enough, this force was generally *lower*, despite the higher puck speed. Second, the puck velocity for slap shots was not directly related to the maximum force produced on the stick. For example, one player exerted a force, recorded by the two strain gauges on the blade, of 13 and 22 pounds, producing a puck velocity of 85 feet/second; for another player, however, the forces for the same two gauges were 11 and 4 pounds, yet yielded a puck velocity of 95 feet/second!

If the power of a slap shot, which is the fastest shot in the game, is unrelated to the maximum forces a player exerts on his stick, what else can possibly be propelling the puck at such lightning speeds?

Using high-speed cinematography (2000 frames/second), René Therrien, the Canadian kinesiologist who studied hockey helmets, appears to have captured the answer on film. He shot pucks from an air gun at 75 mph onto the blade of a stick, which was clamped to a heavy base. The clamps were arranged on the handle in the same way a player would normally hold the stick, and the camera was positioned above the blade, looking down at the impact with the puck just as a player would if his eyes could work that fast.

When the films were developed, Therrien found that within the span of only 83 frames, or within 41.5 milliseconds, the puck danced with the blade, striking it not once but *three times* before flying away *(see Fig. 3.2)*. The solution to the mystery had been caught by Therrien's high-speed camera. Unlike the collision between, say, a rigid bat and a steel ball, where the velocity of the ball is directly proportional to the force applied to the handle of the bat, these photographs revealed that a substantial amount of a puck's velocity is acquired from the *elastic properties* of the wooden stick. As the blade is bent backward after the initial contact, it seeks to regain its initial structural alignment, springing back at the puck faster than a player could ever swing the stick. In other words, players who wielded the stick with a certain technique, which optimally exploited the blade's elasticity, produced a faster shot regardless of their strength or the force they applied to the blade.

Moreover, in several of the filmed impacts, Therrien also observed a tipping motion of the puck, which was initiated when the oscillating blade slammed into the disk at an angle greater

FIGURE 3.2

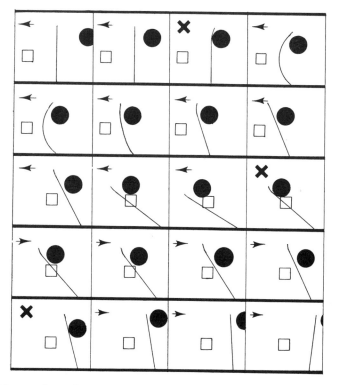

The puck strikes a hockey stick not once, but three times. Us-ing high-speed film analysis (2,000 frames/second), René Therrien investigated the interaction between blade and puck, shooting the rubber disk from an air gun onto a stick clamped to a heavy base. Within the space of 83 frames, condensed above, the puck danced with the blade, striking three times (marked with an "X") before flying away. When the puck first strikes the blade, the wood curves dramatically around the missile, then springs back and loses contact with the puck. For the next nine milliseconds, the puck and blade are moving backward together without touching. Then, a second impact occurs when the blade springs back with a for-ward motion, followed by a second separation as both puck and blade move together without contact. Finally, a third impact oc-curs when the faster-moving blade catches up with the disk and propels it away. The arrows above indicate the motion of puck and blade as they moved together. The small square box repre-sents stationary grid locations against which movement is mea-sured.

*Source: Therrien (1982). (See bibliography.)

than the perpendicular line between handle and blade. In this way, the puck is launched into the air with a higher angle than a player could impart if he were using a totally rigid stick. Moreover, the friction developed between the puck and blade during the brief moments of contact is the only force that can account for the rotation of a puck in flight—a spinning action that causes the disk to curve through the air like a knuckle ball (see "The Aerodynamics of a Baseball," Chapter 6).

These studies have laid the groundwork for a major breakthrough in developing shooting skills in ice hockey. Many scientists and trainers believe that further analysis of the dynamic interaction between blade and puck will soon yield precise information about exactly how a player should hold and maneuver a stick to obtain the puck velocity achieved by Bobby Hull, even if he only has the physique and strength of Wayne Gretzky.

FOUR

BOXING

The Rude Physics of the Sweet Science

When Francisco Kiko Benjines, a twenty-year-old boxer from Mexico, headed into the twelfth round against Alberto Davila in the Los Angeles Olympic Auditorium, he was leading on two of three judges' cards. With a career record of 37–4, Benjines was ranked as the number-three bantamweight by the World Boxing Council (WBC), and on the evening of September 1, 1983, was contending for the title vacated by Lupe Pintor, who had failed to make a title defense within the past year. Davila, a twenty-nine-year-old from California, was the WBC's top-ranked contender with a 52–7 record, but he had failed in three previous title bouts.

Pundits considered the two boxers to be in good condition and evenly matched, but were disappointed by an unspectacular bout in which neither boxer appeared to inflict much damage.

Suddenly, in the last round, Davila caught on fire, opening up against Benjines with a flurry of solid punches. A left-right combination to the head appeared to stun the Mexican and seconds later Davila landed a jab and followed it with a hard right that landed squarely on the top of the chin. Benjines fell to the canvas, landing on the seat of his pants, his back and neck supported by the two bottom strands of rope. With glazed eyes he kept moving his right foot as if attempting to get up, but the referee, Waldemar Schmidt, signaled the end of the fight.

The stricken boxer then slumped sideways and sprawled on the canvas, unconscious.

Schmidt, a seasoned referee who was working his forty-sixth title bout, was surprised, saying later, "I didn't think that he was that badly hurt at first. But this was by far the worst I've ever seen a fighter leave the ring."

As a stretcher was being summoned, the ring physician, Bernhardt Schwartz, knelt beside Benjines and noticed that the unconscious boxer was having slight spasmodic muscle contractions, and that his right pupil was bigger than his left—a black dilated disk, indicating brain hemorrhage. Schwartz was equipped with oxygen and ammonia capsules, but nothing would revive Kiko Benjines. He was finally taken to a local hospital and from there flown by helicopter to the University of Southern California Medical Center.

After confirming Schwartz's initial diagnosis, a team of three neurosurgeons removed a portion of Benjines's right frontal lobe and a blood clot in a delicate, three-and-a-half-hour operation. After surgery, the boxer remained on a respirator, comatose, and died the next day.

For Dr. Schwartz, Benjines was the fourth boxer to die of injuries in the forty-three years he had supervised matches. After the fight, the ring physician said that "nobody could have prevented this. He was a well-conditioned boxer. His head was going forward and the punch was coming at him. There were no signs [he was in danger]."

Benjines was the three hundred fourteenth professional fighter to die of injuries in the past twenty years, and the third to die in 1983, promoting demands by boxing critics, once again, that the sport be banned in all civilized countries. For decades, ring deaths have inspired debate about the merits of the sport and whether it should be subject to stricter regulation or abolished entirely. The controversy is fueled more by moral questions than by an overwhelming death toll: the fatality rate for boxing (0.13 deaths per 1,000 participants) is considerably lower than for college football (0.3 deaths), scuba diving (1.1), mountaineering (5.1), hang gliding (5.6), sky diving (12.3), and horse racing (12.8). But because the boxing deaths appear to have resulted from the intentional infliction of injury, public outcry persists.

One of the first comprehensive books on boxing injuries, written by University of Kentucky physiologist Ernst Jokl in 1941, observed that "the art of the knockout is the one remaining killing skill. . . . The time is coming when boxing, instead of being actively promoted, should be generally banned." This theme has been echoed over the years, most recently by the American Medical Association (AMA), which declared that "boxing, as a throwback to uncivilized man, should not be sanctioned by any civilized society." Months later, George D. Lundberg, the physician-editor of the *Journal of the American Medical Association (JAMA)*, threatened to stop boxing unless reforms were implemented: "Since the medical profession can allow boxing to continue, or can abolish it simply by refusing to participate as ring physicians [as required by most state laws], it is likely that either boxing totally, or blows to the head specifically, will be banned for professionals and amateurs alike. So there it is. For a civilized society, two choices. Either no boxing or no blows to the head."

Notwithstanding the perennial threats of physicians and legislators, it is most unlikely boxing will be banned. As long as athletes wish to box, and there remain millions of avid fans, market forces will prevail over the best intentions of those who believe the sport is a brutal and barbaric spectacle. Moreover, a ban on sanctioned fights might be counterproductive. When asked about this after Benjines's death, Schwartz replied, "If you banned boxing, there'd still be boxing on barges and in garages. And there'd be no way to get medical help to them."[1]

Social forces may not end the sport in our lifetime, but pressure for increased regulation will continue, posing problems for the sports scientist, who usually has mixed allegiances, to balance the aesthetics of boxing against the perceived need to increase safety. The irony, of course, is that regulation is designed to reduce injury and the design of a fighter is to inflict injury. Every new reform reduces the very nature of boxing, and some enthusiasts fear that future pugilists will be relegated to the status of button-pushing laboratory monkeys, displaying ferocious reaction times in response to a stimulus without any true exertion, or even reward for their efforts—a situation more demeaning than the so-called "primitive" condition now ascribed to the sport. If blows to the head are outlawed, others say, boxing would take another step closer to resembling modern fencing. Protected from head to toe, the modern fencer is never scratched by the foil; the contemporary version of this martial art—as most contemporary combat sports—displays the athlete's mental and motor skills only.

Do athletes have an inalienable right to participate in a sport that may cause injury to themselves or to their opponents?

The dilemma between the athlete's desire to express his skills in the ring and the social concern that he doesn't hurt himself in the process might be tempered by the consideration of the possible positive contributions boxing, and kindred sports, make to the public good—social benefits easily obscured by the carnival and commercial atmosphere in which fights are held.

The fact that boxing has endured as a popular activity, in various forms, for so many centuries must be attributed to something other than pathological bloodlust among certain aggressive athletes or the murderous disposition of successive generations of spectators who subsidize this sport. The ancient Greek Olympics were comprised almost exclusively of events that reflected some military activity, and in those days that had immediate implications for survival. The Greeks rarely questioned the utility of expressing forms of combat, from wrestling to the javelin throw, in competitive athletics.

The country cop, the sailor on shore leave, or the modern urban subway commuter will attest that the need to cultivate and demonstrate personal combat skills has not declined or disappeared in today's civilized society. In this regard, is it immoral to perpetuate hand-to-hand combat skills among those who willingly submit to the risk of injury in supervised bouts—or should the art of boxing be limited to the military or to law-enforcement officers?

Although the philosophical questions of the social utility of boxing appear to lie far outside the traditional realm of the sports scientist, part of the burden of resolving these issues has nevertheless fallen upon him. Torn and confused by conflicting social forces, lawmakers and medical policy makers are asking for concrete information to make decisions.

What exactly are the biological consequences of a punch to the head? Is the incidence of concussion higher than the 20 percent reported in football, or is the number of blows to the head in seven sanctioned bouts greater than the 169 head impacts recorded in seven college games by Reid's wired linebacker (see "Collisions and Injuries" in Chapter 1)?

And most important, will headgear significantly reduce acute and chronic brain damage?

HOW THE BRAIN TAKES A PUNCH

From a physiological perspective, the purpose of a boxer is to overload his opponent's body with physical stress until fatigue, exhaustion, and injury force him to throw in the towel or collapse. If neither occurs by the end of the match, judges select a winner based on offensive points. A boxer's body has many stress points, but the head is the target of choice. Boxing is, after all, a showcase for the brain's incredible capabilities—balance, coordination, reflex, memory, instinct, strategy, and creativity. Cripple these functions and the fight is over.

Biomechanists join the investigation by measuring the various forces that can be generated and delivered through the clenched fist. Jabs, haymakers, hooks, upper cuts, straight punches—all possess different forces and exert different effects. These factors are determined by the effective mass and acceleration of the fist, which is related to the athlete's body strength, weight, and height; the length of arm reach; and the distance at which he throws the punch.

It's as true today as in 1941, when Jokl observed that the most frequent knockout is caused by blows to the chin, with oblique blows, such as hooks and upper cuts, more effective than linear blows from the front. In fact, it was Davila's blow to Benjines's chin that sent the Mexican to the canvas. Chin knockouts usually result in an immediate loss of consciousness, whereas Benjines seemed to lose consciousness after being down for a few seconds. In Jokl's day, the mechanics of the chin knockout were not fully understood. One theory was that a special nerve in the chin was damaged, setting the brain into shock; another was that the jaw was jammed back, cutting off the flow of blood in one of the neck's two carotid arteries; a third was that the balance mechanisms in the inner ear were disrupted.

Today, the chin knockout is still something of a mystery. The conventional explanation is that linear and rotational forces that

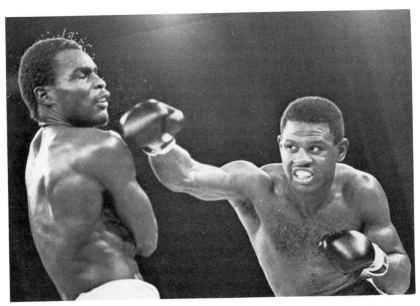

It's as true today as in 1941, when physiologist Ernst Jokl conducted the first medical survey of injuries in boxers, that the most frequent cause of a knockout is from an oblique blow to the chin, shown dramatically here. In fact, most linear blows also have a rotational component, and rotational acceleration inflicts three times as much damage to the brain as a straight punch. Compare to Fig. 4.1 for the internal effects of these oblique blows. (Courtesy of Philip Katz/First Capital Press.)

jar the brain are transmitted more efficiently through the lever action of a blow to the tip of the jaw, producing greater peak accelerations than any other type of punch. Another idea is that blows to the chin transmit a shock wave that travels up the jaw, through the skull, and strikes the *brain stem,* which merges with the spinal cord at the base of the skull *(see Fig. 4.1).* This shock wave may affect the brain stem before the linear or rotational acceleration of the entire brain begins to stretch and twist the brain stem.

This segment of the brain's anatomy is particularly vulnerable to any physical disturbance because all nerve signals to and from the body pass through it. No one has ever tired to estimate the volume of information that flows through this slender braid of living tissue. But considering that the brain is made up of some 20 *billion* nerve cells and that all voluntary activity and most of the autonomic (involuntary) activity of the body is reg-

FIGURE 4.1

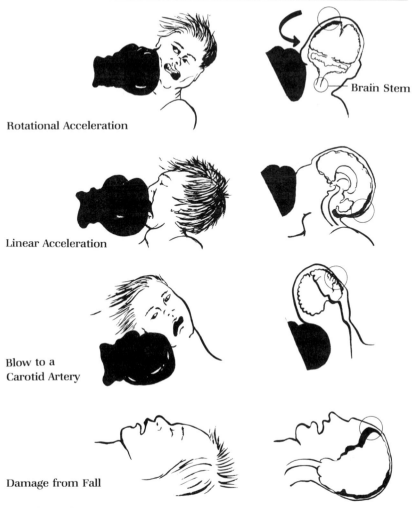

Rotational Acceleration

Brain Stem

Linear Acceleration

Blow to a
Carotid Artery

Damage from Fall

How the brain takes a punch. In rotational or oblique blows, the surface of the brain glides along the interior of the skull, stretching, bruising, and breaking fragile blood vessels. In linear or straight blows, the back of the brain is compressed, often followed by an internal whiplash or "countrecoup" injury at the front of the brain. Rarer is the blow to the neck, which can damage or cut off the carotid artery on the far side of the blow, as well as bruising the brain surface. When an athlete falls to the floor, the damage is similar to the linear blow, with massive damage to both front and back of the brain. In all cases, the slender brain stem is either stretched or twisted, an action thought to account for most knockouts.

ulated by the brain, we can only marvel at its capacity as a carrier of communications. In addition to its role as a trunk line, the brain stem contains nerve centers that set the rhythm of breathing and influence the rate and force at which the heart muscles contract to pump blood. The brain stem also contains an area called the reticular formation, which acts as a switchboard for specific senses, relaying data to specialized centers higher in the brain, and in a related manner it affects arousal and wakefulness.

When any part of the brain is physically insulted, a *concussion* can occur. This kind of brain injury is defined as a temporary impairment of brain activity, which can be observed on EEG tracings, and sometimes in changes in performance or behavior. Some doctors believe concussions do not cause gross or microscopic brain damage. A *contusion*, by contrast, is a bruising injury to the brain. Although this distinction has many uses, neurologists now suspect that all concussions may be accompanied by minute brain damage.

Several years ago, the AMA established its Panel on Brain Injury in Boxing to relate known forms of brain dysfunction to various blows to the head. In doing so they compiled nine levels of boxing concussions, each having its own clinical symptoms.

The first and mildest form of concussion occurs when a pugilist is briefly stunned and may report "seeing stars." There is no impact on motor performance and the recovery tends to be fast and total. The second grade is associated with slower reflexes and coordination, but without any alteration in consciousness. In the ring, this can go undetected, especially in later rounds, when it may be mistaken for fatigue or a change in fighting style. The third level is a total loss of motor control without any loss of consciousness. This rare phenomenon is seen when a fighter's legs suddenly give out following a blow to the head and he hits the canvas, although fully alert. Many so-called knockdowns may be attributed to this level of concussion. The fourth level is a loss of memory without a loss of consciousness or motor control. This can go undetected until after a fight, when the boxer asks his amazed handlers, "Where am I?" The fifth grade of concussion is a groggy state, where there may be mental confusion, amnesia, slurred speech, and a loss of motor control. The fighter in this condition may or may not go down and is often declared "out on his feet," resulting in a technical knockout (TKO), although recovery tends to be relatively rapid.

The sixth level of concussion is the classic knockout. There is usually a loss of consciousness, a loss of muscle tone, and often amnesia. The usual duration of unconsciousness seldom lasts for more than 10 to 30 seconds, and a fighter who stays out longer may be in serious trouble. The seventh and eight grades are variations on the sixth, with symptoms of muscle rigidity, spasms, and convulsions. The ninth and most serious form of concussion is characterized by delayed unconsciousness, the kind of knockout that happened to Kiko Benjines: a boxer takes a blow to the head, but doesn't drop for a few seconds.

The brain stem is usually affected in any hard blow to the head, but the surface and interior of the brain can also be injured, killing nerve cells and splitting blood vessels. The deaths of Benjines, Duk Koo Kim, Willie Calusen, and scores of other boxers resulted from a ruptured blood vessel on or near the surface of the brain, caused by the swirling and bouncing against the interior wall of the skull. As in most forms of hemorrhage, the blood will eventually clot, forming a hard mass of blood known as a *subdural hematoma*. The pressure of this increased mass inside the skull, plus any swelling from the bruised brain, can compress the brain stem, leading to unconsciousness, coma, and even death. As the pressure builds, even if the brain stem appears unaffected, the blood supply to the brain is gradually closed off, which causes further swelling of the brain itself. Even after surgery to remove the blood clot, as in the Benjines case, the brain can continue to swell, effectively strangling its vital supply of blood.

MEASURING THE POWER OF A PUNCH

An interesting study of the mechanical properties of a punch was conducted by Wilhelm Joch, an exercise scientist at the Free University in Berlin, Germany, who turned up information useful for both physicians and trainers. In 1981, he tested seventy boxers on a punch dynamometer, an elastic container resembling a long, cylindrical punching bag, which was filled to capacity with water. The force of a punch was measured in terms of hydraulic overpressure, as the blow caused the water to press electronic sensors in the bag. The dynamometer data was compared to high-speed films as well as to the readings of pressure platforms on which the boxers stood.

Joch found that as a boxer readies to deliver a straight punch, about 80 percent of the body weight shifts to his rear foot before there is any movement in the arms, and for the purpose of the study this was marked as the beginning of the punch sequence, or time zero. As the pugilist prepares to deliver a blow to the bag, there is a backward movement of the arm that takes 400 milliseconds to complete. The delivery or acceleration phase of a punch involves the forward movement of the arm, body weight, and center of gravity, which takes 100 milliseconds up to the moment of impact. Although these times were the average for all the boxers in Joch's study—who were ranked into performance classes according to their experience and proficiency prior to the tests—it demonstrates the startling speed with which a fighter can execute a full punch.

As might be expected, punching force varies with the performance class of a boxer. Highly ranked competitive athletes can deliver an average force of 3,400 Newtons to the target; inexperienced boxers, 2,900 Newtons.[2] These forces were produced when the subjects were asked to find the distance from the bag at which they could punch as fast and as hard as possible. On the average, the best boxers selected a distance of 17.5 inches measured from the tip of the leading foot to the edge of the bag. At the moment of impact the glove velocity was 23 to 26 feet/second.

If Joch's boxers had been striking a human head instead of a punch dynamometer, these central blows would knock the head straight back, imparting a ferocious linear acceleration to the brain, crushing tissue in both the front and back of the brain (see Fig. 4.1). Studies have found that boxers using gloves, but not headgear, can easily impart a force of over 2,500 Newtons in only 10 to 50 milliseconds from either a straight or oblique blow, landing anywhere on the head—a force that one investigator said exceeds the brain's tolerance to injury by a factor

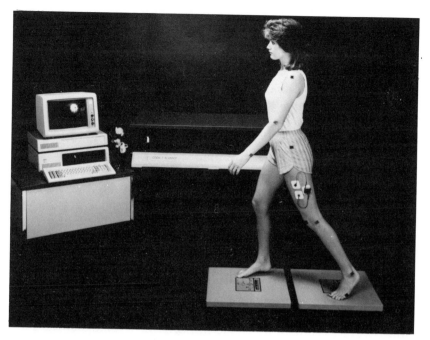

An AMTI pressure platform, which measures the shifts in body mass for an athlete walking, jumping, swinging a weapon, and similar motions. The data can be integrated with an optical recorder, or EMG sensors, both shown here, and the data fed into a computer for an analysis of muscle activity versus efficiency of movement. In Joch's study of boxers, a similar platform was used to detect shifts in body weight before the fighters had even moved their arms to throw a punch. The computer here is an IBM PC. (Photo by Steven Greenberg/AMTI. Courtesy of Advanced Mechanical Technology, Inc.)

of four. Joch's boxers could deliver blows in the range of 2,500 to 3,500 Newtons.

Other research has generated data similar to that of Joch's study, and when the punch forces of all these studies are compared to the forces required to exceed the threshold of brain injury, it leads to the unmistakable conclusion that the gloves of a boxer do not prevent brain damage. Indeed, some die-hards who yearn for the bare-fisted days of John L. Sullivan have argued that gloves do little more than protect the knuckles. A more serious consideration is whether protective headgear, mandatory in amateur bouts since April 1984, offers better protection than gloves.

In theory the beneficial effect of headgear, like gloves, is the cushioning action that lengthens delivery time and absorbs some of the energy of the blow. Published research on the effects of headgear is scarce and it would seem that boxing authorities, like their counterparts in football and hockey, have adopted equipment that has not been subject to rigorous scrutiny. Statistically, it is known that only 0.8 percent of boxing matches in which headgear was used ended in knockouts, compared to 3 to 4 percent without headgear. These numbers sound convincing and are widely quoted, but at this time they appear to be the *only* statistics available.[3] Given that injury surveys are helpful in depicting trends, but are no more than circumstantial evidence in determining the efficacy of protective equipment, questions about the value of headgear in boxing remain unanswered. Some of the vocal opponents of headgear have argued that the reduction of knockouts cited in the survey can be attributed to impaired performance brought about by wearing the new equipment. Like those who were initially against masks in ice hockey, these critics say vision is impaired and the weight is distracting, and they cite the fact that three fights in the 1984 Olympics were stopped several times each by the referees to fix headgear that moved close to the eyes or became snarled in the hair.

The arguments of headgear opponents are shaky at best, but no more so than the lone knockout survey. According to Robert Norman, the kinesiologist who studied protective helmets in football and hockey, "One is forced to wonder what is happening to [boxers] in the absence of adequate information about the level of blows that can be delivered by boxers of various ages and sizes and the blow-absorbing abilities of headgear."

At present, the best evidence of the protection offered by headgear comes from a 1968 study conducted in Czechoslovakia with a helmet design unlike that used in the United States, Canada, or by Olympic boxers. Volunteers were tested, with and without headgear, by swinging a small punching bag at the head at angles that simulated various blows. Frontal blows were delivered at 15 feet/second, side blows at 11 feet/second, and blows to the jaw at 5 feet/second. After sifting through all the data, the researchers concluded that, on the average, acceleration to the head was reduced by 15 to 25 percent when the subjects wore headgear. Impact was also reduced in frontal and side blows, but there was no measurable reduction in head acceleration from blows to the jaw, despite the thick padding that runs along the entire length of the lower jaw and chin in the Czech equipment.

A 15 to 25 percent reduction of the impact force seems substantial, but the velocity of the simulated punches was only *half* of the velocity recorded in Joch's study (presumably the Czech punches were slow due to the use of live subjects). The attenuation of the impact forces that resulted from the sluggish Czech punches probably does not apply to punch velocities in the ring, because the cushioning effect of foams and fabrics tends to decrease with higher speeds. Moreover, it is difficult to imagine a small, free-swinging punching bag possessing the same effective mass as a human boxer laying into his opponent. The Czech researchers (or translators) did not include a physical description of the bag in their report, which is unfortunate, because to calculate impact force accurately, the mass of the striker must be multiplied by its acceleration.

If we imagine for a moment that this study used conventional headgear, that Joch's boxers delivered the blows, that the cushioning did not bottom out at the higher impact speeds, and that the average force was reduced by the Czech maximum of 25 percent, then Joch's 3,000 Newton punches would be reduced to 2,250 Newtons—an impact *three times greater than the threshold for brain injury.*

One can only hope that the American medical community has been putting at least as much energy into headgear studies as they have into their efforts to alert the public about the dangers of head blows in boxing. If so, then the results of these studies should finally settle the question of whether headgear can reduce the 2,500-Newton punch delivered in 10 to 50 milliseconds by 400 percent.

LONG-TERM BRAIN DAMAGE

Shortly after the 1981 retirement of Muhammad Ali, journalists, as well as his business and boxing associates, noticed that the only man in history to win the heavyweight title three times appeared to have aged far beyond his years. At times Ali's speech was slurred and unintelligible, his eye-hand coordination impaired.

After winning the Olympic gold medal in 1960, Ali fought 61 professional fights with 550 rounds, plus an additional 50 known exhibition bouts. In spring 1984, he told the press, "I've taken about 175,000 hard punches. I think that would affect anybody some. But that don't make me have brain damage." Months later, Ali checked into the Neurological Institute of New York's Columbia-Presbyterian Medical Center suffering from symptoms similar to those of Parkinson's disease—speech impairment, transient confusion, unsteady gait, reduced muscle strength, unusual fatigue, and slight tremors.

After examining the champ, physicians denied that he had either Parkinson's disease or *dementia pugilistica*—the "punch-drunk syndrome" seen in many retired boxers, which is linked to chronic and irreversible brain damage. They said, in fact, that his symptoms were "melting away" in response to doses of Sinemet and Symmetrel, drugs that help replenish the brain's supply of dopamine, a substance that regulates many motor functions.

Skeptical of the public denial that Ali was suffering from brain damage, some neurologists speculated off the record that the champ had a condition known as *cavum septi pellucidi,* a cave or space between the two membranes that divide the hemispheres of the brain. Many boxers with this disorder suffer permanently from the Parkinson's-like symptoms that sent Ali to the hospital. This speculation was later confirmed by Ira R. Casson, a neurologist at the Long Island Jewish Medical Center, who had had an opportunity to examine Ali's recent CAT scans, the advanced form of X-ray that looks at the brain or any other part of the body in very thin sections, providing much greater detail than the fuzzy X-rays traditionally seen hanging from light boxes. Casson also reported that the fighter had enlarged ventricles, the cavities in the middle of the brain where the protective cerebro-spinal fluid is produced.

Dementia pugilistica was first recognized as a clinical entity in 1928, and today it's known that its symptoms actually cover a wide range of brain disorders associated with neurological damage from repeated blows to the head. The fact that damage can occur in almost any area of a boxer's brain accounts for the diverse symptoms, from the impairment of fairly simple motor activity to disruption of such higher functions as memory and speech. In fairness to boxers, this diverse lump of symptoms should be renamed to reflect the fact that chronic brain damage due to repetitive head injuries has been observed in athletes from other sports, including football, rugby, professional wrestling, and the steeplechase. The incidence of the punch-drunk syndrome in these sports has not been fully documented, but it would be fair to guess that the rate is not as high as boxing: one study of pugilists who had spent six to nine years in the ring found that 17 percent had symptoms of brain damage.

Many fighters, however, have been in the ring since adolescence, some since age ten. For these individuals, brain damage may accumulate over *fifteen years* or more.

In fact, according to a 1983 AMA report, there are 15,000 boxers, age ten to fifteen, registered in the United States with the National Amateur Athletic Union, who each participate in ten to thirty sanctioned bouts per year. There are an additional 12,000 boxers in about the same age bracket, participating in an equal number of bouts per year, registered with the U.S. Golden Gloves Association. Since few high schools or universities have sponsored boxing squads, there is a large data gap for the fifteen- to eighteen-year-old bracket. From age eighteen on up, there are over 5,000 registered professional boxers in forty-six states. In the ten- to fifteen-year-old group, the AMA report estimates a knockout rate of 5 percent—or over 1,300 young boxers being called for either a TKO, which often indicates a concussion, or being counted out as they lay on the canvas, which is rare.

As the extent of acute injury experienced by a boxer generally depends upon the strength and experience of his opponent, it has long been assumed that young contenders run a very small risk of accruing brain damage; only adults can muster the power to inflict (or acquire) the injuries that ultimately produce the punch-drunk disorders.

That assumption now appears to be false. A study conducted by sports physician Peter Lamperd at the University of

California in San Diego found that repeated blows of low intensity to the head, delivered at or below 23 feet/second, produce more chronic or long-term brain damage than a single intense blow delivered at 26 feet/second or faster. In other words, it's not the thundering knockout punch but the constant rain of light jabs, seemingly innocuous, that permanently impairs the brain of a boxer. In fact, this research concluded that the number of bouts, rather than the number of knockouts, is the best predictor of chronic brain damage.

The tragic irony of the skilled boxer who eludes the haymaker, wins more bouts, and climbs to the top but is doomed to suffer the punch-drunk syndrome from repetitive subconcussive blows is captured in the case of Ali. His condition is considered to have resulted from subtle impact forces rippling through the brain, causing increasing damage in the interior and surface of that delicate organ. The cumulative damage of thousands of low-intensity blows is readily understood by the process known as *cortical atrophy*, the gradual erosion of nerve cells on the surface of the brain as it swirls inside the skull, again and again, literally wearing down layers of brain cells. Similarly, neurologists have discovered microscopic damage to the axons of nerve cells below the surface—the filaments that transmit the brain's chemical messages. Once torn, axons die, and there is no hope of regeneration or repair; yet the cell may still be alive, surviving only as a functionless mute. In areas of the cerebral cortex (the upper portion of the brain), the formation of so-called neurofibrillary tangles, functionless knots of hairlike structures known to accumulate after brain injury, cause widespread nerve damage in boxers. One study reported that damage caused by this neurological debris often exceeds that seen in Alzheimer's disease and senile dementia.

Can young boxers be accelerating what might be called their effective brain age, racing toward senility with every bout? Will the now mandatory use of headgear in amateur fights be effective in preventing chronic brain damage, even though the equipment may be ineffective in reducing acute brain injury?

The studies that show that it is the repeated, low-intensity blows that are responsible for chronic brain damage open the possibility that headgear may actually contribute to the injuries associated with the punch-drunk syndrome. If modern headgear can match the 25 percent maximum attenuation of the Czech equipment, it may protect the wearer against acute brain damage of the 26 feet/second haymakers, reducing the impact force to the equivalent of a 20 feet/second jab—the type of low-level blow linked to long-term brain damage.

Boxing officials and sports equipment manufacturers characterize this kind of speculation as unwarranted and alarmist. Their reaction probably reflects their knowledge that headgear was institutionalized without thorough evaluation. For example, one of the many factors that have not been investigated by headgear manufacturers is the *coefficient of friction*, the quantity of changing slipperiness on a surface. Does the tendency to induce rotational acceleration in the head increase or decrease as the gloves and headgear surfaces become slicked with sweat? Does the increased head diameter of a boxer wearing headgear increase the propensity of punches to rotate the head, as classic physics suggests, or is this effect offset by the greater head mass provided by the helmet? Does the increased weight of headgear produce greater impact forces when a boxer's head falls against the ropes or the mat?

Recent evidence suggests that thirty years from now today's fifteen-year-old boxer could benefit greatly from answers to these and other questions about headgear. Several studies published in 1984 reported that CAT scans found brain damage in young boxers to an extent never before suspected, apparently because the detection of injury was previously missed by EEG, neurologic testing, and other standard prefight medical examination procedures. Alarmed by these findings, the American Academy of Pediatrics promptly urged all "pediatricians to become vigorous opponents of boxing as a sport for *any* child or young adult."

Physicians, especially pediatricians, are unlikely to be persuaded to cease their campaign to ban boxing by arguments about the social utility of this sport or by the assertion that individuals have a right to freely participate in any form of athletic endeavor. As scientists, however, physicians should be able to view boxers, at least adult boxers, as experimental subjects who willingly expose themselves to levels of stress seldom experienced by the general population, thereby producing a staggering amount of useful physiological information that often has direct medical application. In this perspective, a medical researcher would be hard-pressed to condemn boxing without also having to condemn clinical trials of new drugs, artificial organs, and experimental forms of therapy, all conducted on willing subjects who are often paid handsomely.

There are risks, injuries, and even occasional fatalities in clinical research as well as in athletics.

In boxing, the number of injuries and deaths is very low relative to other sports. One unpublished survey of injuries in amateur boxing, conducted over a two-year period, found an injury rate of 1.43 percent from blows to all parts of the body, based on 6,000 bouts involving 12,000 athletes—a rate dramatically lower than the 46 percent reported in 1981 for high school football. A second study, based on 540 bouts held during the 1981–1982 U.S. Amateur Boxing Federation national championships, found the injury rate was 4.75 percent. This incredibly low level of injury reflects, in part, the rigorously controlled environment in which sanctioned bouts are held, where modern referees practice a strict and conscientious policy of "over-call," protecting the combatants while letting them explore their physical and psychological limits.

It may seem simplistic or perverse to think of the ring as a laboratory where individuals participate in a decades-long experiment in human biology, but the metaphor works well enough to make an important point. The sacrifice of many fighters, the meaning of their lives and careers, is tragically diminished if this peculiar process of gathering knowledge of the human body under stress, bought so painfully in countless rounds and bouts, is arbitrarily halted simply because of the high price paid by athletes like Benjines and Ali.

After all, many of the same physicians who call for an end to boxing are also the first to scrutinize the CAT scans and EEG tracings of boxers to learn more about the brain, its disorders and diseases, its susceptibility to injury, and the way it ages.

THE ART OF ANTICIPATION

Perhaps the most interesting finding of Joch's study of boxers whacking his punch dynamometer is that the average execution time to throw a punch was 100 milliseconds, whereas the average reaction time to move defensively was 425 milliseconds—over four times as long as execution. Joch observed that "based on this capacity of reaction, a boxer has little possibility of moving away from an opponent's punch. . . . For an optimal defense, a boxer is dependent not on his capacity to react, but on his capacity to anticipate."

Years of experience, advice from scouts and trainers, and the study of films all help a fighter learn the style of an opponent, but his survival in the ring depends primarily on his ability to anticipate a punch before it's thrown. A pugilist develops this talent with time and tips from seasoned trainers about reading an opponent's body language. In recent years, several new methods of anticipation training have opened up for boxers, although few boxers outside the world-class amateur level use them.

A conservative streak runs through many sports, but nothing like that which prevails in boxing. Anything that sounds like "brain picturing" and isn't an X-ray is shunned without a hearing. Larry Holmes raised eyebrows a few years ago when word got out that he was involved in some kind of stretching exercises. Given the pragmatism of most athletes, which usually tempers highly conservative or highly innovative trends, the reluctance of boxers to get near anything that smacks of the "inner athlete"—even if it applies *directly* to performance—is surprising. The reasons for this are unclear. Sportswriter John Jerome has made a similar observation in his book *The Sweet Spot in Time*, suggesting that the "macho athlete" is threatened by inward, sensual exercises. This may be true, but professional football players have recently shown little inhibition to perform ballet exercises on national television, even if they did look a little silly.

Brain picturing is a form of mental imagery similar to Richard Suinn's method of VMBR, or Visuo-Motor Behavior Rehearsal (see "Shutting Down the Brain" in Chapter 2), and was probably derived from his work. This technique supplements the traditional full-blown visualization of the atheletic event with what might be called VMBR minisessions, which can be practiced before sparring or a fight and can also be used between rounds. The methodical relaxation involved in VMBR can be of considerable help to the corner man who's trying to calm an angry or overaroused fighter. The technique is also useful for giving a boxer instructions between rounds, using the key word *picture* to induce relaxation and visualization of the desired moves and tactics. With practice, upon hearing the words "I want you to *picture* . . ." the boxer recalls the mental processes used in his regular VMBR sessions, opening himself to suggestions that might otherwise be blocked by the tension and stress of the ring environment. In this respect, brain picturing resembles the relationship between a clinical hypnotist and a patient, where the hypnotic state can be induced with only a key word or phrase. Of course, a boxer doesn't need a corner man to use VMBR minisessions before or during a fight.

As the nature of brain picturing is forward looking, it is ideal for improving anticipation. During regular VMBR sessions, a boxer can incorporate images of his opponent throwing a punch and how he would ideally react. Brain picturing has also been suggested as a technique to save a confused or disoriented boxer during a fight, using a knockdown or a standing count as a stimulus to induce imagery, helping the athlete to focus on what he's doing and what he wants to accomplish. Unfortunately, tests of the effectiveness of brain picturing in boxing have not been published in the West, but Soviet sports psychologist Alexander Romen has reported measurable increases in reaction time in athletes using imagery.

Eye training is another new concept in boxing; it increases the speed at which the eyes can move in certain directions. Visual acuity at near and distant ranges and broad peripheral vision are essential for a boxer. Although there is no known method to improve poor peripheral vision, there is evidence that *vergence eye movements*, used to compare near and distant points, and *saccadic eye movements*, used to scan left and right, can be improved through exercise.

One drill recommended for the boxer consists of rotating the eyes in a methodical, circular movement, slowly at first so he can focus and see everything as the eyes travel around the perimeter of the sockets. The speed of the exercise is progressively increased in relation to proficiency. Another method has the athlete push his eyes into a crossed position, then work both eyes outward and away from each other, and repeat the process in reverse. A third exercise involves alternately focusing on near and distant objects, jumping back and forth as soon as the visual targets are perfectly clear, increasing speed with time. These exercises can also be used to help a fighter gather concentration before and during a fight.

In the future, training to track and anticipate the movements of an opponent appears to lie with high technology, a trend that may be adopted more readily than brain picturing. In 1984, East Germany's top boxers started sparring with computerized robots that can be programmed to four different fighting styles, or controlled remotely by the trainer. These human-shaped machines have pressure-sensitive surfaces that measure the impact force of every punch landed. The East German trainers say the mechanical sparring partners improve footwork, punching accuracy, and reaction time.

PAIN RESEARCH

In 1941, Ernst Jokl observed in his book *The Medical Aspects of Boxing* that "boxers who are knocked out by blows to the chin do not necessarily experience any distressing sensations. A well known professional told the writer that he could recall several chin knock-outs as quite pleasant experiences, which he thought to be not unlike those enjoyed by opium smokers."

Jokl hinted that perhaps this pugilist had taken one too many blows to the head, but his anecdote touches on a subject that has no connection to brain damage. In fact, this story is really quite remarkable in light of the recent discovery of natural opiatelike substances found in many locations throughout the human nervous system, a discovery that Jokl could never have anticipated over forty years ago. Today, boxers still occasionally report an absence of pain following a knockout, and others have claimed to have felt no pain in certain rounds in which they received a savage beating that did not result in a knockout. There is no way to verify these statements, and there is a strong possibility that much of their testimony is fabricated, especially by boxers who refuse to accept pain or defeat, or are trying to convince rivals that their best blows are harmless. Nevertheless, the persistence of these reports over the years has aroused the curiosity of researchers in many fields about the possibility of controlling pain without drugs or the impairment of performance.

The perception of pain is a very complex function of the nervous system, modulated by many factors, including emotion and intellect. For centuries the management of pain has relied on various preparations of the poppy plant, such as opium or morphine. Early physicians did not suspect that these drugs act in specific sites in the nervous system intended for the *endorphins*, the body's own opiatelike pain suppressants. Today, endorphins are known to be neurotransmitters located at synaptic relay points on major pain pathways; they act to block or filter the transmission of pain signals to the brain. How much pain is required to activate endorphins is not known, although it appears to vary among individuals. According to research conducted by Glenn Davis, a psychiatrist at Case Western Reserve School of Medicine, the individual differences in pain sensitivity are mediated primarily by endorphins.

The major role of endorphins appears to be the production of stress-induced analgesia. Studies have found that stress increases the level of the opiatelike substances in the blood and spinal cord, but not in the brain. This research has received wide news coverage as the factor behind the phenomenon called *runner's high.*

At Massachusetts General Hospital, endocrinologist David Carr conducted an experiment in which subjects climbed into a stationary bicycle ergometer and pedaled against a graded work load until their heart rate soared to 80 percent of their maximum toward the end of a one-hour workout. Blood samples were drawn before, immediately after, and one hour after the exercise. Carr found short-term rises in the level of endorphins in all subjects during the trials. Similar observations were made by Edward Colt, the medical director of the New York City marathon, who studied the endorphin content in the blood of trained distance runners on thirty-five occasions before and after their runs and found a rise in the natural pain killer in 71 percent. Although the athletes did not report symptoms of opium intoxication, these studies helped to launch the myth of runner's high. Research has shown that exercise does make most people feel good, but the subjective perception of well-being appears to have no link to the production of endorphins.

In sports and medicine, the importance of endorphins rests with their ability to reduce pain. As natural endorphins have been found to degrade quickly outside the body, they're not good commercial candidates, and artificial endorphins produce narcotic addiction just like opiates. At present, applied research is being planned to determine how the body can be manipulated to trip the active release of endorphins. Each of several non-drug techniques for reducing pain sensitivity—including acupuncture, hypnosis, and even placebos—appears to depend on the action of these opiatelike hormones. Other paramedical approaches, such as electrotherapy, ultrasonic therapy, and cryotherapy, may also rely on endorphins.

For boxers, distance runners, and other athletes involved in prolonged and punishing endurance events, research into the mysteries of the endorphins may lead to methods to reduce the pain associated with their sports. But some researchers believe pain is a necessary evil in certain athletic events, an essential component in the acquisition and fine tuning of motor skills, and in the prevention of overuse injuries.

Pain is the most acute sensation any athlete has to detect and gauge the internal levels of stress imposed by his particular sport. If properly used, this most unpleasant of all sensations may actually serve to enhance performance. In fact, one sports psychologist found that, among a large sample of marathon runners he questioned, those who consistently performed the best actively monitored all internal sensations, particularly pain, during a race. Those who performed the poorest denied or ignored their bodies, often daydreamed, or conducted a silent internal dialogue about something unrelated to the race. The runners who monitored their sensations of pain, heat, and fatigue modified their pace or running style accordingly.

If pain can serve a useful function in sports like boxing, then the direction of pain research may shift from the study of analgesia to the development of methods that athletes can use to interpret the unpleasant information from their battered bodies to enhance performance, perhaps to distinguish among different types of pain, to understand what types are dangerous and what types to ignore.

As the product of stress and injury, pain is at the heart of boxing and is linked with the moral objections to this sport. The irony is that over the next few decades, medical science may benefit greatly from pain research involving boxers, research that yields important applications in chronic diseases such as arthritis and cancer.

FIVE

STRENGTH TRAINING

The Science of
Body Sculpture

Despite their reputation for sensationalism, tabloids like the *National Enquirer* contain many authentic anecdotes of incredible feats of human strength. The stories of desperate mothers lifting automobiles off their babies, or strong men pulling boxcars with their teeth are usually based on fact, no matter how much the reporters may have stretched the quotes of eyewitnesses.

Consider the story of Paul Anderson, who, on June 12, 1957, placed a steel safe full of lead on a special table, loaded the remaining surface with heavy automobile parts, crawled under the table, and lifted it off the floor—holding a total of 6,270 pounds in the air. This feat would seem unlikely, or perhaps a hoax, if it were not for the fact that Anderson had been an Olympic weight lifter before he turned pro.

Extraordinary displays of strength pose fundamental questions for sports scientists, who are always searching for new ways to squeeze more power from the human body. What is the maximum power that can be produced by any set of human muscles? What is the maximum tolerance point for tendons and bones before they snap? Does everyone possess superhuman strength that lies dormant until it manifests itself during an emergency? Or can it be tapped with willpower or drugs?

Even the performance of competitive weight lifters poses problems. Consider the short 125-pound body of Lamar Gant, one of the most remarkable strong men in modern times. Gant practices power lifting, an offshoot of weight lifting that involves the squat, bench press, and dead lift. He is one of only three power lifters to have earned more than nine world titles. He has also broken twenty-six world records. And he is the only man ever to dead lift—to hoist a weight from the floor to hip level and lower it by the power of the back—more than five times his own body weight—638 pounds in the 123-pound class.

To those unfamiliar with power lifting, Gant's accomplishments may not seem particularly impressive until they consider his anatomy. His skin is paper thin. Tests at the University of Michigan discovered that only 2 percent of Gant's body weight is fat—3.5 pounds. An average male college athlete, by comparison, has 16 percent body fat. Physiologists believe Gant's metabolism is such that anything he eats is converted to muscle, bone, blood, and guts.

Those who have seen Lamar Gant perform often think their eyes are deceiving them. One reporter from *Sports Illustrated* wrote that when Gant hoisted 500 pounds in the dead lift "his long slim arms appeared to stretch, making him look exactly like a tiny black plasticman." Of course arms can't lengthen, but what does happen seems equally impossible: his back bends and becomes shorter, creating the illusion that his arms are growing.

Gant suffers from a progressive, potentially life-threatening spinal disorder known as *scoliosis,* a lateral curvature of the spine *(see Fig. 5.1).* This disease, which afflicts about 5 percent of the U.S. population, begins in adolescence and is not connected to Gant's lifting. Scoliosis patients usually require a back brace if the lateral curvature is in the 20- to 40-degree range, and surgery at angles over 40 degrees. Gant's curvature is about 70 degrees, yet he leads a normal life without medical treatment.

At the Chicago Osteopathic Medical Center, Gant underwent a series of thoracic X-rays standing without weights and then dead lifting 135 pounds, followed by progressive increments to 425 pounds. The X-rays clearly showed that his spine settled and bent as he lifted heavier loads. While holding 425 pounds his curvature was over 90 degrees.

According to some doctors, the reason he doesn't need a back

FIGURE 5.1

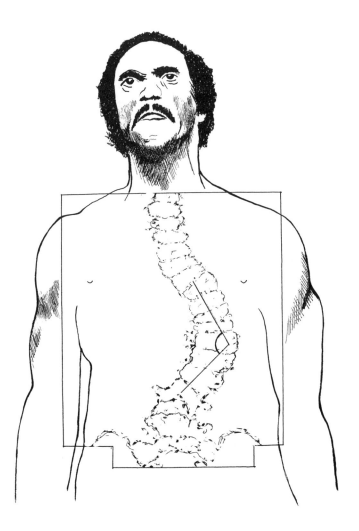

The mystery of Lamar Gant's back. Power lifter Gant suffers from scoliosis, or lateral curvature of the spine. Most victims of this disease with a curvature of over 40 degrees need a back brace or surgery, but Gant's back has a 70-degree curve and he has needed no medical assistance. X-rays have found that when he lifts weights his spine bends an incredible 90 degrees or more. Doctors believe that his highly developed musculature acts as a natural back brace. The sketch above, drawn from an actual X-ray of Gant's back, shows a 75-degree curve as he lifts a set of free weights.

brace to lead a normal life and the reason his spine doesn't break in two as he lifts is the same: his incredibly developed musculature serves as a natural back brace.

Gant is remarkable in other ways. He has phenomenal motivation and dedication, he never misses a training session, and he has never taken steroids or other ergogenic aids. Despite his handicap, his trainers believe if he maintains his level of interest in the sport he could clinch at least twenty world championships before he retires.

THE ADAPTATION OF MUSCLES TO STRENGTH TRAINING

The common denominator between Lamar Gant, Paul Anderson, and frantic mothers hoisting automobiles lies within the chemistry of their skeletal muscles.

Composed of thousands of individual muscle cells or fibers, all arranged in bundles, muscles power all forms of human locomotion by contracting or shortening. Inside each fiber are two types of long, overlapping chemical chains called myosin and actin filaments, locked together by a network of cross-bridges. The contraction of a muscle fiber is due to these two filaments moving toward each other with a ratchet or oarlike interaction as the cross-bridges simultaneously release their grip on the filaments.

The process is initiated by a signal from the nervous system that sets a series of chemical events into motion, ultimately causing calcium to activate the cross-bridges, allowing the filaments to slide together. The sliding itself is powered by ATP (adenosine triphosphate), a basic chemical fuel found in almost all forms of life.

Even at rest the chemical activity within a muscle is conducted at a spectacular pace. The actin and myosin filaments are continually being broken down, as anyone who has had a leg in a cast knows. Within two weeks, all the chemical ingredients of muscle tissue are completely turned over. As actin and myosin break down, they are constantly rebuilt—a process most weight lifters and body builders try to accelerate. When a muscle is stressed enough, it responds by adding more actin and myosin to the fibers, so that the overall diameter of fiber increases, an adaptation known as hypertrophy. The greater the diameter or cross-sectional area of the fibers, the greater the tension a muscle can develop, as there's more actin and myosin either locked together to hold a muscle firm or sliding together to make the muscle contract.

To provide optimal increases in hypertrophy, strength-training programs are designed in accordance with two basic concepts: the *progressive overload principle* and the *SAID* (Specific Adaptation to Imposed Demands) *principle.* Failure to observe the simple rules governing these concepts will waste an athlete's time and effort, and in the extreme, lead to injuries.

The SAID principle refers to the fact that muscles adapt in a very specific manner, responding only to the stresses imposed on them. Push-ups have no benefit for the leg muscles of a runner, nor will stressing the leg muscles in ways that won't be used in running.

Progressive overload refers to imposing ever greater amounts of stress on a muscle so it continues to grow. In strength training, the progression is measured in terms of weight loads and the number of repetitions at which the load is applied. Repetitions, grouped in multiple sets, are designed to physically overload a muscle, producing muscle failure at the end of the sets. Exercising to the point of muscle failure is essential in order to obtain a maximum adaptation.

Optimal strength training balances loads against the number of repetitions, or in the language of the lifter, as work *volume* increases, the load *intensity* decreases. Conversely, as intensity becomes greater, the volume performed is less. Explosive sports, such as sprinting, require high-intensity, low-volume training. Endurance sports, such as distance running, require high-volume, low-intensity training. Other program considerations include work and rest intervals (to allow for the manufacture of new chemical supplies inside the fibers), the training speed (which must reflect the desired speed of limb movement), and the number of workouts per week (to maximize recovery).

The modern athlete faces a baffling array of strength-training techniques and equipment, each backed with its own collection of scientific literature extolling its benefits over all others *(see Fig. 5.2).* Things weren't always so complicated. Thirteen hundred years ago, a Greek wrestler known as Milo of Crotona,

FIGURE 5.2

Five Types of Strength-Training Exercises

Isometric exercise: An isometric muscle contraction occurs when a muscle is stressed, but maintains a constant length. These exercises are usually done with immovable objects, or by pitting one muscle group against another. The effect is to increase strength but only at the joint angle stressed, not throughout the joint's entire range of motion. Athletes sometimes find isometric exercises useful in overcoming "sticking points" or weak joint angles.

Isotonic exercise: This is the most familiar form of strength training; it involves free weights or exercise machines. Isotonic loading techniques include constant resistance exercise (where loads remain constant, as in a power snatch with free weights), and variable resistance exercise (where increasing loads are imposed through the range of limb motion, as with Nautilus machines).

Eccentric exercise: This form of strength training refers to contractions in which the muscle fibers actually lengthen while contracting. The best example is lowering a free weight to the ground. Although eccentric exercises are often used in explosive actions, such as pitching and kicking, they have been associated with muscle pain.

Isokinetic exercise: Also known as "accommodating resistance exercise," this form of strength training controls the rate of muscle contraction throughout the limb or joint's range of motion. This is particularly important, as there are very few sports that require a muscle to contract at a steady rate throughout the range of motion. Isokinetic exercise can be done only with Cybex or Ariel exercise machines.

Neuromuscular facilitation: This form of exercise is done with a partner or trainer. It involves manipulation of limbs and muscles in repeated and rhythmic contractions as well as hold-and-relax movements. Although strength gains are not as profound as those from the exercise above, neuromuscular facilitation is useful for warmups and rehabilitation of injured joints.

with virtually no equipment, used a very simple form of progressive strength training. He worked out by lifting a calf every day until it grew into a bull—and so did Milo, who won three gold medals in the ancient Greek Olympics.

As a wrestler, Milo would have quickly grasped the principles behind the modern *Cybex* machine, also known as an isokinetic dynamometer. The name would have also been familiar: Cybex is derived from the Greek work *kybernetes,* or "steersman," the same word behind cybernetics, the science of control. The exterior of a Cybex looks like a futuristic dentist chair, in which the subject sits and straps his limbs to various attachments. But the external features of the machine can take on any appearance as modifications are made to adapt the Cybex to various sports. Inside the Cybex, a dynamometer measures muscle resistance in foot-pounds of torque (or twist) in the rotation of any limb an athlete selects to use. As the limb works against the machine, a computer analyzes the rapid changes in muscle resistance and provides information about how fast a given muscle produces strength, how quickly the muscles contract, and how fast the muscle fibers are being recruited.

Initially the Cybex was used in sports medicine to diagnose and rehabilitate joint and muscle injuries, especially of the knee. Trainers found it useful, too, because it produced isokinetic exercise, bringing the muscle to its full strength, through the joint's entire range of motion at any preselected velocity—something other forms of exercise cannot do.

Later the Cybex was also used to enhance special muscle functions, such as kicking and throwing. As the machine can be set at training speeds ranging from 0 to 300 degrees per second, baseball pitchers use them to analyze arm strength and learn how to attain the delivery speed of a pitcher like Nolan Ryan. Football punters and soccer players use them in the same way, with different attachments.

Recently, Cybex has been used by sports physicians to prevent injuries. At the Athletic Performance Center in Tulsa, Oklahoma, physiologist Ron Stratton tests athletes with the Cybex to obtain precise measurements of their strength capacity before the season begins. If their muscle strength is below normal for their height and weight, it's a predictor of potential injury during practice or a game. In the leg, for example, Stratton looks for peak strength in the quadriceps (the four-part extensor muscle at the front of the thigh) compared to body weight. For track runners, 90 percent strength is acceptable, but for football players, Stratton wants to see 110 percent strength in the quadriceps compared to body weight because of the extraordinary demands of stopping and starting this game imposes on the knee (see Chapter 10). The hamstring, the tendon group at the back of the knee, is measured next, and its peak strength should be at least 60 percent of the quadriceps. If it's not, Stratton instructs his athletes to do a specific number of hamstring curls to bring power up to the proper level.

In 1972, Gideon Ariel, a biomechanist and consultant for the U.S. Olympic Committee, introduced the principle of *variable strength training*, which led to the manufacture of exercise equipment such as Nautilus machines in 1970.[1] This equipment represented a major improvement over static dumbbell weights, or free weights, since the resistance could be set to increase or decrease as the muscles contracted. But there are many drawbacks to these machines. A critical deficiency is that the speed of limb movement is relatively constant during mechanical exercise, but there are no athletic activities performed at a constant velocity. For a sprinter, this means the exercise machines will improve the overall strength of his legs, but will not increase the speed at which the power is mobilized.

To compensate for the deficiencies, Ariel invented a computerized exercise machine that, for the first time, makes it possible for the equipment to adapt to the user, rather than the user adapting to the equipment. The force, displacement, and duration of every movement can now be monitored *and changed* as the athlete works out, providing the optimal overload. The computer establishes the present strength of a muscle; sets the load, the timing, and the number of repetitions; and also plots an athlete's progress from session to session, modifying the program as his performance improves. The new system, known as the Ariel-4000, requires no special knowledge of computers. A user simply touches the color display screen to select the type of training he needs for any form of athletic activity.

Ken Cooper, director of the Sports Science Institute at Hahnemann University, has speculated that athletes may soon be able to walk into computerized training centers with a personal diskette containing their complete training history, which can be slipped into an exercise machine and program the next session—even if the last session occurred thousands of miles away on another machine.

ELECTRIC STIMULATION OF MUSCLES

In the next decade, athletes may be able to increase strength and endurance using a new and controversial innovation based on a very old discovery. In 1737, Alosio Galvani skinned a dead frog and exposed the large nerve that led to the muscles of the animal's legs. In his anatomy lab in Bologna, Italy, he constructed a primitive electrostatic generator and connected it to the frog's leg with a scalpel. When the generator sparked, the frog's leg contracted. In the centuries that followed, physiologists learned that electric currents simulate the electrochemical stimulation imparted to muscle fibers by excited nerve cells.

In the early 1950s, a Russian physiologist, Jason Kots, reported that electrical stimulation of muscles had the same effect as conventional strength training, increasing the size and strength of muscle fibers. He claimed that low-voltage stimulation at frequencies of 2,500 hertz resulted in strength gains lasting for three months or more. As the electrical stimulation of a muscle is the only known way to induce *all* its fibers to contract, Kots's findings appeared to have found a basis in fact. In the West, however, his work was dismissed as Soviet quackery, at least until some reputable American researchers found that electrical stimulation to the muscles of paraplegics increased the size and strength of those muscles, even though the paralyzed patients had no way to exercise them. Slowly, other studies, many of them with animals, showed similar gains in strength, endurance, and even increases in the number of capillaries feeding the stimulated muscle fibers.

One study, conducted by Terry Sanford, a physiologist at Stanford University, reported that untrained subjects experienced significant improvements in muscle strength following only five weeks of intermittent electric stimulation. The gains included a 21 to 31 percent increase in isometric leg strength and a 13 percent increase in one form of isokinetic leg strength.

The idea of electric stimulation as an adjunct to strength training in athletes is full of promise, but still viewed cautiously by most sports scientists. It is not known how the electric currents might affect contraction force or the recruitment of motor units in the muscle. Further tests are needed to determine if and how this type of research will lead to a whole new approach to enhancing strength and endurance.

To grasp the potential of this research, consider the work being done at Wright State University in Dayton, Ohio, where paraplegics are learning to walk and pedal tricycles. Although they are unable to contract their muscles due to their paralysis, with a computerized electrical stimulation system they are now able to move themselves around. Imagine how this same kind of work could be applied to strength training in a wide array of sports to accelerate hypertrophy as well as improve muscle recruitment in a manner analogous to sprint towing (see "Strength Training for the Rush," Chapter 1).

Coupled with computerized exercise machines, like the Ariel-4000, training time and injury recovery time might be dramatically reduced with Galvani's discovery. Indeed, when we contemplate the future of sports in the next century (see Chapter 12), it may be more than science fiction to think of "wired players" who use electrical stimulation as a supercharger out on the field.

FREE WEIGHTS

The advent of hi-tech equipment is greeted with mixed emotions by many power and weight lifters, who still believe from experience that the best form of training is with the same equipment used in competition. Traditional free weights are cheaper than the $16,000 computerized Ariel-4000, and the SAID principle would seem to suggest that dumbbells are the equipment of choice.

When a new Ariel exercise machine was installed at the U.S. Olympic Training Center in Colorado Springs in 1984, one of the first athletes to test it was Guy Carlton, an elite heavyweight lifter from Philadelphia. After the technicians had fed what they thought was a maximum weight program into the computer's memory, they told Carlton to give it his best lift and he did. A moment later the machine gave off a loud crunch, followed by a whine. Its computer display screen went blank, then flashed one word, *ouch.* Much to Carlton's relief, his lift hadn't broken the machine, but the experience did reinforce his preference for barbells.

Among athletes and scientists alike, there is still some debate as to whether exercise machines are superior to free weights. The most recent studies have found that the machines are more useful for high-volume, low-intensity endurance training, stimulating growth in slow-twitch muscle fibers. Free weights, despite their higher risk of injury, are recommended for developing explosive strength and power. Both types of equipment, however, are generally accepted to be effective in strength training.

Squats have been heralded as one of the most beneficial exercises an athlete can do with free weights, with applications in many sports (see Fig. 5.3). Squats have also been criticized as being among the most injurious of all forms of strength training, particularly for amateur athletes who use free weights without proper supervision. This has led to many myths propagated by coaches, who warn against squats because they ruin the knees and diminish speed and flexibility in the legs.

Early research suggested that squats would stretch knee ligaments, making the joint weak and unstable, and thus prone to injury. Thorough investigation of this claim proved that the opposite was true. The tensile strength of the ligaments is actively improved, especially as they are gradually stretched beyond their normal resting length. Other studies have also found increases in the strength of connective tissues and thickening of the cartilage between the moving surfaces in the knee, all contributing to greater joint stability. Tendons, ligaments, and other connective tissues adapt to stress by thickening in a manner analogous to the buildup of calluses on hands through work. The danger to knees from squats lies in improper technique. Sudden, rapid knee bending under heavy loads will cause ligaments to tear or snap; loads must be applied carefully to allow the tissues to adapt.

Some trainers have recommended partial squats in favor of deep squats to prevent spine injury. The spine cannot tolerate the loads that legs can readily handle in squats, but spine protection can be assured with proper technique. Partial squats do not cause enough stress to the connective tissues to induce adaptation. Additional weights are often used in partial squats

FIGURE 5.3

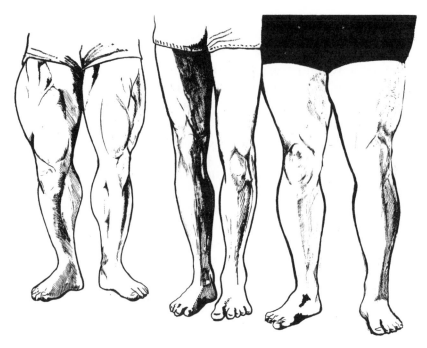

The legs of three athletes, all shaped differently, all from squats. This illustration is drawn from a photograph of three world champions: (left to right) a bodybuilder, a sprinter, and a power lifter. It demonstrates the specificity of adaptation in strength training. Muscles respond to how they are stressed, and they should be stressed in relation to how the athlete will use them in competition.

In the squat, the barbell is taken from the stand to rest across the shoulders behind the neck, while the hands firmly grasp the bar. With head tilted up and feet spread apart, the athlete squats down until his thighs are just lower than parallel to the floor, then stands upright. It's important that the knees are turned outward. The effect, depending on load and repetition, builds the muscles in the thighs.

to compensate, but this only adds to the potential for spine and knee injury.

Unlike machines, free weights are under the total control of the user. The Cybex or Ariel-4000 can be set to move at a fixed speed, but while using free weights an uncontrolled rapid movement resulting from muscle failure can be dangerous. High-volume, low-intensity exercises are generally safe without supervision, but high-intensity exercises should be conducted with spotters (assistants to help lift or catch a free weight during the final repetitions), lifting belts, and other safety equipment in a supervised gym.

THE EFFECTS OF NUTRITION ON STRENGTH TRAINING

Anthropologists have collected evidence from around the world to show that many primitive tribes have a belief in the magical powers of certain foods to produce strength in the body. These diets are usually prepared by the tribal shaman, accompanied by appropriately elaborate rituals. Here in the civilized world, athletes are often entranced by the promise of peak performance from diets dispensed by contemporary witch doctors.

According to Nathan J. Smith, an authority on the nutritional practices of athletes at the University of Washington Medical School, "No population group is more vulnerable to food faddism, cultism, misinformation, and the promotions of the nutritional charlatan than seriously committed athletes. Many coaches and trainers have picked up favorite pieces of nutrition misinformation over the years that they eagerly pass on to their players, convinced it will contribute to that all important winning edge" (see Fig. 5.4).

This is more than righteous rhetoric. A 1983 survey of ninety-three high school coaches in Texas found that virtually all of them thought they should take an active role in advising athletes on their diet, although nutrition had been included in the college training of only twenty-three of these men. It's not surprising that just fourteen of the coaches answered 70 percent or more of the basic nutrition questions in the survey correctly. The average test score was 55 percent—a failing grade at most schools.

What spinach did for Popeye will not work for athletes. There is no evidence that special foods will increase body strength. Diet in itself cannot provide fitness or enhance performance, but poor diet can certainly ruin both (the only known excep-

FIGURE 5.4
Eleven Fad Diets: Summary of Clinical Investigations

Diet	Commercial Claims	Scientific Findings
Banana-Milk Diet	Weight loss through daily intake of 1,000 calories	Protein, vitamin, and mineral supply inadequate
Beverly Hills Diet	Weight loss through special enzymes in certain fruits	Diet has no scientific basis; potential for dehydration
Calories Don't Count	Weight loss through low carbohydrate intake, coupled with special fats that stimulate metabolism	Unsuited for athletes concerned with fluid, sodium, and carbohydrate depletion; calcium and vitamin supply inadequate
Cambridge Diet	Weight loss through daily intake of 330 calories and 33 grams of protein in powdered formula	Protein supply inadequate to maintain muscle mass; this diet can be dangerous when self-administered
Complete Scarsdale Medical Diet	Weight loss through high protein intake with low carbohydrate and fat intake	Vitamin and mineral supply inadequate
Dr. Atkins's Revolutionary Diet	Weight loss through high protein and fat intake, very low carbohydrates	Carbohydrate and vitamin supply inadequate; risk of dehydration; high cholesterol content linked to cardiovascular disease
Dr. Stillman's Inches-Off Diet	Weight loss through high carbohydrate intake, with low protein and fat intake	Protein, vitamin, and mineral supply inadequate
Drinking Man's Diet	Weight loss through high protein and fat intake, with 60 grams of carbohydrates and alcohol	Potential of inadequate supply of vitamins; alcohol and high cholesterol intake linked to cardiovascular disease

124

Diet	Commercial Claims	Scientific Findings
Grapefruit Diet	Weight loss through high protein, fat, and grapefruit intake, with low carbohydrate intake	No scientific basis for claim grapefruit speeds weight loss; high cholesterol linked to cardiovascular disease
Macrobiotic Diet	Weight loss through progressive carbohydrate regimens, especially whole grains	Overt nutritional deficiencies can result if this plan is followed for prolonged period of time
Starvation Diet	Weight loss through low intake of carbohydrates, fats, and protein	Protein, carbohydrate, fat, vitamin, and mineral supply inadequate; appropriate only for hospitalized obese patients

Fad diets don't work for athletes who are trying to lose weight or gain strength and endurance. That's the message from studies conducted at Ross Nutritional Laboratories in Columbus, Ohio, of these and other fad diets. The only known dietary manipulation that enhances performance, and only in long endurance events, is carbohydrate loading (see Chapter 9). The best way to gain strength is to eat a healthy balanced diet. For more, see L.A.P. Porcello (1984), in bibliography.

tion is carbohydrate loading, a dietary manipulation for a very limited number of endurance events, discussed in Chapter 9).

A "winning" diet requires regular meals comprised of a wide variety of foods from each of the basic food groups (dairy products, meats, vegetables and fruits, grains and cereals). Meals should be balanced to provide about 15 percent of the daily calories as proteins, 35 percent as fats and 50 percent as carbohydrates. After moderate training, the body's stores of glycogen—the ready-to-use carbohydrate that helps fuel muscle contraction—can be repleted to normal levels within twenty-four hours with a 70 percent carbohydrate diet.

Despite decades of research, there is still confusion and controversy regarding the protein requirements for athletes undergoing heavy physical training. Proteins are actually composed of an assortment of twenty-two amino acids, which are released into the blood following protein digestion; they are reassembled inside cells to build or repair tissues, such as actin and myosin filaments in muscle fibers.

Because the body's requirement for energy takes priority over tissue building, proteins can be consumed as an energy source, but only if there's an inadequate supply of fats and carbohydrates. In starvation, the body will consume large quantities of its own skeletal muscle. On the other extreme, excessive dietary protein is converted to fat.

The recommended daily allowance (RDA) for protein in normal adults is about 0.8 grams per kilogram of body weight per day. The RDA states that there is no need for additional protein during training, as long as the caloric energy supply is adequate.[2] To insure that athletes do not burn proteins in the absence of fats and carbohydrates, and also keep the ratio of food types balanced, most sports physicians recommend that protein intake should be elevated to 2 grams/kilograms of body weight/day during heavy exercise.

In light of recent data on diet and cardiovascular disease, athletes must exercise caution in the selection of protein foods to keep their blood cholesterol low. Poultry and fish are favored over high-fat red meats; low-fat dairy products should be used only if a lot of them are eaten. Weight lifters in particular have had bad press in the fitness world due to their traditional high-protein consumption and lack of endurance exercise, once thought to be the only form of exercise that helped remove cholesterol from the blood (see Chapter 9). Recent studies now suggest that certain types of strength training can also enhance the removal of cholesterol—even if the athlete does not participate in aerobic activities, such as running or swimming.

In one study, Linn Goldberg, a physician at the Oregon Health Sciences University in Portland, tested fourteen volunteers who had no experience with weights and had not engaged in any form of structured endurance training. First he measured the amount of fats, or lipids, in their blood before and after a strength-training program. Training lasted for sixteen weeks, with the subjects working out three days a week. At the end of the study, the new weight lifters had an increase in one type of blood

126

lipid called *high-density lipoproteins*, known to absorb choles-terol in the blood and remove it from the body. Goldberg also found a decrease of *low-density lipoproteins*, fatty substances known to promote the accumulation of cholesterol in the in-terior walls of arteries; this cholesterol builds up and eventu-ally obstructs the flow of blood through vessels.

This study surprised some researchers, who thought that this healthy ratio of lipoproteins occured only with endurance training. Physicians warn, however, that neither strength nor endurance training is a panacea for cardiovascular disease. Al-though all forms of training may help remove cholesterol, a low-fat diet is also essential.

THE PREGAME MEAL

The pregame meal of steak and eggs, still popular with many athletes, not only produces high blood cholesterol, but it can impair performance during the competitive event. These high-protein meals are particularly popular with football players and weight lifters, who still believe they benefit from extra strength and energy during exertion.

This kind of pregame meal increases the blood flow away from the muscles—where it's needed to power muscle contrac-tion—sending it to the internal organs. A decreased blood flow to working muscles can only promote anaerobic metabolism, increasing lactic acid formation and the early onset of fatigue. Moreover, the high-protein, high-fat pre-event meal takes up to four hours to pass from the stomach to the upper intestine, where the nutritional content is absorbed into the blood-stream. If consumed only an hour or two before rigorous phys-ical exertion such a meal can cause indigestion, nausea, and vomiting, reactions not conducive to optimal performance.

Ideally, pre-event meals should be light, high in complex car-bohydrates (up to 70 percent), low in fat and protein, low in salt, with plenty of fluids to insure proper hydration, especially in the heat (see "Sports Drinks" in Chapter 9). This type of meal can be taken two to three hours before exercise; liquid meals can be consumed one to two hours before exercise, due to their rapid gastric emptying time.

Taking high doses of sugar before athletic events saps strength.

Instead of elevating blood sugar, it lowers it, due to the immediate release of insulin, which removes excessive sugar from the blood. Hypoglycemia, or low blood sugar, will then make an athlete feel fatigued. Some studies have shown, however, that it may be helpful to take in low levels of glucose in the form of fruit juice or a sweetened drink; this takes about ten to twenty minutes to elevate blood sugar slightly.

The most recent advance in sports nutrition is a method of matching the contents of the athlete's training diet, or pregame meal, to the level of key chemicals and nutrients in his blood. This technique, pioneered by Miami nutritionist Robert Haas and outlined in his book, *Eat To Win*, could lead to performance breakthroughs.

In the future, it's entirely possible that a small, inexpensive computerized device could be used by athletes at home to draw a small sample of blood, analyze the contents, compare the data against the individual's normal profile, and calculate what nutrients are needed for a particular game or event, and then recommend the ideal diet. Such an innovation might be particularly useful for athletes who are trying to gain or lose pounds in order to stay in a competitive weight class, or for dietary manipulation such as carbohydrate loading (see Chapter 9).

DRUGS IN STRENGTH TRAINING

According to the *Manual on Doping*, published by the Medical Commission of the International Olympic Committee, "The merciless rigor of modern competitive sports, especially at the international level, the glory of victory, and the growing social and economic reward of sporting success increasingly forces athletes to improve their performance by any means available."

Although the truth of this statement is undeniable, drug use is not exclusively a modern phenomenon. Taking chemical aids to improve performance is known to have occurred at least as early as the third century, when Greek athletes ingested psychotropic mushrooms. In the nineteenth century, chemical concoctions were creative. Marathon runners were given one-sixtieth of a grain of sulphate of strychnine—which in such small doses can act as a potent, if dangerous, stimulant. One preparation consisted of opium, lactose, and ipecac (a medicinal alkaloid). Modern drugs are certainly more effective, and can be just as deadly. The death of Danish cyclist Knut Jensen, who had taken a stimulant in the 1960 Rome Olympics, brought world attention to the problem, prompting stricter regulation by the International Olympic Committee (see Fig 5.5).[3]

Amphetamines continue to be one of the most abused drugs in sports, particularly in contact sports, due to the drug's potency and ready availability. In 1980, Joseph V. Chandler, a physician at the University of South Carolina, reported that athletes given Dexedrine (15 milligrams per 70 kilograms of body weight) two hours prior to treadmill running experienced a 4.5 percent increase in time to exhaustion and a 22 percent increase in knee extension strength. Acceleration in sprinting was also found to increase, but top speed was not affected. A study of athletes at Harvard in 1959 by anaesthesiologist Henry K. Beecher showed that 14 to 21 milligrams per 70 kilograms of body weight, given two to three hours before exercise, improved the speed of runners and swimmers, as well as the distance attained by weight throwers in 75 percent of all the trained athletes. Other studies have reported side effects, such as insomnia, loss of appetite, psychological disturbances, cardiac arrhythmias, and rare cases of sudden death (see Fig. 5.6).

Cocaine, like amphetamines, acts as a central nervous system stimulant, but in sports its use is more glamorous than performance enhancing. Certainly coke produces subjective feelings of well-being, alertness, and exhilaration, and it tends to mask fatigue. Some reports say this drug enhances aggression in contact sports, others disagree. Nasal inhalation of 0.25 gram of street-quality cocaine provides players with a lift that may last thirty minutes. One report indicated that 40 percent of professional football players may have experimented with the drug during their career, and 15 percent may be habitual users. The drug's effects on strength and endurance have not been thoroughly documented.

Butazolidin, or "bute," is an anti-inflammatory agent used by many athletes to reduce the pain and swelling in injured joints and ligaments. Bute is taken orally in doses of 50 to 100 milligrams. Chronic use has been linked to gastric disorders and various forms of anemia. *Cortisone* is another anti-inflammatory drug, but it is used much less than butazolidin.

129

FIGURE 5.5
List of Doping Substances Banned by the International Olympic Committee*

Psychomotor Stimulants	Narcotic Analgesics
amphetamine	Dextromoramide
benzphetamine	Dipipanone
cocaine	heroin
diethylpropion	morphine
Ethylamphetamine	methadone
Fencamfamin	Pethidine
Methylamphetamine	**Sympathomimetic Amines**
Norpseudoephedrine	ephedrine
phendimetrazine	Methylephedrine
phenmetrazine	Methoxyphenamine
Prolintane	**Anabolic Steroids**
Miscellaneous Stimulants	Methandienone (Dianabol)
Amiphenazole	nandrolone decanoate (Durabolin)
Bemegride	nandrolone phenpropionate
Leptazol	oxymetholone (Anadrol)
nikethamide	stanozolol (Winstrol)
strychnine	

Where's caffeine? The common stimulant found in coffee, tea, and some brands of soft drinks, aspirin, and chocolate (check the wrappers) has been shown in several studies to improve strength and endurance, but is not banned by the IOC or any other professional or amateur athletic governing body (see Chapter 9). The inclusion and omission of doping substances has long been controversial, and it's highly likely that substances of great commercial value will remain off the above list in the foreseeable future. Notice how many manufacturers of coffee and caffeine-laden soda sponsor or advertise at amateur and professional sporting events. However, the recent popular aversion for caffeine in foods and beverages may reverse this trend.

*Source: U.S. Olympic Committee (1984). (See bibliography.)

The process of hypertrophy in strength training is accelerated in adolescent males due to the increased secretion of the hormone testosterone. A large number of athletes believe that *androgenic anabolic steroids*—drugs that resemble testosterone—will also accelerate gains in strength, weight, power, speed, and endurance in the adult body. One researcher predicts that it may not be long before athletes also begin experimenting with

FIGURE 5.6
Incidence of Amphetamine Use by 87 Professional Football Players

Position	Yes	No	Sometimes	Dose/game (milligrams)
Quarterback	1	8	0	10–15
Wide receiver	6	5	2	5–15
Offensive line	10	4	0	15–105
Running back	8	3	2	5–25
Tight end	2	2	1	10–30
Defensive line	9	0	1	30–150
Linebacker	5	4	1	10–60
Defensive back	7	4	2	5–20
TOTALS	48	30	9	

The practice of team physicians drugging players with amphetamines was officially banned by the National Football League in 1971, but the rule was not enforced until 1974, in a case against the San Diego Chargers where the coach, team manager, and owner were fined. The team physician, Arnold J. Mandell, was fired, and he subsequently released figures indicating how widespread the use of "speed" was among players, shown in the table above. NFL officials alleged Mandell had given 1,750 pills, 5 to 15 milligrams each, to players over a three-month period. Now that team physicians can no longer prescribe amphetamines, players must acquire their drugs from diet doctors or street sources. A similar rate of amphetamine use has been reported in many other sports, but the documentation has not been as thorough as in professional football. See Mandell (1978), in bibliography.

estrogenic anabolic steroids, drugs similar to the female hormone estrogen. Recent studies have shown that mixing the male and female anabolic steroids is effective in beefing up domestic farm cattle.

Anabolic steroids work by binding to special receptor sites in skeletal muscle fiber and sending a chemical message to the genetic material inside the cell to increase the rate of protein synthesis. As a result, muscle mass has been substantially increased with these steroids in both animal studies and clinical trials, especially in individuals who have a natural deficiency of androgens. A small number of clinical tests of the effectiveness of steroids in athletic performance have produced mixed results, although there is no question of the efficacy in the minds of athletes who have used them regularly. The documented beneficial effects also include an increase in blood volume and in the number of red blood cells that carry oxygen. This is potentially useful for prolonged endurance exercise, as more oxygen can be transported to active muscles, decreasing the role of anaerobic metabolism in exercise and increasing the time it takes for fatigue to set in.

The prevalence of anabolic steroids in sports may surprise even the cynic. Sources suggest that these drugs are used by 80 to 100 percent of national and international body builders, weight lifters, and those who participate in the shot put, discus, hammer, and javelin throws. About half of all professional boxers, football, and hockey players are reported to have used anabolic steroids at some point in their career. Dosage is also high. The male testes can produce a maximum of 10 milligrams of testosterone every twenty-four hours, whereas weight-trained athletes have been reported to take oral doses ranging from 50 to 2,000 milligrams of steroids per day. Terry Todd, a weight lifter turned coach, reported swallowing about 1,200 steroid pills between 1963 and 1967; today, some athletes take higher doses in two weeks than Todd took in four years. The most recent trend is injecting steroids (subcutaneous and intramuscular) to help reduce the toxic effects high oral doses impose on the liver.

Other side effects include changes in personality, infertility, hardening of the arteries, high blood pressure, blood clotting disorders, acne, baldness, and changes in sperm count. Some studies have found hormone imbalances in young athletes using steroids, and a few men experience enlargement of their breasts.

However, contrary to sensational news stories and popular books on the subject, deaths directly linked to the use of steroids in sports are extremely rare. In fact, the actual incidence of side effects among athletes is unknown, and in the absence of hard scientific data, athletes, coaches, and sports physicians are forced to rely on expert opinion and the anecdotes of the few who will discuss their personal use of these drugs. This is unfortunate, because steroids are taken by more athletes and in higher doses than any other drug to enhance performance.

If we were to temporarily suspend the issue of "fair and equal competition," a central guidepost in the regulation of amateur sports, and concentrate only on the medical aspects of steroids, we might be forced to conclude, on the basis of the available evidence, that steroids have significant benefits for athletes. And the risks, despite the uncontrolled, almost reckless pattern of use by thousands of individuals, appear smaller than the list of side effects seems to suggest. Indeed, an argument might be made to advocate the controlled use of steroids in conjunction with various, supervised training programs.

Of course this notion is provocative, but only because so much is unknown about the adverse effects of anabolic steroids in athletes of various ages in different sports. We may get a different perspective on the subject if we recall the development and subsequent mandatory use of certain types of safety equipment in a few sports, where regulation often preempted a thorough investigation—a trend that ought to change as science takes a more active role in athletics.

In the extreme, a lack of data can lead to mistaken assumptions and misguided policies. A few physicians, for example, have written of the need to convince athletes of the dangers of steroids, even though the dangers are not fully known. While the intentions of these doctors are undoubtedly honorable, this approach probably does more harm than good by undermining the credibility of sports physicians, whom athletes must continue to trust if programs to prevent and treat injuries are to succeed. If the risk-benefit ratio of anabolic steroid use is not fully known, as it seems, then concerned physicians might put their energies to better use by organizing a large-scale, confidential study of the adverse effects that have appeared in users, and settle the controversy once and for all.

Human growth hormone (HGH) is the latest drug in the athletic pharmacopoeia. At present, it's not listed on the International Olympic Committee's list of banned drugs *(see Fig. 5.2)*, in part because the benefits are entirely unknown and because this substance occurs naturally in the body, making foolproof detection of HGH doping almost impossible.

HGH is a hormone secreted by the pituitary gland that promotes normal growth throughout the body. In a healthy adult, HGH appears to be secreted at different times of the day, opening the possibility of increasing the natural supply of this hormone by tinkering with the body's biological clock (see "The Frontier: Chronobiology" in Chapter 11). Dwarfs have been found to be lacking in HGH, which is now administered to help stunted HGH-deficient children grow to a normal height. Originally, HGH was extracted from the pituitary glands of human cadavers and was very expensive; it can now be manufactured in vastly larger quantities with genetic engineering technology. On the black market HGH can be obtained today for about $100 a dose.

Like anabolic steroids, HGH stimulates protein synthesis and also accelerates the breakdown of fats, while decreasing the amount of carbohydrates burned by the body. As far as can be determined, athletes who have secretly used HGH to gain height have done so in vain. After adolescence the bones of the body become fused and can't grow any longer; however, adults who use HGH develop thicker bones and more soft tissues. Rumors of increasing HGH use abound but the benefits in performance are all anecdotal.

It is possible that an insanely ambitious parent could feed a growing child HGH in the hope of producing an adult with the stature of an NBA basketball player. As abominable as this may sound, some forward-looking sports scientists believe the present clandestine experimentation with HGH and steroids will seem trivial once genetic engineering begins to revolutionize the pharmaceutical industry—and in the distant future allows a new breed of athletic trainer to insert genetic programs into their athletes. Formidable challenges lay ahead: now is the time to establish new protocols to assess the use of drugs and other offspring of biotechnology in sports, gathering sufficient data in the laboratory lest athletes test them on themselves in the field.

DRUG TESTING

The science of analytic chemistry made headlines in the summer of 1983 when drug monitoring uncovered unexpected widespread use of banned substances at the Pan American Games in Venezuela. Sixteen athletes tested positively for steroids and three were found to have taken stimulants. Another dozen U.S. athletes, terrified of what the tests might reveal in their own bodies, returned home without competing. Recent challenges in court about the reliability of breathalyzers, blood tests, and urinalysis for detecting drugs in employment screening and law enforcement raise questions about the accuracy of modern drug screening in sports medicine. Are careers being ruined by false positives, or are the methods used absolutely reliable?

The analytic techniques used at the Pan Am Games were, in fact, not as discriminating as the press reported, nor as discerning as some of the athletes might have feared. Manfred Donike, a chemist from Cologne, West Germany, who was responsible for organizing the drug-testing lab in Caracas, denies the reports that his equipment could detect drugs taken a year before the games. He said that, at best, there were some drugs that could be spotted three months after application, but others could be traced back only two weeks. As a rule, oral anabolic steroids are usually not detectable fourteen days after their last use, but injected steroids can be traced up to two months after last use. Cocaine and amphetamines are usually flushed out of the body forty-eight hours after consumption. There's evidence that some athletes take diuretics, drugs that increase urine output, to accelerate the flushing of drugs before a test, but the effectiveness of this procedure is not known.

To detect such stimulants as cocaine and amphetamines, a method known as *gas chromatography* is used. After a urine sample is prepared for analysis, it is injected into the chromatographer, where it is vaporized and driven by an inert gas through a column coated with chemicals that separate the different compounds in the sample. This technique is considered very accurate, but to double check, a second analysis is made by passing urine from the original sample through a *mass spectrometer*, where it's fragmented into its constituent parts, and a chemical's unique "signature" is taken and compared to known signatures for the various banned substances. Both of these machines are used widely in many fields of science and are generally accepted as highly reliable. But where there are humans there will also be error. In world-class competitions, such as the Pan Am Games or the Olympics, the sampling procedure is very rigorous and it's difficult for an athlete to cheat. In professional sports, however, where management seems more concerned with a clean image than clean athletes, sampling procedures can be a bit sloppy. There are stories of drug-free urine samples being smuggled to tests in plastic bags held under the armpit, and of players swapping samples in the locker room.

In the 1980s, black-market manufacturers of illegal street drugs, such as heroin and amphetemines, confounded the authorities by creating so-called "designer drugs." These substances are more difficult to detect in the body of a user with routine screening techniques because the chemists who've created these hybrids have subtly altered their molecular structure. Moreover, because "designer heroin"—and there are at least six different designs—is not specifically covered by the law, the drug remains legal until state lawmakers amend existing legislation. In this way, illegal drugmakers can always stay one step ahead of the law. Given the large size of the sports market, it will probably be just a matter a time until designer drugs become available to athletes.

The use of *ergogenic aids*—any substance or device that boosts strength or endurance—will advance and spread at a pace set by developments in biotechnology. Genetic engineering, for example, has brought the once prohibitive cost of a dose of HGH down to the cost of a single gram of cocaine. Moreover, new discoveries, like blood doping was in 1975, will lead to abuses if there is even a remote possibility they will enhance performance.

In this regard, progressive developments in biotechnology will eventually challenge the definition and standards of "fair and equal competition." At present, if one weight lifter takes steroids to increase his strength through accelerated hypertropy and his rivals do not take steroids, there is obviously no fairness or equality in competition. But consider the weight lifter who can afford to use an Ariel-4000, although his competitors can only train with Nautilus machines. And what about the future use of electrical muscle stimulation?

Where should the officials and governing bodies of amateur and professional sports draw the line between fair and foul use of various new and existing ergogenic aids?

Power lifter Lamar Gant is very proud of the fact that he is a "natural athlete," by which he means he has never taken drugs to boost his strength—a claim that he substantiated with a lie-detector test in 1981. However, the term "natural" raises interesting philosophical questions. In relation to the human body, most people believe "natural" means the original biological state of the organism, which grows, develops, and performs untouched and unaffected by the external or artificial influences of man. This include drugs as well as training and technology.

To look at the issue from another perspective, jump forward about fifty years in time, when the sports scientist is confronted with athletic twins, one of which, by some fluke, has a lower output of testosterone or HGH than his brother. This scientist might conceivably argue that competition between the two would not be "fair and equal" unless the deficient brother is given, say, readily accessible genetic therapy to correct his condition.

In the final analysis, "fair and equal competition" cannot rest on vague notions of the "natural athlete," because the very essence of all forms of training is to tamper and tinker with the human body, sculpting profound changes in its anatomy and physiology—changes that would not occur if the body had developed naturally.

To cope with the recent developments in biotechnology, those who govern sports will eventually have to focus on the more fundamental issue of the risks and benefits of ergogenic aids, and then, if the benefits far outweigh the risks, ensure *equal access* to these aids for any athlete who wishes to use them. Only then can there be "fair and equal competition."

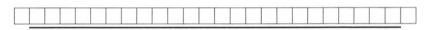

SIX

BASEBALL

How to Throw a Lamb Chop
Past a Hungry Wolf

After the 1946 midsummer All-Star game in Boston's Fenway Park, Ted Williams, the greatest slugger to stand at the plate for the Red Sox, made an extraordinary claim.

In the course of the game, Williams hit two singles, two home runs, and drew a walk in five trips to the plate. His performance was remarkable in that the pitcher was Rip Sewell, whose celebrated "blooper pitch" was one of the most difficult to hit in baseball—a soft lob thrown in a high arc that fell through the strike zone at a steep angle. Until Williams came to bat that day, no one had ever hit a home run off Sewell's blooper.

When asked by sportswriters in the locker room how he could hit such a wide variety of pitches, including the phenomenal blooper, with such consistency, Williams simply replied, "I keep my eye on the ball from the moment it leaves the pitcher's hand until the moment it strikes the bat."

Coming from such an authority, the earnest scribblers never doubted the truth of this statement and dutifully filed their stories for the next day's edition. Today, despite the persistent exhortations of coaches to "keep your eye on the ball," scientists believe it is impossible for the human eye to follow a pitched ball all the way to the plate, let alone as it hits the bat.

Every American knows that a major league baseball player, especially a Hall of Famer, would never tell a lie, so what exactly did Williams mean, or more to the point, what did he *see*? For years there has been some debate about whether or not the sharp break of a curve ball or the hop of a fast ball is an optical illusion. Could Williams's eyes have been playing tricks on him, or did he develop a unique form of visual tracking that could be learned by any aspiring batter?

THE SCIENCE OF PITCHING

The essence of the confrontation between a pitcher and a batter is deception. If a pitcher threw only fast balls down the middle, an experienced batter would have little problem putting one ball after another out of circulation. It's for this reason that the old catapult-style "Iron Mike" mechanical pitchers are no longer used in batting practice. Modern major league clubs use a twin-wheel pitcher that can hurl a curve, slider, fast ball, even a knuckle ball at any part of the strike zone, at various speeds, to keep batters alert for the unexpected.

The pitching fraternity succeeds in confounding batters (and catchers) by conspiring with the laws of gravity, ballistics, and aerodynamics to shape the trajectory of the ball. And in the case of the mysterious knuckle ball and spitball, they let the properties of the atmosphere randomly affect a ball's path to the plate in such a way that no one knows where it will go, including the pitcher.

The ritual begins when the pitcher kicks the rubber slab, 60.5 feet from home plate, and leans forward as if myopic to read the catcher's sign. He may shake his head once or twice in protest, but eventually nods, however slightly, before he goes into the stretch and windup. A catcher's traditional role in calling the pitch is based on his unique vantage point: he is the only defensive player facing the field and the alignment of all players. In modern baseball, a catcher's contribution to the pitch has become much like a quarterback calling an audible—it's a sudden deviation from the game plan.

The brains behind the contemporary pitching strategy are made of silicon: computers are now able to tell a hurler which balls are most likely to slip past any slugger. When Davey Johnson took over as manager of the New York Mets in 1984, he installed an IBM personal computer in his office, adjacent to the locker room. (In the same year Johnson installed his computer, more than half of the twenty-six major league teams had a

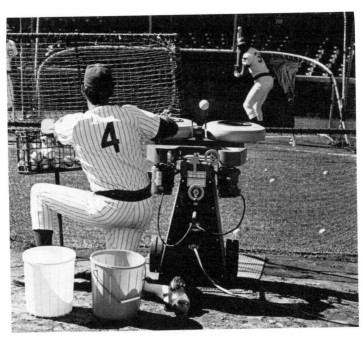

*If a pitcher threw only fast balls down the middle, an experienced batter would have little problem putting one ball after another out of circulation. It's for this reason that the old catapult-style "Iron Mike" mechanical pitchers are no longer used in batting practice. All major league clubs now use a twin-wheel pitcher that can hurl a curve, slider, fast ball, even a knuckle ball at any part of the strike zone, at various speeds. Here the "Curvemaster" twin-wheel pitcher is being used in practice by the Chi-*cago Cubs. (Courtesy of Sports Equipment, Inc., Curvemaster Division, Greenville, IL.)

computer in the dugout. At Dodger Stadium, manager Tommy Lasorda has one sitting between the water cooler and the bat rack.) Armed with a degree in mathematics, a love of computers, and eighteen years as a professional baseball player, Johnson designed a special program to store and display all individual and team statistics, including hit-by-hit records of each batter's drives, showing the distance and placement of each ball. Before every game, Johnson calls up the pertinent data, which are updated daily, and makes changes and adjustments to give the Mets a better chance. If an opposition batter has consistently hit, say, Johnson's starting pitcher's slider, then he'll brief the hurler to avoid the slider in critical situations against that batter.

The pitcher, now knowing the best ball to give the slugger, prepares to throw with the windup. The purpose of the windup is to confuse the batter, as well as to start a rhythmic motion in the pitcher's body, setting the limbs in a position to attain the maximum distance over which the ball can be accelerated. The object of most pitches is to obtain a linear (forward) velocity between 80 and 140 feet/second, a range in which various aerodynamic forces can move the ball up or down, left or right, while minimizing the time it takes to reach the plate. The faster the ball, the less time a batter has to focus on it, study its spin and trajectory; and move, or not move, the bat.

The launch speed of any ball is determined by the pitcher's ability to rotate various segments of his body with increasing velocity. (This applies equally to the overhand throw of a football, basketball, or javelin.) Studies have found that about 50 percent of throwing speed is the result of body rotation and 50 percent is the result of muscular strength of the upper body, especially in the muscles that extend between the elbow and the wrist.

Pitching strength can be measured and technique adjusted using a Cybex machine (see Chapter 5). When the pitcher grabs a special arm of the Cybex and rotates it with his pitching motion, the dynamometer inside the Cybex measures the muscle resistance; when EMG leads are attached to his shoulder and pitching arm, they measure the electrical activity in the muscles as they contract. A computer integrates the information and provides a physiological portrait of the maximum amount of resistance the hurler can handle without causing an injury. If, at the beginning of the season, the pitcher's arm looks weak to the computer, which predicts that fast-ball deliveries will eventually lead to an arm injury, specific forms of strength training will be prescribed to get the arm back into shape. In this way, a healthy player can alter his throw or build his strength to prevent injuries; an injured player can learn to alter his throw to accommodate an injury.

As strength is half of throwing speed, the Philadelphia Phillies have connected their Cybex to the team computer to assist in making on-the-field decisions of when a pitcher is ready to be pulled off the mound. Other teams have added a second lever, a "Sagedahl axis," to the Cybex. With the axis, named after University of Minnesota pitching coach Steve Sagedahl, complex motions of the shoulder, elbow, and wrist can be measured more accurately to help hurlers throw their fastest.

After the windup, the actual delivery of a pitch basically involves stepping forward and revolving the throwing arm around the shoulder as a radius of a circle. The greater this circle, the greater the launch speed. Biomechanic studies of pitching technique have found that this larger circle can be created by keeping the pitching elbow up and extended at release point (see Fig. 6.1). A second advantage of a high elbow is that the pitcher is able to throw on a downward plane to the plate, and thus stay "on top of the ball," facilitating easy vertical spin, which is essential to controlling the ball's path through the air. From a manager's vantage point in the dugout, a tired pitcher will display a marked drop of his elbow during delivery, indicating that it's time to call his relief pitchers to start warming up in the bullpen.

The final force of delivery is in the whiplike action of the throwing arm. This is acquired by letting the ball hand trail the wrist, forearm, and elbow; as the elbow is advancing in front of the forearm, the ball is pulled through the first phase of the delivery. At the point where the throwing arm reaches its highest position, the ball is released with a forceful vertical snap of the wrist. The ball actually leaves the hand (in the overhand throw) at a point on a line with the bill of the pitcher's cap—at this point, the linear velocity of the ball is the greatest.

As delivery technique varies from pitcher to pitcher, and may even vary for an individual during the course of a game, a batter has no idea what kind of ball is going to approach the plate. Some batters say they can read a pitch by watching a pitcher's feet; high-speed film analysis of top pitchers has shown this claim to be dubious.

The motion of the ball in flight is set just as the ball is released, the wrist and fingers imparting the precise angular rotation, or spin. Here lies the real magic of—as sportswriter Bugs Baer once said—"throwing a lamb chop past a hungry wolf."

A landmark investigation of the behavior of a baseball in flight was conducted by Carl Selin at the University of California at

142

FIGURE 6.1

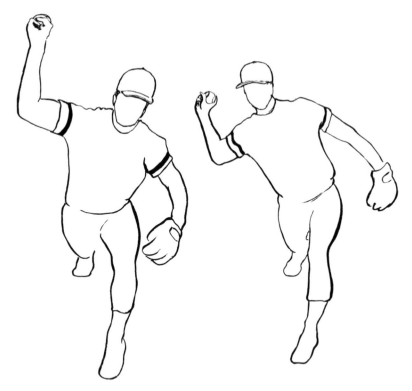

A tired pitcher tends to drop his elbow and lean toward the ball. This illustration, drawn from photographs of fresh and tired hurlers, both with identical overhand pitches, shows the pronounced drop of the elbow in the tired pitcher (right)—a clear signal for the manager in the dugout to have relief pitchers warm up in the bullpen.

The delivery of a pitch involves stepping forward and revolving the throwing arm around the shoulder as a radius of a circle. The greater the circle, the greater the launch speed of the ball. This larger circle is created by keeping the elbow up and extended at the point of release. Throwing with a dropped elbow, also known as side arming or short arming, produces a shorter radius of motion and a slower ball, which is easier to track and hit.

Riverside in 1959. Using high-speed cameras mounted above and to the side of pitchers, he found that each pitch, no matter what type, had either a vertical or horizontal deviation, or both, from a true straight line of flight in gravity—none of the pitches followed the course of a freely falling sphere. From this Selin and other early investigators concluded that something other than gravity was acting on all the balls.

Assuming for a moment that a ball is thrown horizontally, it should descend at the rate of 32 feet/second squared due to gravity, a rate of acceleration that applies to everything not anchored to the surface of the earth. Because the pitcher strides forward by about 6 or 7 feet during delivery, the ball is actually released at about 54 feet from home plate: at this distance a 100-mph pitch should drop about 2 feet before it crosses the plate. But as Selin discovered, few do. Some drop more, some rise. As wind-tunnel tests have now shown, the defiance of gravity is due to the interaction of the ball with the surrounding air.

THE AERODYNAMICS OF A BASEBALL

The basis of all aerodymanic phenomena lies in the properties of the air. Although the atmosphere seems intangible or frictionless to human senses, it is really a fluid medium with a measurable density (almost 3 pounds per cubic yard) and viscosity, which offers considerable resistance to a ball in flight.

When a ball is placed in a wind tunnel and air is forced to flow past it, two simultaneous effects are produced. First, the direction of the air near the ball is altered so that it can pass around the obstruction; second, the airstream closest to the surface of the ball, called the *boundary layer,* slows down as a result of friction. This second effect, known as *drag,* reduces the speed of the ball. At high speeds, the boundary layer of air no longer travels around the ball in a smooth, orderly manner, called *laminar flow,* but becomes violently jumbled, developing into a *turbulent flow.* This causes the boundary layer to tear away from the surface. The torn layer of fast-moving air is known as the *wake* and trails behind the ball *(see Fig. 6.2).*

If aerodynamic drag acted on the entire surface of the ball uniformly, the effect would be simply to reduce its speed and the ball would sink even faster toward the ground on its way to the plate. But because the surface of the ball is not uniformly smooth and because the ball spins in flight, surface drag will be more pronounced on some areas than others.

144

FIGURE 6.2

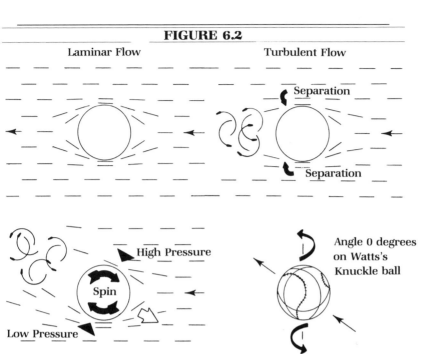

Laminar Flow   Turbulent Flow

Separation

Separation

High Pressure

Spin

Low Pressure

Angle 0 degrees
on Watts's
Knuckle ball

*Simulated wind tunnel tests showing the aerodynamic prop-
erties of a baseball. The illustration top left, shows the* laminar
flow, *where the air travels past the ball smoothly, without turbulence. Top right shows the* turbulent flow, *where at higher
speeds the boundary layer separates from the surface of the ball,
producing a wake. Bottom left shows how the spin of a ball alters
the wake and produces a curve, the ball deflecting in the same
direction it's spinning. Bottom right shows the position of Watts's
knuckle ball in the wind tunnel at the position he called angle zero.
He slowly began to spin the ball counterclockwise around its vertical axis and observed left-to-right deflections as the boundary
layer selectively skipped back and forth over the stitching.*

As a ball spins, about half of the surface area is going to be
revolving against the air flow, and the other half with the air
flow. According to Bernoulli's principle, as the speed of the air
increases, the pressure exerted on the ball's surface decreases.
In this way, the pressure of the faster moving air on one-half of
the ball will be less than the pressure exerted by the slower
moving air on the other half. This effect is known as *lift,* which
is slightly misleading because lift always occurs at right angles
to the drag force, even if that means left, right, or down relative

to the flight path. (A more descriptive term might be deflection or deviation.) Thus, the lift of a rotating ball, referred to as the *magnus effect*, will deflect a ball with a clockwise spin to the right, counterclockwise spin to the left, backspin will cause it to rise, top spin to sink in flight. In all cases, *the ball will deviate in the direction it's spinning.*

A pitcher can cause a ball to jump or swerve as much as twenty inches by exploiting these basic aerodynamic principles. The most dramatic results are produced by spin: the greater the speed of rotation, the greater the deviation.[1]

THE MYSTERY OF A KNUCKLE BALL

The knuckle ball is something of an anomaly. It's thrown with little or no spin, but it still curves and hops. Pitchers say it's the most difficult ball to throw; batters say it's the most difficult to hit.

The contemporary champion of the knuckle ball is Phil Niekro, the forty-six-year-old Yankee pitcher who, at the time he joined the New York club in 1984, had won 268 games, lost 230, and struck out 2,912 batters in 4,619 innings. Only eight other pitchers in the history of the game have struck out more batters. Niekro credits his success to his fingertips: by digging the fingernails of the forefinger and middle finger of his right hand into the stitched seams, he is able to release the ball with a stiff wrist, inhibiting spin.

"I do it 85 to 90 percent of the time," says Niekro. "The ball will wobble, drop, and break unpredictably. It's so effective managers have told me to go out and throw nothing but knuckle balls, even if it means walking the whole ball park."

The knuckle ball baffled scientists for decades because of its lack of spin; the magnus effect had to be ruled out as the cause of its eccentric behavior. The mystery seems now to have been cracked by Robert G. Watts, a mechanical engineer at Tulane University, who placed regulation baseballs in a wind tunnel and attached strain gauges to detect lift and drag forces. He also glued fine wool threads to the rear of the ball to observe the action of the wake.

When the ball was set up, Watts forced air to flow past the suspended sphere at speeds between 40 and 70 feet/second, slower than most pitches but within the range of knuckle balls recorded by radar guns. With the ball facing the wind in a position he called angle zero *(see Fig. 6.2)*, the air glided by without causing any deflection. He then turned the ball slowly around its vertical axis and began to observe lateral (sideways) forces of 0.1 pound toward the left or right. At angles of 140 and 220 degrees, there were *jumps* in the lateral force of about 0.08 pound in one direction to 0.08 pound in the opposite direction. Then at angles of 52 and 310 degrees, there was a pronounced instability in the air flow that caused the lateral force to *alternate* from left to right with an amplitude of 0.18 pound once every 0.5 second.

According to Watts, "This alternating force occurred when a portion of the strings was located just at the point where boundary layer separation takes place . . . it resulted when the point of separation changes from one side of the strings to the other." The effect on an actual pitch would be to deflect it one way or the other, depending on the orientation of the stitched seams.

Watts concluded that the erratic fluttering flight of the knuckle ball could be attributed to two mechanisms. First, if there is no spin on the ball, the fluctuating lateral force is caused by boundary layer separation skipping from one side of the strings to the other at certain locations on the ball. But this would require that the ball be released into the air with a precise initial orientation so that the special angle of the strings interacts with the air. The second, and far more likely mechanism, is that the ball spins very slowly as it approaches the plate (between a quarter to full revolution), exposing the ball to varying lateral forces as the position of the strings changes. Here lies the difficulty of the pitch: if the ball is given too much spin there will hardly be any lateral deflection. For example, if a knuckle ball is thrown at 60 feet/second and undergoes two complete revolutions before it reaches the batter, it will experience a peak lateral force of 0.08 pound, moving it only 0.048 feet to the left or right—an easy ball to track and hit.

Without the surface roughness of the stitches, the effects of the knuckle ball would not be as pronounced. Any roughness on a sphere will affect its drag curves. In fact, there is undeniable evidence that pitchers go to great lengths to alter the aerodynamic properties of the ball to obtain eccentric deflections in their standard fare. A well-known example is the spitball, which was outlawed in 1920, although it is still used surreptitiously by some pitchers. In 1982, Gaylord Perry of the Seattle Mariners was suspended for ten days because he "doctored the ball." This can be achieved by applying saliva, perspiration, hair grease, or by cutting or scuffing the ball's surface. Legal ways of altering the ball include working the surface with fingers and thumbs, or roughening some of the strings along the seams with the fingernails. It is for this reason that umpires frequently inspect balls during a game, checking on surface roughness that might unfairly affect the aerodynamics of a pitch, and promptly eject any ball together with the hurler suspected of illegal tampering.

In recent years, these findings have been embraced by pitching coaches who encourage their charges to always grip the ball for any type of pitch in the same orientation relative to the seams. This insures that a pitcher can consistently apply the same forces to the ball over the initial portion of its trajectory to keep the batter guessing. It also allows a pitcher greater control over when and how a pitch will "break."

A uniform release will result in the changes in the spin axis occurring in a standard manner until the boundary layer stops separating from the surface of the ball as the pitch slows (by about 10 mph in most cases) to the critical velocity, and the ball makes the transition from turbulent to laminar flow. At this point there is a sudden change in the forces affecting the ball, causing it to dramatically curve or hop. As noted earlier, drag increases as the linear speed of the ball decreases, causing a sharp change in the curvature of its trajectory. Thus a batter is not the victim of an optical illusion, as some claim, when he sees a ball break; he is witnessing a projectile whose lateral deflection is changing at an accelerating rate.

VISUAL TRACKING IN BATTERS

This brings us back to the question of Ted Williams's perception of a pitch, which he claimed he could track along the entire flight from pitcher to plate.

From the moment the ball is released by the pitcher, a batter has about half a second to evaluate the pitch and swing the bat. Experienced batters do more than focus on the ball; they concentrate on the red stitched seams to detect spin, knowing that the direction of the spin dictates the direction in which the ball will break. The longer a batter has to evaluate a pitch, the more likely he'll make the correct decision. Studies of fast balls (traveling at over 100 feet/second) have found that major league hitters with a batting average below .300 take an average of 0.26 second to evaluate a pitch and 0.28 to swing. Ted Williams took an average of 0.31 second to study a pitch and 0.23 to swing. The 0.05 second difference may not seem like much, but it's the margin that distinguishes great sluggers. Mickey Mantle and Willie Mays took a leisurely 0.33 second to evaluate and 0.21 to swing. Stan Musial, known to have some of the "quickest wrists" in the game, studied a pitch for 0.35 second and swung the bat in an astonishing 0.19 second.

Of course the batter is trying to track the ball during both the evaluation and swing phase. Whether the eyes can actually stay with the ball is determined by his maximum gaze velocity over a given set of angles. A catcher can keep his eyes on the ball without difficulty because it is coming directly at him. A batter, however, is standing at a right angle to the pitcher and he must swivel his eyes and head to follow the ball (see Fig. 6.3). A 100-mph fast ball, for example, has an angular velocity greater than 500 degrees/second as the ball passes the batter, whereas most humans cannot swivel eyes and head faster than about 100 degrees/second.[2]

How, then, could Williams see the ball hit his bat? Or, for ordinary mortals, if a ball is too fast to follow, how can anyone hit it?

All batters integrate three basic types of eye movement to hit a ball: *saccadic*, used for scanning left to right; *vestibulo-ocular*, used to lock onto a target while the head is moving; and *smooth-pursuit*, used to follow a moving target. Each of these distinct movements are controlled in three separate areas of the brain, and each system has its own maximum response and movement times.

To assess how these systems work together for baseball batters, A. Terry Bahill, a bioengineer at the University of Arizona, set up an experiment that monitored the eye movements of a

FIGURE 6.3

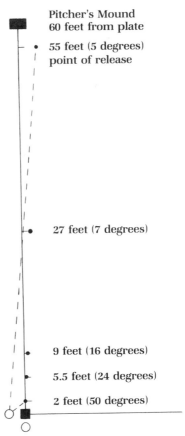

Pitcher's Mound
60 feet from plate

55 feet (5 degrees)
point of release

27 feet (7 degrees)

9 feet (16 degrees)

5.5 feet (24 degrees)

2 feet (50 degrees)

If a ball is moving too fast to track it, how does anyone hit it? Terry Bahill found that the visual tracking system of a baseball batter operated at a 90-degree angle between mound and plate and forward relative to the batter's box. In one test, Brian Harper, an outfielder for the Pittsburgh Pirates, was able to follow the pitch until it was 5.5 feet from the plate, which corresponds to a visual angle of 24-degrees. When the ball was 2 feet away, at the 50-degree point, Harper could no longer see the ball—which had traveled the distance between those two points in 67 milliseconds.

batter tracking a simulated fast ball. He attached a white plastic ball to a length of fishing line stretched 60.5 feet, the distance between the pitcher's mound and home plate. The line was connected to a pulley and motor so the ball could travel to the batter at speeds between 60 to 100 mph. When the line crossed the plate it was fixed at 2.5 feet from the batter's shoulders to simulate a high outside fast ball thrown by a left-handed pitcher to a right-handed batter, a relatively easy ball to track. By controlling the motor's speed and counting the shaft rotations, Bahill could calculate the exact position of the ball at every moment in time, enabling him to compare the position of the ball to the position of the batter's gaze.

Monitoring the batter's eye movements was more complicated. Bahill devised a pair of goggles that aim invisible beams of infrared light at the borders of the iris of both eyes and installed photodetectors to measure the amount of reflected infrared light as the eyes move. Head movements were measured with a video camera mounted above the batter; three small lights were fitted on the subject's head, providing coordinate points to compute yaw, pitch, and roll angles. The experimental batters included university students who did not play organized baseball; students who played on varsity teams; and Brian Harper, an outfielder for the Pittsburgh Pirates.

As the experiments proceeded, Bahill found that Harper kept his eyes on the ball longer than any of the students. He was able to follow the ball until it reached 5.5 feet from the plate, and then he lost it. At 2 feet from the plate, the ball was 16 degrees off his fovea, the functional center of sight of the eye, too far off to track.

In real pitches, the 100-mph fast ball would have slowed to about 90 mph as it neared the plate due to air resistance, and one might think it would be easier to track; the difficulty in following a pitch is that the angle *increases* as the ball approaches the plate. When a ball is 9 feet in front of the plate it has covered only 16 of the 90 degrees between pitcher and batter; when it is 2 feet in front of the plate it has covered the angle between 16 and 50 degrees in 67 milliseconds—traveling at 507degrees/second compared to the batter's maximum gaze velocity of 100 degrees/second.

It turns out that Ted Williams, and presumably other sluggers who have made the same claim, developed a method of visual tracking that is subjectively perceived as uninterrupted to the moment the ball hits the bat, but that in fact is discontinuous. The trick lies in a visual operation known as an *antic-*

ipatory saccade, something done unconsciously, but that may be learned through conscious effort.

A saccade is a very fast, horizontal eye movement. You are using it right now to read these lines of text. It is a critical visual function in many sports, such as basketball, and for visual tracking by the judges of, say, a tennis tournament, who sit on the sideline watching the ball travel left to right (see Chapter 7). For a batter, an anticipatory saccade involves moving the eyes ahead of the fast-moving pitch and letting the ball catch up to the eye movement. A batter who uses this strategy will track the ball for over half its trajectory—during his evaluation phase—then jump ahead as he executes the swing, enabling him to actually see the ball strike the bat.

This may sound as if the batter knows he is not keeping his eyes on the ball, but he is unaware of the jump due to a phenomenon known as *saccadic suppression,* which prevents him from seeing during saccades. This suppression of vision, a "blackout" that is never consciously perceived, extends to about 20 milliseconds after the saccade.

Unfortunately, there are no studies comparing the batting performance of players who use an anticipatory saccade to those who lose the ball 5 to 6 feet in front of the plate. It's possible that individual sluggers can use either tracking strategy and have the same batting average. More research is required to determine which strategy is best and whether batters should be taught to jump ahead of the ball.

This raises the question of whether there is any advantage to watching the ball as it crosses the plate. Certainly, there is no way the batter could use the visual information to correct his swing. The bat is already in motion, swinging at over 60 feet/second, potentially able to connect with the ball with a force of up to 1,500 pounds. In the milliseconds remaining before impact, it's impossible for his relatively sluggish nervous system to calculate the changes necessary in the bat's movement, transmit the signal to the relevant muscle groups, and initiate contraction of the muscle fibers—he's committed.

Bahill suggests that a batter who uses anticipatory saccades uses the information to discover the ball's actual trajectory, whether or not it is coincident with the position of his bat. In this way he is *learning* how to predict the location of different pitches as they cross the plate, programming his kinesthetic memory to enhance his performance in the future (see "Putting: Programming the Skill" in Chapter 8).

For batters who lose the ball in front of the plate, they are experiencing an effective "down time" of 60 to 70 milliseconds, a period during their swing time comparable to the time it takes the anticipatory batter to make his saccadic eye movement (40–50 milliseconds) and recover from the subsequent saccadic suppression (20 milliseconds). Regardless of visual strategy, both types of batters have already made the mental calculations, set their muscles in motion, and are operating with blind faith in their autopilot.

Or as Yogi Berra once confessed, "I can't think and hit at the same time."

THE BIOMECHANICS OF BATTING

"Hitting a baseball," the late Charlie Lau of the Chicago White Sox often said, "is supposed to be the most difficult thing to do in sports. But the real challenge is to hit the ball consistently, game after game."

Lau knew this from experience. Over his eleven major league seasons, mostly with the Baltimore Orioles, his batting average was only .255. As a catcher, however, Lau had an analytic eye that studied the batting techniques of countless sluggers who stood before him. He parlayed this experience into a career as one of the best and highest-paid batting coaches in professional baseball.

Without the aid of high-speed films and computers, Lau developed his own "absolute laws" of good hitting. His advice to batters included how to shift their body weight back in their stance to increase forward momentum during the swing; striding forward with the front foot's toe closed relative to the pitcher; keeping the head down to increase the chances of seeing the ball as it crossed the plate; and letting the lower bat hand dominate during the swing, so that the weaker arm pulled the bat around while the stronger arm controlled its position.

The biomechanical analysis of any athletic activity seldom starts from scratch. The legends, lore, anecdotes, and firsthand observations and experience of men like Charlie Lau are the starting point for any comprehensive study of sports. In baseball, for example, the claim that batting is the most difficult feat in any sport is a tempting challenge to investigate, but whether or not it's true, its analysis will usually yield new insights and techniques to enhance performance.

At Stanford University, physicist Paul Kirkpatrick was one of the first researchers to thoroughly study the problems of batting. He discovered that the state of a baseball bat is defined by thirteen independent variables, all subject to the batter's control. These are the three position coordinates of any point on the bat, three coordinates of angular orientation, three of linear momentum, three of angular momentum, and one time coordinate.

Of course, a batter can misjudge any of these variables by too much or too little, so that there are twenty-six separate ways to err. He also found that the margin of error in batting is small. In the time coordinate, a swing that starts about 3 milliseconds too early or too late results in a strike—even if all the other coordinates are correct. The coordinates in space are equally exacting; to connect a stick of white ash, 2.75 inches in diameter, with a cowhide sphere, 2.88 inches in diameter, requires coordination that must be accurate within about 0.8 inch. To make a fair hit, the batter has to meet the ball within 15 degrees of either side of the right angle between the pitch and the plate, which translates to a point somewhere along an arc of only 24 inches in a swinging bat.

The highly vaunted motor skills of a batter are augmented by the power a batter can develop in his swing. The rate and force of muscle contraction can make the difference between a home run and a pop-up to the second baseman. The power of a swing is fed to the bat by the coordinated torque of the shoulders, elbows, wrists, and also by the forward motion of the torso as the batter strides forward into the pitch. The surge of power actually starts at ground level and rises upward in fluent coordination, starting with the muscles in the legs and ending with the muscles in the arm.

The batter initiates his swing with a step forward. The purpose of this stride is to start moving the body weight forward *before* pulling the bat around toward the pitch. Studies have found that the timing of the stride is essential: if the forward foot has not lifted off the ground by the time the ball has left the pitcher's hand, the batter will miss the ball.

The direction of the stride has been the subject of some controversy. Some batting coaches believe sluggers should change the direction of their stride according to whether the ball is heading for the inside or outside of the strike zone; others advise batters to stride consistently into the same position for all pitches. Which is right? One study, based on the analysis of thousands of feet of film of hundreds of major league batters, found that the top sluggers—including Hank Aaron, Mickey Mantle, Willie Mays, Stan Musial, and Ted Williams—all placed their striding foot in the same spot, whereas poorer hitters were not consistent. Placement and length of stride (the optimal range is between 3 to 12 inches) is one of the most important biomechanical attributes of outstanding batters. Studies such as this highlight the important contribution biomechanical analysis can make to the science of coaching.

The successful application of overlapping torques from ground up can provide as much as 1,500 pounds of force to a bat in about 0.25 second, bringing the weapon across the plate at up to 100 feet/second. Upon impact the ball is crushed to half its regulation diameter, as the momentum of the bat is transferred to the ball. The ball recovers its original shape in little over 1 millisecond and begins its return flight at 130 feet/second or more. With the proper angle, a ball hit at 150 feet/second will usually clear the outfield fence.

It's somewhat surprising that the speed of a batted ball is not necessarily faster than a fastball. In fact, the fastest batted ball ever clocked with a radar gun was 179 feet/second (hit by Lee May of the Baltimore Orioles). One of the reasons a baseball doesn't fly off the bat at greater speed has to do with its sluggish return to its normal shape after it's crushed by the bat. The tendency of a body to regain its original shape once it has been deformed differs from one body to another, a property physicists call *elasticity*.

The most practical measure of elasticity is to drop an object onto a hard floor, measuring its speed before it hits and after it rebounds. If a ball rebounds at half of its preimpact velocity, physicists say it has a *coefficient of restitution* of 0.5. A perfectly elastic ball will have a rebound velocity identical to its preimpact velocity and thus its coefficient of restitution (COR) is 1.0. A baseball's COR is 0.53. By comparison, a basketball's is 0.76, a tennis ball's is 0.67, and a lacrosse ball's is 0.62. If baseballs were made with the same COR as a basketball, they would fly off the bat 23 percent faster.

The measure of elasticity in a ball, bat, racket, playing or running surface, even in safety equipment affects performance in all sports. If a designer can increase the COR in critical pieces of athletic equipment, speed and distance can be substantially increased. In baseball, there is good evidence that the elastic properties of the ball have been altered at various times during the history of the game, sometimes by the sport's authorities and sometimes by teams looking for an extra edge.

TAMPERING WITH THE ELASTICITY OF A BASEBALL

In July 1965, the Chicago White Sox were playing the Detroit Tigers at Cominskey Park in a bitterly contested five-game series in which both teams were in the running for the American League pennant. During the series, the White Sox charged that the Detroit team had illegally cooled the baseballs.

"All the balls were ice cold," said Hank Aguirre, the Tiger's pitcher. "Freeze a ball and it won't go anywhere."

Indeed, in the course of the series, both teams together made only 17 runs, without a single homer.

Al Lopez, manager of the White Sox, denied the charge and accused the Tigers of heating the balls in their 4-game series the previous weekend. During those games there were 53 runs, including a phenomenal 19 homers.

The charges were never substantiated, although one young amateur scientist, Dorel L. Baila, set up an experiment to see if heating or cooling a baseball would significantly affect its COR. To cool the balls he placed them in a household freezer for one hour; to heat them he used an oven at 225 degrees Fahrenheit for fifteen minutes. When he dropped the test balls onto a hard floor from a height of 60 inches, the heated balls bounced 19 inches, the cooled balls only 13 inches, representing a significant increase in the COR of the heated balls. If this increase in elasticity is extrapolated to a ball pitched at high speed, the results could account for the discrepancy in runs and homers in the two Sox-Tigers series of games.

Around 1920, the number of home runs hit in the major leagues increased dramatically and led to questions and accusations that material changes in regulation baseballs had produced a "lively ball." Although there is no scientific data comparing the COR of balls prior to 1920 with modern balls, the former period is referred to by pundits almost universally as "the dead ball era."

The *official* baseball is made of a composition-cork core, wrapped in two thin layers of rubber, surrounded by 363 feet of tightly wrapped blue-gray wool yarn, 135 feet of white wool yarn, 159 more feet of blue-gray yarn, 450 feet of fine cotton yarn (apparently any color), a coat of rubber cement, and the cowhide jacket, held together with 216 slightly raised red cotton stitches. In theory, altering any of these materials (except the color of the yarn) will change the COR of a baseball, and it could be done without detection because only the *surface* of balls are inspected before and during a game. Indeed, many knowledgeable baseball enthusiasts believe the materials in the ball have been changed many times, either unintentionally by manufacturers or intentionally at the request of the major league clubs. These charges are denied by both parties, who explain the increase in home runs in modern baseball as a result of bigger, stronger, and better-trained batters.

In recent years, investigators have measured the COR of balls produced in 1927, 1930, and 1961, and found that *the elasticity could vary by 20 percent.* The fact that the materials in balls have been changed over time, including recent years, has been substantiated by the ball surgery of suspicious players, like Tom Seaver, who early in his career started taking the jackets off baseballs and comparing their guts to official specifications. Changes were found in the lining of the cork center (some were hard plastic, others soft rubber), in the glue used to attach the cover to the cotton yarn, and in the methods of winding the yarn. It's too bad that balls from the dead era haven't been found so similar tests could be conducted to settle the dead-versus-lively-ball question once and for all. Surely, the Smithsonian must have one of these relics, which they could donate to the cause of sports science.

Long before Seaver's ball surgery and COR tests were conducted, Earnshaw Cook, an accomplished statistician and the first man to use computer analysis in baseball, believed that the only plausible explanation of the "lively ball era" was some kind of change in the ball's elasticity. In his classic book *Percentage Baseball*, he wrote, "Diagnosis of the home run syndrome requires a decision between improbable muscular dystrophy in the Ruthian era and the increased elasticity of the ball. . . . When impotent pitchers and bantam-weight infielders begin dunking the old apple into the bargain seats, something other than a new race of supermen is responsible for the plethora of round trip tickets to the plate."

All told there are six factors that affect the speed of a batted ball: the mass of the bat, the mass of the ball, the velocity of the bat, the velocity of the ball, angle of incidence (striking angle), and the ball's COR. In practical terms this means the greater the mass of the ball, the smaller its launch speed; the faster a ball is pitched, the faster it travels away from the bat. Similarly, the greater the speed and mass of the bat, the greater the speed of a batted ball.

A batter has no control over the mass or velocity of a ball, but he can select the size of his bat, which in turn will affect the speed at which he can swing. Heavier bats will transfer more momentum to the ball, but require more strength to swing; lighter bats can be swung faster, but transfer a fraction of the momentum of a larger bat. The tradeoff between mass and speed is tricky, prompting some sluggers to try all kinds of cunning machinations.

TAMPERING WITH A BAT'S MASS

The mass of a bat can be increased, regardless of the wood's inherent size and weight, through effective manipulation of the batter's muscles. Biomechanists have discovered that a bat, in the hands of a slugger, strikes a ball with a mass greater than if the bat was swinging freely on its own. This is the concept of *effective mass*, which treats the limbs of the body as rigid segments, each contributing additional mass to the weapon. Studies have found that effective mass can be increased in a bat by maintaining a very tight grip on the handle at impact.

The tighter the grip, the greater the effective mass of the bat. With strength training, the muscles in the lower arm can increase grip tightness, hence the speed and distance of a batted ball, regardless of any other factors. But don't run out and try this in golf or racket sports: until recently it was thought that the concept of effective mass applied to all sports using a ball and a hand-held weapon, but it's now known this is not true (see "Death Grip versus Light Touch" in Chapter 7).

In selecting the best bat, the two objectives of maximum mass and maximum swing velocity are mutually exclusive. So, given a choice, which is more effective, swinging a heavy bat at low speed or a light bat at high speed? Assuming for the sake of argument that a batter produces a fixed power output for every collision with the ball, it turns out that more momentum will be transferred to the ball if the available torques and forces are used to produce high speed rather than accelerate a large mass. In which case, calculations show that the ideal bat would weigh only 20 ounces. Regulations, however, state that bats must be made of solid wood, so our ideal weapon would be either too short or too thin for effective use. Consequently, players must compromise or resort to subterfuge.

There have been cases where players have been caught hollowing out the barrel of a bat and filling it with cork, thereby obtaining light weight with effective size. Unfortunately for these players, these doctored bats break easier than solid white ash, and when the cork filling starts to fly around the infield they are suspended without pay.

A legal fix in amateur baseball is provided by the aluminum bat, which is hollow and can be manufactured in a wider range of weights and lengths than the traditional wooden bat. From an economic point of view, aluminum bats do not break when they strike a fast ball, and despite their high initial purchase price are used almost exclusively by university and amateur leagues, where equipment budgets are limited.

Major league baseball prohibits aluminum bats because they would alter the complexity of the game, shifting the odds in favor of the batters, an idea that has been hotly disputed by the makers of metal bats, who claim baseballs rebound off aluminum and wooden bats at the same speed. At the University of Arizona, home of one of the best collegiate baseball teams in the West, engineers decided to investigate which party was right. Using a radar gun to compare the launch speeds of balls off both types of bats, they found that line drives from an aluminum bat were about 4 mph faster than those hit with a wooden bat—corresponding to a 10 percent increase in the distance the ball travels.

Statistically, there has been a phenomenal rise in batting averages and a drop in pitching effectiveness among university teams using aluminum bats, which should come as no surprise in light of the study at the University of Arizona. If major league clubs adopted metal bats, the time-honored records of baseball heros would be rapidly eroded, and there would be many confusing changes in both offensive and defensive strategies—especially if the faster balls were fielded on faster artificial playing surfaces, like Astroturf.

BASEBALL BY COMPUTER

Baseball is a game of odds and the whole point of the game, in one sense, is to beat the odds. This principle was first harnessed by Earnshaw Cook, the baseball mathematics pioneer. Cook set about his task by feeding 750,000 statistics from over 12,000 major league games into his data processor. Using the results and applying elementary probability theory, he claimed that any manager could add 270 runs to a normal season total. That's enough to disinter a dead club rotting in the cellar and resurrect it to the glory of the first division.

Cook advised managers to scrap the intentional walk and the sacrifice bunt; prohibit pitchers from batting for themselves without a comfortable lead; arrange the batting order in descending rank of batting average; platoon pitchers so the "starter" delivers the middle five innings, with relievers opening and closing the game. Although Cook's statistics were scientifically sound, they ran contrary to decades of established opinion of how a ball club should be run. At the time his work was published, managers were disposed to propel a wet gob of chewing tobacco toward the shoes of anyone with the temerity to invoke Cook's theories. He was twenty years ahead of his time.

Certainly, baseball is an enterprise steeped in conservative traditions, and one of those traditions is extensive record keeping and the divining of statistical probabilities. It is therefore somewhat surprising that clubs were not quicker to adopt the very tool that could help the most—the computer. Although some managers—Steve Boros of the Oakland A's, for example—have made extensive use of computers to select the best lineup of batters for every game, Yankees manager Billy Martin has often insisted he doesn't need one. "It's all up here," he told one reporter, tapping his cranium.

Computers are presently making the transition from being simply electronic actuaries to being active baseball coaches, and this fact undoubtedly accounts for some of the resistance. Today, a California software company, Pacific Select Corporation, has a computer program called EDGE 1.000, which dispenses visual coaching advice for batters with the aid of computer-generated color graphics. Sluggers can review their own performance at the plate, studying the hit zone, which is displayed on the computer screen as a nine-cell grid, and watch as the trajectory of any pitch comes to the plate. They are also able to see when and where they are swinging in relation to the pitch. The ideal position at which they should connect with the ball, the "honey spot" (not to be confused with the physical "sweet spot" on a sports weapon), is displayed as a red dot; teaser zones are displayed with blue shading. By reviewing a long record of their hitting performance, batters can use this program to see if they have mastered one pitcher's fast ball, but have, say, consistently swung too late on the curve ball. According to one batting coach, the computer is presenting readily digested feedback, which players tend to understand as well as believe more than the verbal critiques from the staff—and it eliminates the ego problem.

In the next few years, the marriage of computers to video will turn conventional batting practice on its head. Donald S. Tieg of the Connecticut-based Institute for Sports Vision is working on a revolutionary system that will project a three-dimensional holographic image within screens, which a batter will face and watch major league pitchers throw their best balls. The sluggers will hold an electronic bat of the same size and weight they ordinarily use, which will be covered with a light-sensitive chemical that registers a hit when the bat intersects an invisible laser beam projected from the rear screen. A computer coordinates the position of the laser beam with the 3-D holo-graph of the projected ball. The system will accept ordinary videotape recordings of any pitcher; a second computer will translate the video image into a program to control the 3-D projection.

This system will enable batters to practice against pitchers they've never met before a big game, or improve their perfor-mance against old opponents. Ultimately, Sports Vision will provide a display of ball trajectory and placement to be re-viewed after an "electronic hit" or, in the case of a strike, to show what went wrong.

The science of baseball computing has come a long way since Earnshaw Cook and has lent new meaning to Casey Stengel's old adage "You can look it up." But Stengel was never a man to be awed by statistics and was famous for doubting whatever they implied.

Baseball managers and coaches have no need to fear com-puters and will embrace them as useful tools as soon as it be-comes apparent that computer technology is light-years away from building a machine or writing a program with the cun-ning and intuition presently possessed by the human biocom-puter. As long as baseball is played by human beings, there will be a need for flesh-and-blood management.

Besides, computers will never be able to spit tobacco juice.

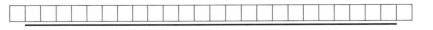

SEVEN

TENNIS

The Pursuit of the Sweet Spot

For a champion he has a peculiar list of attributes: he's sometimes shy, possibly makes more money than any American athlete in history, claims "I've never spent more than a couple hours a day practicing in my life," and seldom smiles. Scientists say, "biomechanically he's so perfect it looks like magic." Considered a mad genius, John McEnroe is perhaps best known for his loud service grunts and, of course, his theatrical temper tantrums.

He's certainly a very audible player, but does any of the noise help his game? Is his grunt service more deadly than his silent service, or is it just a ploy to psyche out the opposition? Does verbal intimidation of the officials produce favorable or more accurate calls?

Linesman means nemesis to McEnroe. It usually starts with, "Wait just a minute, that ball was out by a mile! Are you blind? Are you crazy!" Imagine if you were yelled at like that in front of millions of TV viewers. There has to be some internal urge to fight or flight, and the emotional arousal should have some impact on judging performance.

Presumably linesmen do make mistakes. Low pay, long hours, fatigue, and eye strain can't help. The competence of linesmen and other officials is also challenged on the grounds that no tests are administered (other than 20/20 vision) to determine the ability of these officials to track a ball moving at up to 140 mph, landing on or near a 2-inch line for only 3 milliseconds, and then caroming off in another direction. For his part, McEnroe is convinced tennis officials have visual deficiencies: "I have zero percent doubt that I see balls better than they do."

THE VISUAL ACCURACY OF TENNIS OFFICIALS

To settle the dispute of whose eyes are better, the U.S. Tennis Association subsidized a study to determine exactly what players and officials can and cannot see. Headed by Gideon Ariel, the biomechanist who invented the computerized exercise machine, the subjects were eight experienced officials, twelve teaching pros, and one man who had no experience with calling balls or the rules of the game. Ariel organized the study so that on-court subjects could record where they thought balls landed in games they played against an opponent who also recorded where he thought the ball landed, shot by shot. Off-court subjects called the shots from seats overlooking the game at twenty different angles and distances. Some subjects were positioned in the traditional judge's seat and at the lines. At the conclusion of the experiment, Ariel combined all the estimates and compared them to actual ball positions as recorded by high-speed film.

It turned out that accurately placing the position of the ball was more difficult than anyone expected. The least accurate observations were made by the *players*, who admitted that almost 40 percent of the time their calls were only guesswork. Players returning a high-speed serve were found to misjudge a call by up to 3 feet. Moreover, those pros who forced themselves to track the ball while they were playing made less accurate strokes, implying that a player can't watch the lines and play a good game at the same time.

Observers in the traditional umpire's chair missed only *half as many* calls as players. Subjects seated around the court, in many of the same positions normally occupied by spectators, scored as well as the umpire, unless the ball approached from angles outside their line of sight.

The most surprising result of the study showed that the unblinking television camera had the same problems of perspective as the human observer. The court would have to be covered from every angle to obtain accuracy on TV, and even then the standard commercial equipment is not able to slow the ball's

flight enough to pinpoint the location of impact during re-
plays.

The real shocker, at least for the usual protesters, was that
the subjects who did the very best were standing in the normal
linesman's position—including the man who had never made
a call before in his life. The linesmen missed only 50 percent
as many calls as the umpire and 25 percent as many as the
players.

Of course, this study was not conducted in the pressure-
cooker conditions that accompany a real game, especially a
championship match, where many types of stress could impair
linesmen's accuracy.

The question of whether an observer's powers of visual dis-
crimination could be affected by the behavior of aggressive
players wasn't addressed until 1983. Richard H. Cox, a psychologist at Kansas State University, found that it could. Using
66 university physical education students, Cox conducted his
study with a series of 128 slides depicting tennis balls landing
in or out of bounds, flashed on the screen at 8-second intervals. Thirty-two of the slides were shown four times each to
check the consistency of the calls. The results were interesting.
Compared to their ability to judge balls without any feedback
from observers, scores deteriorated when the novice judges were
told they had made a bad call, and became worse if they received an electric shock for bad calls. Cox found that under
"nonabuse" conditions, his judges could give different responses to the same pictures on separate occasions. Because
this study was not conducted in a live environment as Ariel's
was, it's difficult to project what the real-life results would be,
but the findings do confirm the suspicion that negative feedback from players can impair judgment in game officials.

Cox's study suggests that McEnroe's outbursts, whether or
not they are intentionally orchestrated to throw his opponent
off tempo, adversely affect decisions that concern his own shots.
He might be better off if he saved his venom until after the match.
Moreover, McEnroe watchers say he loses more games when
he has a tantrum, and not just because of bad calls.

What about McEnroe's controversial grunts?

In 1983, as a third of a million people consumed 10 tons of
strawberries and drank 17,000 bottles of champagne at Wim-

bledon, Dennis Lendrem, an animal behaviorist from the University of Nottingham, studied McEnroe as he grunted his way to the men's singles title. On his way to the finals, McEnroe's grunts were recorded by Lendrem when he faced Sandy Mayer, Ivan Lendl, and Curtis Lewis of New Zealand. Against these three, McEnroe logged about 300 serves and grunted audibly on more than two-thirds of them. Sandy Mayer received grunts with 82 percent of McEnroe's serves, Lendl got 65 percent, and Lewis 67 percent.

Lendrem first looked at McEnroe's grunts to see if they were a sign of exertion, reflecting possibly a more powerful serve than those delivered in silence. He did this by comparing grunts on first services, which are usually more powerful, to those on second serves, which tend to be safe shots, expecting to find a higher proportion of grunting in the first. It turned out there was no difference. Similar comparisons of grunt versus silent serves soon eliminated any link between grunting and exertion.

Did McEnroe's grunts accompany good serves, regardless of cause? Lendrem found that the silent serves were almost twice as successful as grunt serves. Moreover, grunt serves were usually followed by a protracted struggle, whereas silent serves were followed by short rallies in which McEnroe quickly dispatched his opponent's return. In fact, it turned out that his grunt service was consistently less accurate, resulting in more faults, lets, and net faults than the silent variety. The topper is McEnroe served almost twice as many silent aces as grunt aces.

On the basis of these studies it would seem that noise in McEnroe's game, from simple grunts to tempestuous tirades, adversely affects his performance.

How can he possibly be number one in men's tennis and do so many things wrong? His practice hours are minimal, his slight build suggests he shuns extensive strength training, and in one respect, his motivation appears low for a world-class competitor. He recently told a reporter from *Sports Illustrated*, "I don't love the game as much as I should."

In tennis, the extreme contrast to McEnroe is Martina Navratilova, who is wholly dedicated to the game and faithfully follows a highly structured training program—in fact, it's been said she is virtually plugged into a computer. For every opponent, she works with her coach and a computer to figure out a game strategy. She has a special reflex trainer who gives her special drills to improve reaction time.

Navratilova's diet system, which was designed by Miami nutritionist Robert Haas, has received a great deal of attention. Haas takes small samples of Navratilova's blood and uses a computer to organize her daily menu, integrating her diet with some of her strength and endurance training schedules. Couriers occasionally fly thousands of miles to bring specially prepared foods to her hotel room in locked briefcases.

Haas explained to a sportswriter, "Martina suddenly wanted to do this diet and exercise program 100 percent every minute of her existence."

Navratilova and McEnroe are light-years away from each other in their attitudes toward tennis and in their styles of training, yet both will probably remain at the top of the field, or close to it, in the near future. And this makes it very tempting to imagine how they would both fare if they swapped roles at this point in their careers. Could Navratilova make it without the high-tech training? Could McEnroe still play without grunts and tantrums?

Perhaps a more fundamental question is how much does training and technology affect world-class players—and how much of their game is really an extension of their personality and stylized behavior?

A role reversal between the two stars is, of course, out of the question. Both are locked into their own styles. In fact, when McEnroe was asked recently whether he'd like to try the Haas diet, he replied, "I prefer the Häagen-Dazs diet."

DESIGNING A PERFECT TENNIS RACKET

When Howard Head, the inventor of the first successful metal skis, sold his stock in the Head Ski Company in 1969, he planned to retire with his fortune and enjoy the good life, indulging in leisurely activities such as tennis.

As a novice, Head had a hard time learning the game, especially because the racket had an annoying tendency to twist in his hands when the ball struck the face off center. As his patience came to an end, so did his retirement.

In 1972, back at his drawing board, Head began to think of ways to reduce the disturbing torque produced by off-center hits. Scrapping all preconceptions of a racket, he looked at the weapon purely in terms of collision mechanics. Unlike a baseball bat, the large face of a racket provided more margin for error when meeting the ball, but if the collision occurred at a location other than along the vertical axis running from the handle to the tip of the frame, the racket would twist and the return would be soft and wayward. In principle, Head knew that this type of angular acceleration could be reduced by increasing the rotational inertia. This was fundamental physics: a body at rest tended to stay at rest, and the greater the mass the more the racket would resist motions imposed on it by the ball. At first he tried to increase the inertia by adding weights to the rim of the racket. Not only was this particular design ineffective in reducing torque, but the racket broke when he hit a fast ball. (Years later, the Wilson company perfected this idea by adding tungsten weights to a durable frame's perimeter.)

After stewing over the problem some more, Head woke up in the middle of the night with the solution: he could effectively move mass away from the racket's center by making the head and face larger. So it came to pass that he designed a 10.5-inch-wide racket, 2 inches wider than the conventional racket, and gained a 50 percent advantage in the moment of inertia. To prevent the wider racket from being too top heavy, he also enlarged the frame longitudinally, bringing the string area down about 3 inches closer to the handle. The larger prototype was legal, as both U.S. and international tennis authorities placed no restrictions on the weight, size, shape, or materials used in a racket.

In tests, however, the old problem soon emerged again. The wooden frame could not support collisions on the larger face without cracking or collapsing. Adding more wood only made the racket too heavy. In the end the answer was to use an extruded aluminum alloy for the frame, which was stronger and lighter than laminated hardwood.

In setting out merely to reduce the torque resulting from off-center collisions, Head accidentally realized a tremendous bonus. By elongating the face toward the handle, the center of the racket also coincided with the *center of percussion*. This is the point on any bat or racket where the energy of the swing is most efficiently transferred to the ball because it produces no reaction—or painful jar—at the pivot point in the handle. This is well known, especially to baseball players. A ball striking near the tip of the bat or near the throat of the bat sends a dreadful shock to the hands grasping the pivot point. A ball hit at a point far from the center of percussion will not travel as far, but an impact at the center of percussion maximizes the momentum transferred to a ball in tennis or baseball, and feels effortless.

On a conventional racket there was no perfect place to hit the ball, as the center of percussion was about 2 inches below the center of the face. With the hand in the normal position, hitting the ball on the low center of percussion felt good, but accuracy was sacrificed.

Although the new racket had the same overall length and balance, the 20 percent increase in string area more than doubled the center of percussion, known to some people as the *sweet spot.* Thus Head's invention provided accuracy and power, as well as "more forgiveness" on the errors of novices.

Head did not appreciate what he had done until he took the prototype to a sports lab, clamped it to a stationary vise, and shot tennis balls at it. He compared the results with balls rebounding off a conventional racket using high-speed films. At speeds of 38.5 mph he discovered that the maximum coefficient of restitution (COR) for the new design was 0.67, compared to the standard maximum of 0.57 (see "Tampering with Elasticity" in Chapter 6).

Excited by the prospects, Head and Princeton University physicist Kenneth Wright started mapping the surface areas that produced the maximum COR on both rackets and discovered the phenomenal difference *(see Fig. 7.1).* He subsequently patented his invention and granted production rights to the Prince Manufacturing Company in New Jersey, a long-time maker of ball machines used in tennis schools. The oversize Prince racket has since enjoyed a reputation for having the largest sweet spot of any known racket and today captures about 25 percent of the market.

Subjectively, every player knows the location of the sweet spot as the area where collisions feel smooth and effortless. Objec-

FIGURE 7.1

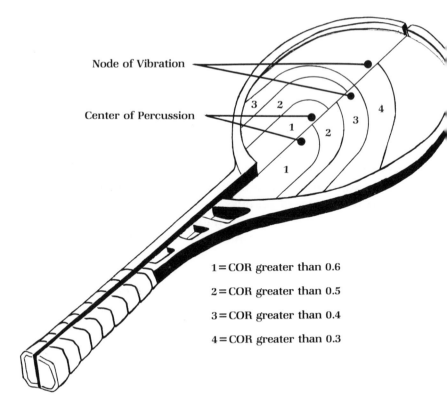

Node of Vibration

Center of Percussion

1 = COR greater than 0.6

2 = COR greater than 0.5

3 = COR greater than 0.4

4 = COR greater than 0.3

Which is the real sweet spot? When Howard Head designed a larger racket to reduce the twisting effect produced by off-center hits, he accidentally created a racket that put the center of percussion, the node of vibration, and the areas of highest COR nearer to the center than existed on the conventional racket. No one can agree on which of these three points is the true sweet spot, but a ball struck on any of them certainly feels like the real thing.

tively, the location and definition of the sweet spot is much more elusive. At the University of Pennsylvania, physicist and tennis player Howard Brody believes he has found *three* sweet spots on a racket, or at least three definitions of the sweet spot. In the advertisements and patent for the Prince racket, Howard Head defined the sweet spot as those areas of maximum COR observed when a racket is clamped to a vise. A second definition, used by many physicists, has the sweet spot at the center of percussion. A third definition claims the sweet spot is a vibrational dead zone where, after the ball strikes, the resulting higher-frequency vibrations are at an absolute minimum. All three of these factors, regardless of which is called the sweet spot, are essential ingredients in the future design of the perfect tennis racket.

Hitting the ball on the dead zone, or *nodes of vibration*, is considered very desirable by good tennis players because impacts outside this area lead to vibrations, which cause a loss of ball control, an increase in arm fatigue, and an unpleasant feeling. Nodes are detected in the laboratory with accelerometers and oscilloscopes, but out on the court the human hand, a very sensitive detector of vibrations, is an adequate substitute to find the location and size of the nodes on various rackets. By holding the racket face up, parallel to the ground, and dropping a ball from a height of about 8 inches onto different locations, the area of least vibration can be detected. Marking or painting this area and trying to align service balls and returns with it may lead to improved control and comfort.

The elasticity of any structure, from baseballs to skyscrapers, is its inherent ability to recover its normal shape after being deformed. The strings of a tennis racket have a tendency to whiplash during the recovery of their original shape after being struck by a ball. This occurs in most elastic materials, the to-and-fro vibrations, like that of a pendulum, displaying a "periodic time," which is unique to every material. The frequency of vibration is the number of complete to-and-fro movements, or cycles, the strings make per second (measured in units of hertz, where 1 cycle/second equals 1 hertz). The fundamental mode of vibration in a tennis racket is between 25 and 40 hertz.

The elastic properties of a tennis racket produce some very interesting results at the moment of impact with a ball. As soon as ball and strings meet, some of the impact force is absorbed by the deformation of the ball, which flattens almost completely. The remaining energy is absorbed by the deformation of the strings, which move away from the ball like a trampoline and actually cause the frame of the racket to bend slightly in the direction of the ball. It's the action of the ball and racket snapping back to their original shape, releasing the stored energy of deformation, that gives the ball its initial 150-mph ve-

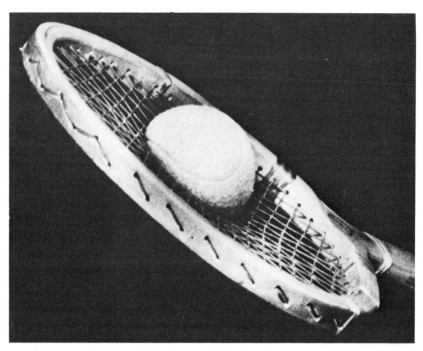

The elastic properties of a tennis racket produce some very interesting results at the moment of impact with a ball. As soon as ball and strings meet, some of the impact force is absorbed by the deformation of the ball, which flattens almost completely. The remaining energy is absorbed by the deformation of the strings, which move away from the ball like a trampoline and actually cause the frame of the racket to bend slightly around the ball. It's the action of the ball and strings snapping back to their original shape, releasing the stored energy of elastic deformation in milliseconds, that gives the ball its initial 150-mph velocity, re-corded in the service of top players. (Courtesy of Harold Edgarton/Science Photo Library.)

locity, recorded in the service of top players. Without these elastic properties—imagine a ball with the consistency of a light, fluffy sponge—the ball wouldn't make it to the net, no matter how fast the racket is swung.

Since the amount of time the ball and strings remain in contact during the collision is only 4 to 5 milliseconds, there is nothing further a player can do to affect the flight of the ball while it is sitting on the racket. Some tennis coaches tell students to impart spin or make trajectory changes during impact, but this is quite impossible. Not only can the human body not recruit motor units and make muscle contractions within this short period of time, but studies have found that the launch speed and trajectory of the ball are determined *entirely* by the angle and force of the strings as they recover from elastic deformation—as if the player did not exist.

THE ELASTIC PROPERTIES OF THE RACKET

String tension is a matter of some debate among players. It is often said that increasing the tension will produce a higher ball velocity, but some players swear they obtain faster balls with low string tension, even though this sounds crazy.

According to Howard Brody, string tension in any racket affects the length of time the ball remains in contact with the strings and the velocity at which it rebounds. In a simpler world, the COR of a tennis ball would remain constant under all conditions. Brody has discovered, however, that the COR of a tennis ball *decreases* as the impact velocity increases; similarly, the COR *decreases* as surface stiffness increases, so that about half of the kinetic energy of a moving ball is lost when it strikes clay or asphalt. The racket strings, on the other hand, lose relatively little energy when they are deformed.

Brody juggled these factors and discovered that if strings can be made to absorb more of the impact energy, the ball will deform less and lose less energy, receiving more rebound energy from the strings, and fly off at a higher speed. The only way to get strings to absorb more energy is to make them *looser*. The more the strings are allowed to deform, the more elastic energy they will return to the ball. In the available range of 35 to 75 pounds of tension, less is more—up to a point. Brody suggests that this lower limit is the point where the strings begin to trampoline sideways, parallel to the face of the racket. As elasticity is also affected by string length, string gauge, spacing of the strings, and the size of the head, players will have to experiment with lowering string tension on each racket they own, progressively decreasing tension until ball velocity peaks.

The strings of a racket are able to transfer their elastic energy to the ball because they spring back into shape before the ball has left the racket under its own speed. However, this does not apply to the relatively sluggish recoil of the racket frame, which recovers its original shape about 15 milliseconds after the ball has gone. Because the frame plays no direct role in the velocity or angle imparted to the ball, impact energy is wasted if it is absorbed by the deformation of the frame. By making frames stiffer, they deform less. This principle has led designers to hunt for new materials that are strong, stiff, and lightweight.

There is evidence that wooden paddles with a striking surface strung with sheep's gut were used in court tennis in the sixteenth century, and materials of very similar composition were used in the first lawn tennis tournament at Wimbledon in 1877. As the game became more vigorous, wood lamination was introduced in the 1920s, and from that point until the 1960s racket technology remained at a standstill. The first of the stiffer frames came in 1967, with the introduction of the steel tube design, followed by Head's aluminum frame. The mid-1970s brought graphite and fiberglass frames, and recently, boron frames.

Boron is six times as stiff as steel and five times stronger than aluminum. Unfortunately, boron does not exist independent of other elements in nature, and the extraction and conversion to a useful metal is an expensive process, resulting in a cost of about $250 per pound, five times the price of graphite. Accordingly, boron rackets retail at over $400. This metal, which can withstand stress up to 40 million pounds per square inch, reduces frame distortion better than any other known substance. Frames of the future may be made of ceramic fibers (a blend of silicon, boron, and aluminum in an epoxy matrix) or super-reinforced fiberglass.

With millions of dollars at stake, the major sports manufacturers are in hot pursuit of the perfect racket, blending the physics of the game with materials science. In theory, the ultimate hybrid would be designed so that the center of percussion, maximum COR, and vibrational node all overlap and cover the largest possible area coincident with the center of the racket—possibly spread over the entire face. The racket frame would be almost totally inelastic. Impact vibrations would be absorbed by foam and other fillers in the frame's hollow core;

further damping could be achieved with a third or fourth prong leading from the frame to the handle. The final shape may not be round or oval, the face may not be entirely flat.

When Howard Head came up with a new prototype, he carried it out to the court and played with it until it broke. Field testing of new equipment will always accompany research and development, but the preliminary testing of prototypes can now be done by computer. A design technique known as *finite element analysis*, borrowed from old-fashioned finite graphs in mathematics, takes a new design idea, breaks the components down into many finite, or limited, line segments and angles, and displays the new racket on the computer screen. Strength, stiffness, and other factors have already been programmed, so various stresses can be applied to the design by the computer operator, and the machine calculates the impact of these forces on structural elements of the racket. If the design proves to be faulty, the prototype "breaks" on the screen, saving considerable time and energy in physical testing. When the physics of researchers such as Howard Brody are added to the program, structural elements can be rearranged on the computer screen to determine how various materials and designs affect ball velocity.

Since the governing authorities of tennis place few restrictions on the shape, size (a racket may be as large as a player can wield), or construction of a racket, designers have a free hand to pursue the perfect model as long as they don't adversely affect the flight of the ball. This restriction is very new, resulting from the introduction of the so-called spaghetti racket a few years ago by a German inventor. The frame of this racket did not differ from conventional models, but the face was equipped with double strings and elaborate tubes woven between the strings. The strange-looking racket was able to produce so much spin on the ball that it was almost impossible to return. In one sense the racket was too successful. When Ilie Nastase used a spaghetti racket against Guillermo Vilas, the Argentinian stormed off the court in frustration, and the ensuing furor led to a hasty ruling by the International Tennis Federation prohibiting any attachments on a racket that altered the ball's flight.

DEATH GRIP VERSUS LIGHT TOUCH

When the game of lawn tennis was institutionalized at Wimbledon over a century ago, there was no right way to hold the racket. You just picked up the weapon and that was your grip. Modern players not only have to choose from a baffling array of racket designs, but must also decide which grip to use—Eastern, Continental, Western, or variations thereof (*see Fig. 7.2*). Now the confusion has multiplied with conflicting reports on grip firmness.

In baseball, a power hitter grips the bat as if he wants to strangle it. The purpose of a viselike grip on a bat is to increase the weapon's *effective mass* by making it an extension of the human body. For years the same principle was thought to apply to the tennis racket, and players were advised to grip the handle tightly on impact with the ball. Some top players, however, found that a tight grip was uncomfortable and that they could obtain more control of their stroke with a light touch.

Although such hard-hitting pros as Vitas Gerulaitis and Brian Gottfried squeeze the racket or "lock through the stroke," the biggest revolution in the game today is the soft or flexible wrist with a light, loose grip. Watch John McEnroe. He holds the racket like a toothpick; his fingers are hardly touching the handle. As a result he has essentially one grip for all strokes and he enjoys more control than Gottfried or Gerulaitis. Ivan Lendl and Ilie Nastase have light grips, flexible wrists, more control, and as much power as the wrist lockers.

The acceptance of a new grip, like the adoption of many techniques, hinges on the greatness of the champion who uses it. When Chris Evert, at the tender age of fifteen, beat Margaret Court, countless novices adopted the two-handed backhand (particularly because it's beneficial for young or weak-gripped players). Similarly, the Western grip was shunned until Bill Johnson used it to lick Bill Tilden and win the U.S. Nationals in 1915 and 1919. Now the light touch is rapidly becoming popular, but more than champion endorsement and anecdotal evidence is required to establish the efficacy of a new sports technique.

At the University of Iowa, biomechanist John A. W. Baker conducted an experiment that, at first, seemed impossible to

FIGURE 7.2

Eastern   Western   Continental

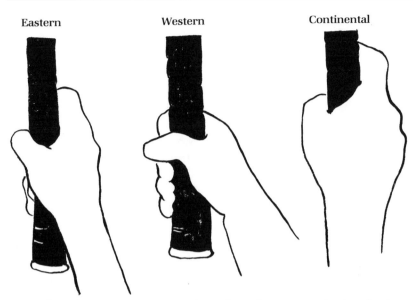

Three basic grips on a tennis racket. The Eastern forehand grip provides a fuller, freer swing, generating more power; it also allows a ball to be hit with more top spin. The Western grip is ideal for the backhand, which provides a lot of top spin, but it's difficult to hit low balls. The Continental grip is ideal for both forehand and backhand, and thus is known for its great versatility, but there is a loss of power, since the ball is met at the player's side instead of front, and there is considerably less top spin than with the other two grips.

believe. The purpose of his research was to compare the rebound velocity of a tennis ball when it struck a tightly clamped and a freestanding tennis racket. Using multiple stroboscopic photographs of the ball approaching, impacting, and rebounding from both rackets, he found that the effect on the ball was *practically identical* under these two extremes of "grip firmness." Fairly accurate measurements can be made with strobe photography: by setting the strobe light to flash at precise intervals with an electronic timer, the ball's velocity before and after impact can be computed by measuring the distance it has traveled between flashes. Baker's photographic findings were remarkable because they showed that, contrary to all expectations, a racket standing unsupported on the butt of its handle could return a ball at the same speed as a clamped racket.

Although the photographs were conclusive evidence that grip firmness and effective mass of a tennis racket played no role in the rebound of a tennis ball, the physics were hard to explain. After the ball hit Barker's freestanding racket, the racket fell over, so some of the ball's momentum was obviously transferred to the racket. The lost energy, however, should have been reflected in a slower rebound. Had there been a violation of the basic laws of physics?

Intrigued by Baker's experiment, Y. King Liu, a materials engineer at the University of Iowa, used mathematical models to quantify the physical forces involved during the impact of ball and racket, reasoning that numbers do not lie. He obtained data for the mass and velocity of the ball, the mass, dimensions, and moment of inertia of the racket, the duration of impact, and the COR between the ball and strings. He mixed these factors together and arrived at a very satisfactory explanation.

The key ingredient in Liu's calculation was the impact time. Since the ball remained in contact with the strings for only 4 milliseconds—during which the elastic materials in each deformed and sprang back to their original shape—the relatively ponderous 15-millisecond deformation of the stiff frame precluded any involvement of frame with the ball. The dramatic difference in elasticity between the frame and the strings allows them to act as if they were two independent systems, at least during the fleeting impact time. If the frame does not contribute rebound energy to the ball, neither does a player, regardless of his grip.

There had been no violation of physics. The energy that eventually toppled the freestanding racket was imparted equally to the clamped racket, which reacted by vibrating. The toppling or displacement of the freestanding racket does not begin while the ball is on the strings due to the rapid exchange of energy between ball and strings, which is over before the shock wave can effectively move the whole racket.

Years before Baker and Liu tortured the problem of grip firmness, tennis star Bill Tilden wrote, "The greatest tennis motto I know is 'Let your racket head do your work.' Just swing your racket head through the ball at the place you want it to go."

The soft-touch grip technique does just that—it lets the racket do all the work, as long as the player can connect it with the ball.

TENNIS ELBOW

In 1968, Robert Nirschl, an avid tennis player, developed a sharp pain in his elbow, which flared up usually when the joint was moving or bearing the weight of an external load, like a tennis racket. When he sought medical attention, physicians advised him to quit tennis or have surgery. Reluctant to do either, Nirschl began reading through the available research on tennis elbow. Although the ailment had been known as a clinical entity since the first tournament at Wimbledon, he discovered that little was known about what provoked the pain, and the treatments all appeared to suppress symptoms without removing the cause of the affliction. After physicians injected cortisone into the elbow, the pharmaceutical fix would remove the pain, the patient would resume tennis, and return with the same problem months later.

Today, as medical director of the Virginia Sportsmedicine & Rehabilitation Institute in Arlington, Nirschl has treated over 3,500 cases of tennis elbow. His diligent research has led to methods of treatment that do not require surgery, except in rare cases. It's ironic that he has spared thousands of patients from the knife even though he is an orthopedic surgeon by training. But this hasn't ruined business. Recognized internationally as an authority on tennis elbow, Nirschl is in constant demand as a consultant and lecturer, and still maintains a heavy caseload. Tennis players of all calibers are interested in Nirschl because the main thrust of his work is based on the *prevention* of the disorder through proper tennis technique.

The high interest in tennis elbow reflects its prevalence. One study found the disorder occurred in 2 percent of the general population, ages thirty-four to seventy-four, which is high for a noninfectious disease. The incidence among tennis players, however, is truly staggering. According to a survey conducted by James A. Priest, associate director of the Institute for Athletic Medicine at the University of Minnesota, 31 percent of 2,600 players at a tennis college in California developed tennis elbow at some time during their career. And contrary to expectation, the pain isn't confined to novices: Nirschl has estimated that between 20 and 30 percent of pros have or will experience tennis elbow.

One reason for this may be that the overriding factor in the development of the disorder appears to be the frequency of play. Priest's data show that 45 percent of those who played daily acquired symptoms, compared to only 7 percent of those who played two to three times a month.

Like headache, the term "tennis elbow" has been used loosely to describe the discomfort associated with a wide range of specific orthopedic maladies from pinched nerves to arthritis, but Nirschl prefers to translate the term as *tendonitis*—an inflammation of the tendons that run over the bulbous stump of the humerus bone (the lateral or medial epicondyles in *Fig. 7.3*). The inflammation results when mechanical forces on the arm converge at the stump of the humerus, stretch the adjacent tendons beyond their usual limit, and produce microtears. Tendons can adapt to moderate overloads incurred in training or exercise, but sudden and repeated overloads outstrip the reparative processes with an accumulation of microtears, and the new replacement tissues are defective, slow to heal, and painful.

The magnitude of the mechanical forces that traumatize the tendons at the elbow can be appreciated by considering the kinetics of the racket arm during a serve. The sequence of arm movements is almost identical to those in a baseball pitch: the arm is rotated around the shoulder in a wide circle to obtain maximum velocity before the racket strikes the ball, which is met above and in front of the head. Peak racket velocities before striking the ball have been measured between 300 and 350 mph. On impact, however, much of the kinetic energy of the swing is absorbed in the elastic deformation of ball and racket, and the weapon is abruptly slowed to 150 mph. The tremendous forearm momentum built up in the swing tends to keep the arm moving while the racket's velocity has been cut in half within only a few milliseconds. The racket hand is prevented from ripping right off at the wrist by the eccentric contraction of the muscles of the forearm, which are connected to the humerus above the elbow by firmly anchored tendons. As the

FIGURE 7.3

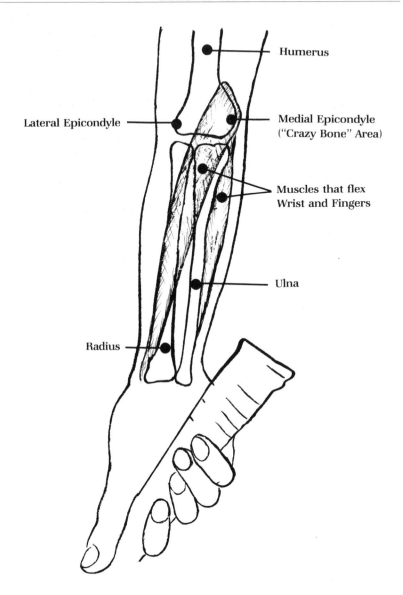

Anatomy of the elbow. Tennis elbow is thought to occur when the lateral and medial epicondyles (the tendons that run over the bulbous stump of the humerus) sustain microtears from stretching overloads. With repeated overloads the tissue healing is impaired and tendonitis results, causing pain and reducing the range of motion.

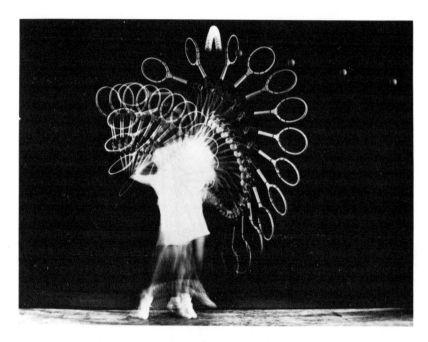

In a tennis serve, peak racket velocities have been measured before impact between 300 and 350 mph. On impact, much of the kinetic energy is absorbed by the elastic deformation of ball and racket, slowing the weapon suddenly to 150 mph. The strain of the sudden deceleration has been linked to some cases of tennis elbow. (Courtesy of Harold Edgerton/Science Photo Library.)

muscles can stretch much more than their connective tissue, microscopic tears are produced in the tendons.

While the hard service causes medial tennis elbow (tendon damage on the "crazy-bone" side of the elbow) frequently in pros, lateral damage (on the "thumb side" of the elbow in *Fig. 7.3*) is five times more common and is associated with backhand returns in novice and average players. This observation is supported by a biomechanical study of the backhand by Arthur M. Bernhang, a professor of orthopedics at Stony Brook Medical Center in New York. By wiring rackets and players with strain gauges and EMG leads and correlating these signals to their actual movements recorded by high-speed photography, Bernhang identified a specific backhand technique that produced the crippling forces in the arm.

In good players, including local club champions and one world-class player, the backswing just prior to hitting the ball

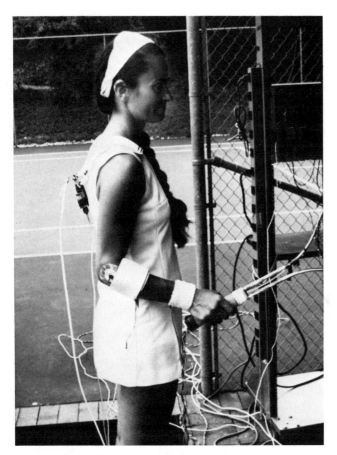

A "wired" tennis player who participated in orthopedic sur-geon Arthur M. Bernhang's investigation of the causes of tennis elbow. Disposable leads at the player's elbow are sensitive enough to pick up electrical activity of the muscles beneath the skin. These EMG signals are relayed via a free-hanging cord to an oscillo-scope and chart recorder on the sidelines. Measurements of the pressure a player exerts on the handle are made with a fluid-filled plastic tube wrapped around the handle and connected to a pres-sure transducer from an F-14 jet fighter. (Courtesy of A. M. Bern-hang, M.D.)

was characterized by the racket shoulder dropping, the arm remaining straight, and *the tip of the elbow pointing toward the ground.* Players with a history of tennis elbow consistently dis-played a different technique, which Bernhang calls "the lead-ing elbow." In this condition, the racket shoulder is raised, the

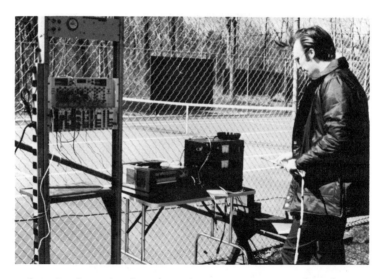

The wired tennis player's actions are transmitted to the portable EMG computer shown up on the rack at the left, which drives a high-frequency galvonometer mounted in a CEC oscilloscope recorder, shown on the table. Bernhang discovered that the backhand delivered with a "leading elbow" is a major cause of one form of tennis elbow. (Courtesy of A. M. Bernhang, M.D.)

forearm slightly flexed, and *the tip of the elbow is pointing at the net.*[1]

Where the power for the backhand stroke in good players was supplied by the lateral shift of body weight and the shoulder muscles, power in afflicted players was supplied by abduction, a pulling away, at the shoulder in concert with a partial straightening of the arm. Not only does the "leading elbow" technique produce less power, its pulling effect on the arm (through the abduction of the raised shoulder) occurs during impact, so that the tendons at the elbow are stretched in opposite directions at the same time.

Bernhang's study is a good example of the relationship between injury and efficiency of motion and how biomechanical analysis can be used to diagnose the cause of injuries and to improve technique. Poor technique, however, is often a compensation for a more basic problem. Favoring an old injury or shifting the body around to make up for a weak muscle group can lead to motions that unduly stress joints and muscles. For example, some researchers have speculated that players who have a poor backhand technique (other than the "leading el-bow") do so because weak knees get them to the ball late, forc-ing them to overcompensate.

Bernhang's data suggest that "leading elbow" may be a com-pensation for a lack of grip strength. In healthy players, the av-erage pressure on the racket handle was about 4.5 pounds per square inch stronger than players with a history of tennis el-bow. However, the likely explanation may be that the weakness is related to the tendonitis and these players may have had stronger grips prior to injury.

Another study, by Alan M. Strizak, an orthopedic surgeon at the UCLA Medical Center, suggests that the tennis-elbow syn-drome may be associated with a failure to develop the usual levels of arm strength seen in better players. As a result of test-ing regular players, nonplayers, and tennis elbow players, Stri-zak suggests that one approach to preventing this affliction is to increase the flexibility of the muscles and tendons around the elbow through manipulation and stretching exercises (see "Stretching Exercises" in Chapter 4). Alternatively, he suggests strengthening the muscles in the forearm.

Nirschl is reluctant to pinpoint any one cause of tennis el-bow, although he has said poor technique would be near the top of his list. He emphasizes that training errors, massive overloads, multiple repetitions, and deficient strength or flexi-bility are often the main culprits—and these are all correctible before injury develops. He adds that age, hormone imbalances in some women, and other factors that may not be detected before symptoms appear can also produce tennis elbow.

The truly remarkable advance is in conservative treatment when prevention fails. The widely used surgical procedure de-veloped thirty years ago has been conducted on only 3 percent of Nirschl's 3,500 patients and then only as a last resort. He ad-vocates rest and moderate exercise so that muscles and ten-dons are stimulated but not to the point of abuse. He also uses ice to reduce swelling, high-voltage electric stimulation, and ultrasound to promote healing.

When the symptoms subside, players are put on total body strength and flexibility programs until the muscles in the racket arm are 5 to 10 percent stronger than in the other arm as mea-sured with devices like the Cybex machine. If there is no pain without medication, Nirschl then lets his patient-players back onto the court. His final dose of medicine is to remind aggressive individuals that there are only 128 world-class tennis players in circulation, so instead of heading for the very top, they should relax, avoid extreme overloads, and learn to *enjoy* the game.

EIGHT

GOLF

Thinking in Fast Twitch

One week before the 1960 U.S. Open, Arnold Palmer, a thirty-one-year-old challenger who had won five of his thirteen tournaments that year, told Will Grimsley of the *Saturday Evening Post*, "Ever since I was able to walk I have been swinging a golf club, and ever since I was big enough to dream I have wanted to be the best golfer who ever lived."

It was great copy from this newcomer to professional golf, but was it just so much show talk to psyche out the opposition or a hint of special hunger?

The sincerity of Palmer's words was demonstrated days later during the tournament, held at Cherry Hills, Denver. Pitted against the likes of Ben Hogan and Mike Souchack, he seemed at first to be in the wrong league. When it came to the fourth and last round of the Open, Palmer may have wished that as a five-year-old boy back in Latrobe, Pennsylvania, he had never climbed off his father's links tractor to try his hand at golf—and get hooked on the game. Trailing in fifteenth place, he was no longer a contender in the tournament. One sportswriter's dispatch said Palmer had no more of a chance "than the man operating the hot dog concession."

Never one to hide his emotions, Palmer was visibly agitated as he prepared for the first hole tee-off in the final round. A handful of professionals simply smiled at him when he said, "If I'm going to win, I've got to go out and shoot a 65." After scoring a disastrous 72–71–72 on the first three rounds for a total of 215, any bookie would take money that a 65 was out of the question.

187

Then, as Palmer addressed the tee facing the troublesome first hole, something happened. All the boyish hopes and dreams welled up, something clicked, something kicked in. He stared at the ball, drew his club over his shoulders, and *pulled*. The impact sounded like the landfall of lightning in the split second before thunder, as the ball climbed into the clear Colorado sky, impossibly high and long, landing on the green with legs that ran within 30 feet of the pin.

Suddenly, the smug smiles vanished. All bets were off. Starting with that par-four *346-yarder*, Palmer assaulted the Cherry Hills course as if his life hung in the balance, with booming drives and pinpoint chips. He shouted at putts and danced as they dropped. He birdied six of the next seven holes—one stroke under for each. He was unstoppable, and the competition sensed it. Even the unflappable Hogan was unhinged, landing in a moat on the seventeenth and in a lake on the eighteenth. Unlike anything seen in the history of the U.S. Open, Palmer had called his shot and come from behind with a 65 for a winning total of 280, the challengers folding in the presence of a miracle.

His astonishing performance echoed the prophetic words recorded days earlier: "I get myself more keyed up when an important title is at stake. . . . When I get on a hard, exacting course, I feel as if I am wrestling a bear."

Golf is often portrayed as a lazy man's sport, stereotyped with images of middle-aged men navigating the club around their bellies. The reality is that a powerful drive, such as Palmer's 346-yarder, requires the generation of a phenomenal amount of energy delivered to the club within a fraction of a second. A rough calculation shows that his drive took over 3,000 watts of power, more than an Olympic sprinter generates in the first second after the gun. It's easy to understand why, after winning the Masters Tournament in Augusta, Georgia, that same year, Palmer remarked, "I hadn't been this tired since I worked in the steel mills and I kept telling myself, What a way to make a living."

THE PHYSICS OF THE DOWNSWING

Golf has received more scientific scrutiny than just about any other sport, and one of the reasons is to crack the mysteries of the full-shot swing. Although the explosive power behind drives like Palmer's 346-yarder is certainly baffling, the elusive nut is exactly how players manipulate their bodies to transmit this power to the ball, and whether design changes in the club can increase the range of a drive.

Those who do not play golf may wonder what could possibly remain unknown in such an uncomplicated sport, one that has been around for over 500 years. But the simplicity of the game is deceptive. The act of accelerating the head of a golf club to over 150 feet/second and squarely striking a 1.68-inch ball, to propel it 200 to 300 yards down the fairway, is arguably one of the most difficult motor skills in sports. Despite the wealth of scientific data collected on the motions of a golfer, there remains considerable uncertainty about how he should wield the club.

In the absence of expert consensus on the optimal technique, improving performance in the game relies on the opinions of professionals, who often advocate one method while unwittingly using another. The uncertainties also carry over to the design of equipment. If golfers are told they can improve their driving range by using a heavier club head or a more flexible shaft, manufacturers respond by producing whatever the market demands, even if these factors are known to have no effect—or a negative effect—on performance.

One of the first breakthroughs in the biomechanical analysis of golf came with the invention of the stroboscope, which permitted a moment-by-moment breakdown of the downswing, which until then had remained too blurred to observe. In fact, the inventor of the stroboscope, Harold Edgerton, was the first man to freeze the motions of professional golfers on film. The multiflash image of Bobby Jones taking a shot, probably the most widely published picture of the founder of the Masters Tournament, was taken by Edgerton over forty years ago and is still used to dissect the technique of golf's "mechanical man." In recent years both multiflash and high-speed films have been digitized and the data fed into computers for rapid analysis, comparing the movements of one golfer to another to build an electronic portrait of the perfect swing.

This process was made possible, in part, by the Golf Society of Great Britain (GSGB) which in 1962 sponsored a six-year investigation of various shots and techniques. This study was the first concerted effort to establish exactly what forces were exchanged between the player and the ball. Although some of the research was less than definitive, one of the many positive results was the discovery that each golfer has what might be called a unique "swing signature." This individual pattern of movement can be identified with strobe photography and similar techniques by measuring the angle of the arms and club in each film exposure and plotting these movements over time in terms of the rate of acceleration, torque, and total power.

This method can be very instructive when considering extraordinary performances, such as Palmer's drive at Cherry Hills. In the absence of a gale-force tail wind, the displacement of a golf ball over 346 yards requires an initial launch speed of about 285 feet/second, a momentum obtained from the collision with a 7-ounce club head moving at 197 feet/second. By breaking Palmer's lightning swing down into discrete frozen frames of reference, it's possible to get some idea of how he generated this ungodly speed and compare his technique to that of less successful golfers.

In some ways, a full-shot swing in golf is akin to an Olympic hammer throw, where the athlete uses an angular motion to increase the velocity of the equipment. The hammer thrower whirls three or four times in a circle at an ever-increasing rate before letting the hammer fly, but the golfer is confined to accelerating his club in a single swing, which follows an arc of about 270 degrees, although most of the power is produced when the club head is within only 90 degrees of the tee. As the basic motions of the downswing are similar for all golfers, the question is how and where in the swing to apply muscle power to obtain a club speed that will transform the usual 200-yard drive to a spectacular 300-yarder.

It is unfortunate that Harold Edgerton or biomechanist Gideon Ariel wasn't at Cherry Hills to record Palmer's blast, because this high a level of swing power has never been documented in laboratory studies. Enough data has been collected, however, to enable us to recreate that drive as if we had sent our own high-speed film equipment back through time. The "stickman" in *Figure 8.1* is a rough approximation of Palmer addressing the first-hole tee; the positions of his arms and club

FIGURE 8.1

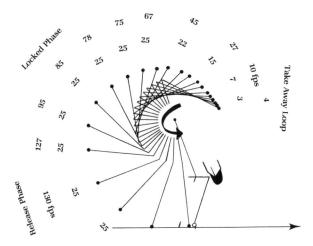

Arnold Palmer's 346-yard downswing. If we went back in time and took film exposures once every 0.01 seconds of Palmer's tremendous drive at Cherry Hills, the image might look similar to that drawn above (compare to photo on p. 228). The values closest to the golfer represent hand speed during the downswing; the values farthest from the golfer represent the club head speed. Note how the angle between the club and the golfer's arm remains constant through the Locked Phase, then gradually opens up during the Release Phase, as it would in a mechanical double-hinged pendulum. Compare the angles of this smooth shot to those in Fig. 8.2.

are shown frozen in imaginary film exposures taken once every 0.01 second during his downswing. *Figure 8.2* shows data recorded at the same time intervals for the average duffer's 200-yard drive, with a similar swing time.

After visualizing the shot and addressing the tee with both feet planted on a line parallel to the ball's intended line of flight, the golfer begins his *backswing.* This is equivalent to the windup in a baseball pitch, setting the arms in a position to obtain the longest possible arc through which to accelerate during delivery. It differs in that it's almost a mirror image of the downswing. Every motion in the backswing is designed to obtain the maximum amount of power in a drive, which means recruiting the largest number of fast-twitch fibers in the major muscles of the body. In the average 160-pound body, about 43 percent or

FIGURE 8.2

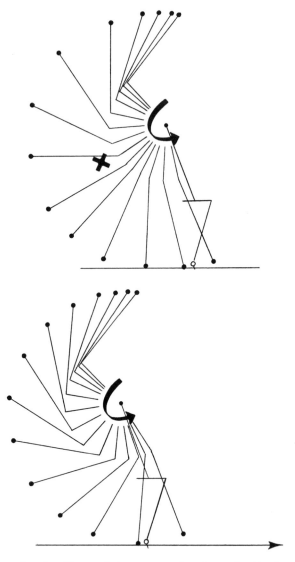

The weekend golfer can't be expected to have the flawless swing of Arnold Palmer. The illustration on the top shows what happens when the golfer tries to push on the hinge at the wrists between club and arms: a badly timed sequence results. The illustration on the bottom shows a weak action at the wrist hinge as a result of a delayed uncocking. Both swings can result if a golfer attempts to interfere with the natural opening of the wrists due to centrifugal force.

70 pounds is muscle, but 37 pounds of it is located below the waist. (Selective strength training in certain sports can substantially increase muscle weight in the upper body, but this is seldom seen in golfers.) Ben Hogan and Jack Nicklaus both proclaimed the virtues of "hitting the ball with your legs" and the distribution of musculature certainly supports this idea.

From above, the motions of the backswing look like the golfer is twisting himself around an invisible vertical axis winding a spring from the ground up. The process begins with a clockwise rotation of the hips to a point about 40 degrees off the flight path, the shoulders continue this rotation to 90 degrees, and finally the hands and club are wrapped above and around the head. Studies have found that the motion of the legs, hips, and shoulders are remarkably similar in seasoned golfers, but the final position of hands and club vary a lot between individuals and appears unrelated to drive power or accuracy.

During the last stage of the backswing the wrists are "cocked" or bent laterally toward the thumb side of the forearms (ulnar deviation), a maneuver that facilitates the extreme angle of the *takeaway point*, the position where backswing becomes downswing. Here lies one of the most perplexing problems in a golfer's stroke. Most pros and scientists believe that as the club is swung down toward the ball, the player imparts an extra boost of power when the wrists are uncocked, applying leverage on the handle by pushing down with the right wrist. A minority opinion says a golfer should let the club force the wrists back to their neutral position, and that any attempt to apply leverage can impair performance. Researchers who have examined the problem have come up with conflicting results.

All investigators do agree that the point at which the backswing ends and the downswing begins is characterized by the shoulders, arms, wrists, hands, and club being locked together, moving as a single unit. (In *Fig. 8.1* this area is shown as the locked phase.) Since the wrists are locked, the angle between the club and arm remains constant through the entire locked phase of the downswing.

It's difficult to pinpoint where the backswing ends and the downswing starts, as various body segments appear to be moving in two directions at once. In fact, the club head does not stop and start on the same plane, but describes a small loop as it alters course. Pros advise there should be no hesitation at the peak of the backswing before pulling down on the club. This fluidity of motion reversal has been caught on high-speed films and probably accounts for the absence of any measurable jerks on the club despite the rapid acceleration. The GSGB study found that the forward movement of the hips begins about 0.1 second *before* the club head reaches the peak of its backswing.

As the hips lead the shoulders, arms and club through the locked phase, the acceleration of the club is relatively slow, attaining a velocity of about 5 to 10 feet/second. Then as the velocity of the club head begins to exceed that of the hands— because it's traveling in a wider arc than the hands—the wrists must uncock. Otherwise when the arms were at their lowest point, perpendicular to the ground, the golf club would still be in the air. The uncocking of the wrists marks the beginning of the *release phase* of the downswing. Here the angular momentum built up in the legs and hips is transferred to the shoulders and arms, which now all begin to swing in unison, causing the club head to accelerate from 10 feet/second to 195 feet/second in under 0.2 second. As *Figure 8.2* shows, bad timing at the start of the release phase can ruin the stroke.

THE PUZZLE OF WRIST ACTION

Should the golfer push down with his wrists during the release phase or just pull along the shaft and let the accelerating club lead the wrists through their uncocking motion?

David Williams, an engineer at Britain's Royal Aircraft Establishment and a former consultant to the U.S. Golf Association, used strobe photographs and mathematical models that, he claims, show that the outward centrifugal force of the club compels the wrists to unlock. The GSGB study, on the other hand, concluded that "the obvious way to add speed to the club head is by applying effort at the hinge [of the hands]." They suggest that the right arm should *push* down and straighten the elbow to provide extra speed with a lever effect. Williams believes that the predominant action should be to *pull* the shaft through the downswing.

In the reconstruction of Palmer's downswing, through the entire release phase, the club head can be seen picking up speed

reduced the velocity of the club head from 143 to 140 feet/second. Budney calculated that without interfering with the natural out-swinging of the club, this golfer's final head speed would have been 175 feet/second—which means an extra 15 yards on the fairway.

If this evidence is not enough, Williams challenges players to try an experiment of their own to prove that the centrifugal force of the double pendulum is responsible for the uncocking of the wrists. If the hands do apply 10 to 15 pounds of force to the shaft during the release phase through wrist pressure, he suggests that nonbelievers fit their club head into a vise, or wedge it against a door frame, and quickly apply 10 to 15 pounds of leverage to the handle—a force similar to that you might use yanking on a car's hand brake in a sudden emergency. Unless the shaft is made of a space-age alloy, the lever effect will either break the shaft or bend it out of line.

Williams invites golfers reluctant to try this test to inspect a strobe photo of the downswing of a top player. They will observe no backward bending of the shaft, which is the whole principle behind the application of wrist pressure. If anything, some strobe photos show a significant *forward* bending about 0.01 second before impact, the opposite of what would be produced by positive leverage. It's unlikely that this forward bending is caused by a braking action in top golfers so late in the swing. Rather, it's probably due to the club head rushing toward the ball faster than the shaft due to centrifugal force—the club leading the uncocking action of the wrists.

Despite all this, almost all of the instructional books on golf, written by famous pros, advocate wrist pressure late in the downswing. In his fascinating book *The Science of the Golf Swing*, David Williams observes that "The wrong idea persists even among the top names in the world of golf [but] such wrong notions may not affect their own game because their practice has little connection with their theories."[1]

PUTTING: PROGRAMMING THE SKILL

In the highly competitive world of professional golf, the majority of present-day tournaments are decided on the putting surface, because players at this level of the game usually get to the green within more or less the same number of strokes. Although putting seems easier than driving, players at all levels seem to have a more difficult time moving the ball several feet than hundreds of yards.

Putting demands precise control of fast-twitch muscles—many of the same muscles involved in the explosive drive—without requiring any considerable strength or endurance. From the point of view of power, everyone—man, woman, child—stares at the pin as equals. It's the nervous system that counts, but in the inevitable "this putt for the game" situation, the nervous system can betray the player, even on the easiest shots. For this reason, the green has become the stage for major drama, where masters can go astray and dark horses pull out front.

During the 1960s, Arnold Palmer was one of those who could sink the impossible putt and make the crowd crazy. The press said, "Palmer is the man who can deliver miracles." Fans demand miracles of their heroes because this kind of unexpected, impossible performance upsets the predicted outcome of a game, topples villains, turns an afternoon of passive observation into an event of a lifetime, but perhaps most of all, a sports miracle reaffirms their faith in the unfathomable reserves of the human body. After all, if it can happen to a guy who was given as much chance to win as the hot dog vendor at the edge of the crowd, then it can happen to *anybody*.

From an athlete's perspective, the aftermath of an extraordinary finish on the green may have an unsettling effect. Once he's home at night, mulling over the inexplicable shots of the day, mixed in with the joy, gratitude, and I-knew-I-could-do-it glow, there's the inevitable question, "Why can't I play like that all the time?" The occasional Doug Flutie Hail Mary pass, the Franco Harris immaculate reception or the Larry Bird last-second swish from the opposite end of the basketball court is certainly awesome, but a sustained peak performance, like pitching a no-hitter in baseball or Arnold Palmer's last round at Cherry Hills, is a different breed of miracle. If luck, odds, and fate have to be ruled out in a sustained performance, the question is, If this level of potential talent is there, what internal buttons do successful players push to activate *all* their talents?

The opposite effect occurs in sudden performance slumps. Consider Ben Hogan at Cherry Hills. As Palmer came from behind going into the last two holes, apparently destined to clinch the winning score of 280, Hogan needed only *two pars* to make 280. Yet he put one ball in a moat and the other in the drink. One sportswriter called it "the collapse of Hogan." Another wrote, "The old master lost his touch completely." But all the sports jargon boils down to: his nerves got the better of him.

Peaks and slumps in putting are notorious among golfers, occurring even when their drives remain consistent. Because performance on the green is such a raw act of nerves, "the other game" has always been a fascinating laboratory to test theories and techniques designed to enhance the acquisition and control of basic motor skills. In 1908, Arnold Haultain was the first writer to give putters psychological tips in his book *The Mystery of Golf.* In *Better Golf without Practice* (1940), Alex Morrison advocated a visualization system similar to Richard Suinn's method of Visuo-Motor Behavior Rehearsal (see Chapter 2). The 1980s brought Timothy Gallwey's popular manual *The Inner Game of Golf.* Today, sports psychologists are examining the process of learning motor skills for clues about how these programs are stored in the nervous system and what factors are involved in blocking or retrieving them.

The theories of motor learning come and go with startling regularity, but there are some broad outlines that adequately explain the many disparate experiments concerning memory, recall, attention, arousal, feedback, and other factors. Basically, the acquisition of a new skill seems to be broken down into separate, but overlapping processes. For a novice golfer equipped with a general understanding of the purpose and goals of a putt, the moment he steps onto the green and addresses the ball with weapon in hand, he is aroused by the challenge of the new situation and presumably his desire to master it. As arousal increases, so does his level of attention on the task—up to a certain point. If he becomes too excited or aroused, attention, learning, and performance will deteriorate. Following arousal there is an internal comparison of the actual movements required in a putt against those movements he has already mastered. Then there is a covert rehearsal of the new task, where the required movements are unconsciously segmented into muscle groups. Studies have shown that when people think of movements, the brain thinks in terms of muscles. This is followed by the first trials, discrepancy reduction, and corrections.

So far, all of these factors have been initiated and monitored consciously. When conscious monitoring of physical movements stops, a motor skill is said to have been acquired. In fact, whenever the conscious mind begins to monitor and attempt to control an acquired skill, performance falls dramatically. No one thinks twice about walking, but once they do, pace slows, steps become awkward, and there may be stumbling.

The observation that beginners compare the required movements to those they have mastered in the past is linked to a notion called *transfer*, where the skills of one task are used to perform another. If the novice putter is a seasoned baseball player, he would likely grip the club with the baseball grip as opposed to the Vardon or interlocking grip, unless specifically taught otherwise. Similarly, swimming instructors have observed that novice swimmers who have mastered the sidestroke will frequently substitute the scissors kick of that stroke when first learning to swim the breaststroke. This raises interesting problems for instructors and coaches: sometimes a previous skill can be successfully adapted to a new one. But in different activities these previous skills may retard learning because the beginner prefers to use the known skill to obtain quick results at the novice level—although that technique may prove to be inefficient or even injurious at higher levels of performance.

Countless observations of the transfer effect and related phenomena support the theory of *general motor programs* in the central nervous system. These are the general instructions for the 200-odd basic movements involved in all human activity. New skills, in this case putting, are stored, recalled, and in many ways controlled by these programs. No two putts are the same—each is a slightly new experience—but the learning process is not repeated in every putt.

In the absence of a wiring diagram of the human nervous system, psychologists can only make educated guesses on how and where programs are stored. It is tempting to think that athletic practice reinforces a motor program by cutting a deeper groove. It appears, however, that the programs are not stored in one central memory bank, but are dispersed throughout the brain. The *redundancy* of motor programs was discovered years ago when neurologists were trying to find the center of memory in the brains of rats who had been trained to do a specific skill, like run a maze for food. Progressive slices of brain tissue were removed in the hope of finding memory, but in the end, when so much tissue had been removed that the rats could hardly walk, they still struggled through the maze. This work was paralleled by neurologists who electrically stimulated the brains of conscious patients undergoing routine brain surgery for various ailments; they discovered that memories were widely distributed in the brain and in some rare cases found more than one site for the same memory.

Some of the most basic motor skills may be stored in the spinal cord. Records on guillotine use during the French Revolution indicate that some victims ran away from the block after they had been decapitated. The gruesome phrase "running like a chicken with its head cut off" alludes to the spine's central role in locomotion.

The old pediatric homily that anything an infant does once becomes a habit is another way of saying that what goes into the "blank" mind of an infant comes right out again. With age and the accumulation of motor skills, this tendency disappears, and many psychologists believe the sorting and assembly process among the large number and complexity of motor programs can be visualized in terms of competing sets of instructions for a single activity. This gives rise to dominant and inferior programs, where dominance is determined by frequency of use and subjective reinforcement of success.

In this sense practice is only the replay of a motor program, and if that program is a set of instructions for a faulty technique, continued practice without correction will lead to a faulty skill. Practice is only practice. In learning a new skill, dominance has not been established, and correct performance feedback is essential for the student to enhance the dominance of the correct movements, by sending an immediate message to the brain: "*That* was the right move."

Manipulation of feedback signals is one of the more promising areas in the search of methods to enhance the acquisition of motor skills. Almost all studies have found that learning rate increases as amount and accuracy of feedback increases; and performance declines dramatically when feedback is removed. The question is what kind of feedback? Visual or verbal?

Golfers have known for decades that the head movements involved in looking back and forth between the hole and the ball are disastrous in putting, and this has led some researchers to wonder whether golfers might not be better off if they didn't look at the target at all after the preliminary setup; others believe that visual input may be a distracting factor in learning how to putt.

Vision is such an important sensory factor that it's hard to conceive of athletic performance without it, but research has found that *proprioceptive sense*, or muscle sense, is much more important in learning and running motor programs. In sports it's no exaggeration to say that your muscles see more than your eyes: a larger portion of the central nervous system is devoted to receiving and integrating sensory signals from muscles and joints than is devoted to the eye and ear combined.

While experimenting with the effects of different types of feedback on the skill of putting, Gwendolyn Aksamit, a physical education researcher at California State University, discovered that the *elimination* of vision enhanced learning. A separate study found that blindfolded putters performed as well as those who looked at either the hole or the ball, but the performance of the blindfolded students surpassed the open-eyed putters once the blindfolds were removed. Similar findings have been recorded in basketball shooting and darts, two activities that depend on eye-hand coordination.

Like strength training, where athletes discover there is an optimal number of repetitions of certain loads at a given speed that's best for gaining strength for their particular athletic activity, motor skill acquisition is enhanced with optimal levels of arousal, feedback, and practice. *Massed practice* refers to programming sessions in which the rest period between performance trials is less than the duration of each trial. *Distributed practice* describes sessions in which rest periods are equal to or greater than the duration of each trial. In some sports, massed practice impairs learning in a manner analogous to overtraining; in others distributed practice does not provide enough stimulus to adequately define or set dominance among motor programs. Some studies have found that in quick, discrete tasks such as putting, massed practice does not impair or enhance learning. The search for "quality practice" programs is a goal of learning research in all sports.

The speed at which a putter can obtain feedback is as important as the amount and accuracy of performance feedback. The importance of speed rests in a phenomenon known as the *proprioceptive trace*, the inner perception of the muscular feelings associated with every movement. This trace is stored in short-term memory and lasts up to 30 seconds. In this short period of time, an athlete must be able to reinforce the motor program by reaffirming that the trace is associated with the proper movements, otherwise the movements will not receive optimal dominance over competing movements for the same activity.

The computer is rapidly becoming a tool that will revolutionize the acquisition of motor skills in golf and many other sports. In 1927, a sportswriter described the famous flawless swing of Bobby Jones by saying, "They wound up the Mechanical Man of Golf yesterday and sent him clicking around the East Lake Course." The 1984 PGA tour was accompanied by another kind of mechanical man, an R2-D2 lookalike, which was observing the movements of top golfers, programming itself to become the world's first computerized golf pro.

Known as Sportstech, the same name as the Connecticut company that created it, the computerized pro holds up an instant performance mirror for any golfer immediately following his shot, displaying many of the characteristics the GSGB study found in each golfer's "swing signature." The central sensor is a pressure platform, which in this case is disguised as a grasslike carpet on which the golfer stands. After each swing, a computer display—and print-out, if required—provides accurate data on weight distribution during the stroke, path of the club head away from and through the ball relative to the intended flight path, position of the club head at the peak of the backswing and at the moment of impact, and similar factors. A Sportstech costs about $20,000, and there are about thirty prototypes in use across the United States.

The future training technology will capitalize on the same principles of instant feedback with accurate, objective feedback. Computer-controlled 3-D "fairway screens" similar to those being developed by Sportsvision for baseball batters, and previewed in the science fiction motion picture *Outland*, may be available by the 1990s.

Until the advent of ideal learning programs or widespread use of computerized golf pros, golfers will have to follow the example of Bobby Jones, who, emerging from a seven-year slump, explained that he improved his game simply because "I kept on hammering at the pesky ball until I found a way to make it behave."

NINE

ENDURANCE TRAINING

The Fate of Pheidippides

The story of the original marathon has particular significance today because of the increasing number of conflicting reports on the risks and benefits of intense endurance training.

The word *marathon* is derived from a narrow valley in Greece, where, on September 12, 490 B.C., the Athenians, under the command of General Miltiades, pinned down a superior Persian expeditionary force and proceeded to slaughter every man who couldn't flee from the valley. The Persians lost 6,400 men in the Battle of Marathon, whereas the Greeks lost only 192.

Fearing that the city of Athens might surrender to a Persian naval assault if unaware of the Marathon victory, Miltiades dispatched his fastest runner, Pheidippides, to carry the good news home. After having already run to Sparta and back, the exhausted Pheidippides raced over 26 miles to Athens, cried out, "Rejoice—we conquer!" and fell dead.[1]

The death of Pheidippides was not in vain. Athens was saved and the Persians retreated to Asia. But the tragedy of this young athlete of 2,475 years ago periodically returns to haunt many of the 20 million Americans who regularly participate in some form of structured aerobic exercise or endurance training—particularly since the ironic death of running guru James Fixx.

On July 20, 1984, the best-selling author of *The Complete Book of Running* was stricken on a back road in Vermont while out alone on a 10-mile run. At age fifty-two, Fixx had inspired thousands to improve their health, and presumably prolong their lives, through jogging. Fixx, who had once been an overweight, two-pack-a-day smoker, appeared to be in fine physical condition at the time of his coronary. His friends and family said he never mentioned any pain or discomfort, even when exercising strenuously.

The autopsy, conducted by Eleanor N. McQuillen, Vermont's chief medical examiner, raised disturbing questions about what role exercise played in protecting against coronary heart disease. McQuillen found that all three of Fixx's coronary arteries were impaired by *atherosclerosis*, a leading cause of death in the United States. Only a trickle of blood could pass through the pinholes in his left circumflex coronary artery; 80 percent of his right coronary artery was blocked; and half of his anterior descending artery was blocked in places. Although the disease left the arteries that fed his brain unaffected, his aorta and the arteries in his legs were damaged. In short, his cardiovascular health was poor and it's surprising that his heart had supported the 80 to 90 miles Fixx used to run every week for so many years.

Clearly, the physiological benefits of distance running vaunted by James Fixx had to be amended: exercise alone does not confer immunity to heart disease. Indeed, some runners began to fear that intense training might even precipitate heart attacks.

The impact of Fixx's death was somewhat eclipsed by the Los Angeles summer Olympics, a celebration of health, fitness, and vitality that seemed to reaffirm the medical advantages of athletic endeavor—until the agony of Swiss marathoner Gabriella Andersen-Schiess. Staggering deliriously through the final lap at the Coliseum before millions of TV spectators, she collapsed into the arms of officials after crossing the finish line. Within days, newspaper reporters began filing stories about the incidence of death and injury among people who exercise regularly. Physiologists were interviewed about the risks and benefits of endurance training. Psychologists spoke of an epidemic of "compulsive runners" who escaped from anxiety and depression by running themselves to ruin. Even TV aerobic dance exercise came under the shadow.

Perennial reports of the dangers of intense training and competition may be welcomed by sedentary loungers, but for the athlete who occasionally wonders about the extreme, even masochistic, nature of training, they provoke doubt and anxiety.

Like strength training, where the skeletal muscles are stressed to the point of failure (see Chapter 5), endurance training pushes the body to the point of exhaustion to obtain maximum adaptation in aerobic tissues, from the heart and lungs down to the microscopic mitochondria, or energy factories, in muscle fibers.

Are these extreme and painful efforts really safe and effective? Is the fate of Pheidippides an inherent risk of maximum exertion?

THE PHYSIOLOGY OF ENDURANCE TRAINING

Basketball, tennis, soccer, cycling, and swimming are sports that use endurance training to stretch the aerobic capacities of their athletes. Distance runners have served for decades as living laboratories for exercise physiologists, who study and experiment with the adaptations produced through training. The lone runner can be scrutinized without adjusting for performance variables such as equipment or team interaction. Treadmills allow measurements to be taken in the lab and compared to performance in the field. The uniformity of movement coupled with the large number of runners has made it possible to amass a tremendous amount of information on oxygen uptake, the role of the heart and circulation in transporting oxygen around the body, and the combustion of metabolic fuels within the muscle fibers.

In strength training, the object is to increase the explosive power of muscles through hypertrophy of fast-twitch fibers. Endurance training does not elicit the profound changes seen in the physique of body builders and weight lifters, but on a microscopic level the adaptations are just as dramatic. Muscle core biopsies and computerized axial tomography, an advanced form of X-ray also known as a CAT scanner, have shown that slow-twitch fibers do not undergo significant hypertrophy as a result of endurance training, but there is a threefold increase in the number of mitochondria, the specialized tissues that use oxygen to produce the fuels of muscle contraction. There is also a 30 percent increase in the number of capillaries that feed slow-twitch fibers, an increase that can occur after only three to four weeks of vigorous training in various aerobic activities.

By increasing the mitochondrial content and blood supply in these fibers, the energy for muscle contraction over long periods of time is produced with less dependence on anaerobic metabolism. Anaerobic activity produces higher levels of lactic acid, which causes the onset of fatigue. This idea is supported by blood samples of conditioned athletes who have finished marathons and show little if any elevation of lactate over normal levels.

To cope with the increased oxygen demands of such strenuous aerobic activities as marathons, adaptations occur in the lungs, heart, blood, and circulatory system. These adaptations improve both the maximum amount of oxygen that can be consumed, or VO_2max, and the amount of oxygenated blood that can be transported through the body.

One of the first measurable effects of endurance training is an increase in blood volume. After the first few days of training the amount of blood can increase by as much as 400 milliliters. This larger volume of blood is an immediate response to the need for more oxygen and the increased volume actually helps the return of blood to the heart without causing an increase in blood pressure. The normal blood volume in the body is 5 liters, but the circulatory system has a capacity for 25 liters. Blood pressure remains normal in a healthy body by selective dilation or enlargement of the blood vessels.

There is also an increase in the number of red blood cells, which carry oxygen from the lungs to the tissues. Red blood cells live for about 120 days and are manufactured at the rate of 2 *million per second*. This phenomenal rate of production allows the bone marrow, where red blood cells are created, to respond rapidly to any shortage of oxygen in the body, an adaptation dramatized even in sedentary individuals who travel to high-altitude environments (see Chapter 11). At sea level, as a rule, the increase of red blood cells in response to training is usually proportionate to the increase in blood volume.

The increase in blood volume, coupled with the demands of exertion, does make the heart work harder, and this causes its musculature to grow. In turn, the additional size and strength of the heart allows it to pump more blood per beat, or stroke.

Stroke volume can be increased by 20 percent through weeks of intensive endurance training, and higher levels have been observed in elite athletes. The increased stroke volume reduces the resting heart rate by up to ten beats per minute, sometimes more, and heart rate can be decreased by about three beats per minute during exercise. (*See Fig. 9.1* for a summary of key adaptations to endurance training).

The lungs appear to adapt by increasing the amount of oxygen that can be transferred from the alveoli, or air sacs, to the blood. The evidence of this change is inconclusive as well as difficult to explain. In nonathletes, the hemoglobin is already 95 percent saturated with oxygen, binding about 1.34 milliliters of oxygen per gram of hemoglobin, so that further saturation is difficult to imagine. An increase in the number of alveoli is also unlikely. In a normal adult, the alveolar surface, if it was to be spread out flat, would cover about 50 square yards—half the size of a singles tennis court. Now if you imagine trying to spread a half liter of blood—the volume present in the lungs at any given instant—over this surface, it becomes apparent that the ratio of alveolar surface area to blood volume is already disproportionately large. (In fact, it's this large surface area that enables cigarette smokers to clog their lungs with tar and other by-products of combustion and still lead apparently normal lives.) It could be that the increased lung blood volume of endurance athletes accounts for the apparent adaptation of the lungs, but this increase of 30 to 40 milliliters does not fully explain the report of a doubling of the amount of oxygen moving from the lungs to the bloodstream.

Regardless of the exact nature of changes in the lungs, it is known that oxygen uptake and transport is improved through training, and the minimum level of endurance exercise required to induce adaptations has been firmly established. According to the American College of Sports Medicine (ACSM), endurance training must involve at least 50 percent of the body's muscle mass in some form of rhythmic activity for at least 30 minutes a day, three to five days a week. The level of exertion must be between 60 and 90 percent of the existing maximum heart rate, and between 50 and 85 percent of the existing VO₂max to obtain measurable conditioning effects.

These guidelines, first published in 1978, were formulated to

FIGURE 9.1
Adaptations to Endurance Training

Functional Change	Resting Degree of Change	Maximum Exercise Degree of Change
Heart rate (beats/minute)	−15	−5
Stroke volume (milliliters/beat)	+8	+15
Cardiac output (liters/minute)	0	+2
Blood volume		
plasma (liters)	+0.2	+0.2
Blood flow		
to heart (milliliters/minute)	−10	+40
to active muscles		
(milliliters/minute)	−45	+2,400
O_2 uptake (milliliters/kilogram-minute)	0	+7
Respiratory rate (breaths/minute)	0	+9

Dramatic changes in cardiovascular and pulmonary function after endurance training are shown in table above for an average 150-pound male. Physiological adaptations can be even more pronounced with more intense and prolonged training. These changes are typical following ten to fifteen weeks of moderate exercise.

address the question of how much exercise is enough to develop and maintain fitness in healthy adults. The ACSM guidelines do not address, however, questions about how much training will produce maximum adaptations for competitive athletes or how much training is too much.

To probe the limits of human adaptation to extremely intense endurance training, Kevin A. Mikesell, a physiologist at Ohio State University, conducted an interesting experiment with seven well-conditioned distance runners. To sedentary individuals the intensity of training in this experiment might seem impossible.

The athletes trained six days per week for a six week test period. Part of the training consisted of running as far as possible within 40 minutes with the intention of gaining greater distance in successive runs. They also performed 5-minute rides on stationary bicycle ergometers, separated by 5-minute intervals of jogging, then more time on the bicycles with the cranking resistance increased in session after session to induce peak oxygen uptake. The purpose of Mikesell's study was to push these athletes to exhaustion to prompt adaptation, and as soon as the adaptations appeared, to push them further and further to determine if and when VO_2max leveled off.

Prior to Mikesell's research it was well established that substantial increases in VO_2max, about 20 to 40 percent, can occur after only one week of strenuous endurance training, and 44 percent increases have been observed after only nine weeks of training. These numbers are discussed almost casually between athletes and scientists, but a few minutes of reflection about what they imply—a 44 percent increase in the amount of oxygen the body can extract from the air after a mere nine weeks of exercise—boggles the imagination.

On the basis of prior studies, Mikesell and his coworkers had expected that if the intensity of training is increased relative to improvements in VO_2max, the increases in oxygen uptake would level off as each subject approached his own genetically determined upper limit. The surprise was that adaptations appeared to have no ceiling in the test period. On average the weekly increase in VO_2max was 0.11 liter of oxygen per minute—an increase that continued unabated.[2]

Despite the apparent limitless nature of this adaptation, VO_2max correlates poorly to performance times in long-distance swimming and running, which means there's more to endurance than the measure of oxygen that can be extracted from the air. A more important factor seems to be an athlete's ability to use a large fraction of his VO_2max during a competition. The greater the percentage of VO_2max that can be used, the farther and faster an athlete can run without calling on his anaerobic reserves. Studies have found that endurance training improves total VO_2max as well as the fraction that can be used during exercise.

On an average, marathon runners have been found to use 75 percent of their VO_2max during a race, although this may vary between 65 to 90 percent among highly trained individuals. In other words, it's possible to have two runners with an identical VO_2max, but who differ in their ability to use a given fraction of their aerobic capacity.

To demonstrate this point, David L. Costill, a runner and physiologist at Ball State University in Indiana, published a study citing the example of Australian marathoner Derek Clayton (best marathon time: 2 hr, 8 min, 33.6 sec), who had a maximum aerobic capacity of about 70 milliliters per kilogram per minute (ml/kg-min), and used 86 percent of this capacity. By contrast, another runner tested by Costill had a higher aerobic capacity of about 78 ml/kg-min, but was able to use only 64 percent of his VO_2max. Pitted against one another, all other things being equal, Clayton would probably win the race, since he could deliver about 60 milliliters of oxygen to every kilogram of body weight per minute, whereas the other competitor could deliver only 50 ml/kg-min. Even though milliliters are minuscule quantities of oxygen, it only takes an extra few per minute to make a champion.

Another factor that affects endurance performance is the efficiency of motion (see "Training for the Rush" in Chapter 1), which can also be measured by oxygen consumption. Consider two distance runners who possess similar maximum aerobic capacities (65 ml/kg-min) and use the same fraction of the capacity (85 percent VO_2max) in their best races, yet one consistently runs 10 percent faster than the other. This is a clear signal that the slower runner's physiology may be in top condition, but the mechanics of his gait, his stride length and stride frequency, or height of foot and knee lift, are somehow inefficient. Inefficient motion requires more energy, and this is reflected in oxygen consumption.

Treadmill analysis can show that the efficient athlete may consume, say, 3 liters of oxygen per minute in the first mile of an event, whereas the inefficient competitor uses 3.3 liters per minute. In football, the biomechanic analysis of rushers is used to acquire a gait that produces the fastest possible output of power without regard for oxygen consumption; in distance runners, speed is a function of aerobic capacity, and strides are adjusted to attain maximum distance within an athlete's ideal VO_2max.

For decades, exercise physiologists have been in disagreement about which body system puts an upper limit on performance in endurance events. Some believe the limiting factors lie with the output of the heart and lungs, others say the limits to performance are within the skeletal muscles. One interesting idea is that the limiting factor may be the arterial circulation, the vital link between heart and lungs and the peripheral muscles.

Even without endurance training, healthy lungs can oxygenate more blood than they receive due to the tremendous alveolar surface area. Healthy hearts are capable of pumping all the fresh blood they receive from the lungs, and even at maximum cardiac output, the blood from the lungs is 95 percent saturated with oxygen. At the other end of the pipeline, the mitochondria in both untrained fast- and slow-twitch muscle fibers have a capacity to consume much more oxygen than the blood supply delivers (the principle behind blood doping; see Chapter 2). As endurance training greatly increases the aerobic capacity of both these central and peripheral systems, the process of elimination would make it seem as if the arterial circulation might limit oxygen transport.

This possibility was first suggested in 1970 by Dan Tunstall Pedoe, a cardiologist at St. Bartholomew's Hospital in London and chairman of the British Association of Sports and Medicine. He proposed that, in accordance with the principles of fluid dynamics, blood flow at rest travels through arteries with a laminar flow pattern, but with increased cardiac output in response to exercise, blood velocity will become sufficiently high to produce turbulent flow patterns—with large losses in pressure (not unlike the aerodynamics of balls in flight; see Chapter 6).

There is, however, some adaptation in the circulatory system. As Pedoe points out, greyhounds have much larger arteries compared to more sedentary dogs of similar size. Athletes are also known to develop larger aortas than nonathletes, and the vessels serving active skeletal muscles increase in size as the capillary network in those muscles becomes denser. It seems likely that larger arteries can handle larger blood flow without incurring turbulence, because only small increases in vessel size yield disproportionate increases in volume: a vessel with an interior radius of 4.2 millimeters will deliver 5 cubic centimeters of blood per second, whereas a vessel with a radius of 5 millimeters will deliver 10 cubic centimeters of blood per second.

Pedoe's proposal is further mitigated by the fact that during strenuous exercise the muscles can receive more than 85 percent of the total cardiac output, although they comprise only

40 percent of the body's tissues. This is achieved during exercise by selective dilation and constriction of the arteries. The vessels are also known to dilate to accommodate the increased blood volume that results from training. All told, it would seem that the adaptability of the circulatory system can accommodate the changes caused by endurance training, but Pedoe's theory remains interesting and deserves further investigation.

The evidence available today suggests that endurance is not limited by the mechanics of oxygen transport—ventilation, cardiac output, and arterial distribution—which seems capable of handling any load, even under the artificial and extremely intense conditions imposed on the athletes in Kevin Mikesell's study. But there is obviously a limiting factor somewhere, and today it appears that factor is the supply and use of basic metabolic fuels, particularly glycogen, in the muscles.

THE HEART OF AN ATHLETE

Endurance training can transform a healthy heart into an enlarged, misshapen organ. The muscle of the heart, or myocardium, responds to increased work loads from endurance training like skeletal muscles to strength training. Cardiac and skeletal muscles both have fibers containing actin and myosin filaments, which contract when stimulated, and undergo hypertrophy as an adaptation to overload. Cardiac muscles differ in that contraction is not stimulated voluntarily; the fibers are bundled so that the stimulation of one cell fires the whole group, and the fibers are shorter than skeletal muscle fibers.

During exercise, feedback from active muscles relayed through the nervous system, coupled with changes in blood flow and chemistry, increases the rate and force of myocardial contractions. In addition, the ventricles of the heart (see Fig. 9.2) are stretched when they receive more blood and contract more forcefully as a result. When the right atrium is stretched, the heart rate can be elevated up to fifteen beats per minute. Through these mechanisms, progressive increments in training present the heart with the overload stimulus that brings about the peculiar structural changes associated with increased cardiac output.

According to David Costill, Australian marathoner Derek

FIGURE 9.2

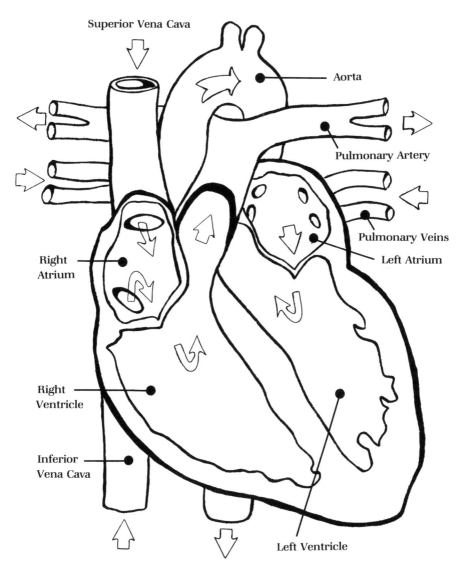

Superior Vena Cava

Aorta

Pulmonary Artery

Pulmonary Veins

Right
Atrium

Left Atrium

Right
Ventricle

Inferior
Vena Cava

Left Ventricle

Anatomy of the human heart. The blood returns from the tissues through the venous system, pouring through the superior and inferior vena cava, into the right atrium, past the tricuspid valve, into the right ventricle, out through the pulmonary arteries to the lungs, where it picks up fresh oxygen, returning by the pulmonary veins, into the left atrium, the left ventricle, and back to the tissues through the aorta.

Clayton had a maximum cardiac output estimated at about 35 liters of blood pumped per minute, compared to an average 23 liters per minute for normal, active men. During competition, distance runners will use over 90 percent of their maximum cardiac output for two to two and a half hours, exerting considerable stress on their hearts. In two and a half hours, Clayton's heart would pump over 4,700 liters of blood—enough to fill an automobile's 15-gallon gas tank about 75 times—contracting between 160 and 175 times a minute.

For a healthy, oxygenated heart, this work is accomplished without incurring damage or discomfort, but hearts with clogged coronary arteries will receive an insufficient supply of blood to fuel contractions. This form of *exercise ischemia* can induce chemical alterations in the heart muscle, causing abnormal and potentially fatal irregular heartbeats, or *arrhythmias*. Larger insufficiencies of oxygenated blood will deprive the muscle fibers of the ability to contract, often precipitating cardiac arrest. For this reason, individuals involved in endurance training, especially the middle-aged and elderly, are often given regular heart examinations, using electrocardiograms (EKG) to detect arrhythmias during exercise, and echocardiograms, a diagnostic technique using ultrasound to produce an image of the heart, to observe changes in the heart's structure. It should be noted that, according to family accounts, Jim Fixx had not had these tests for years before his coronary.

By conventional medical standards, many joggers, distance runners, and swimmers have "abnormal" hearts. Training often produces an enlarged heart, and a very slow resting heart rate, sometimes with arrhythmias on the EKG tracings, even if the heart is receiving an adequate supply of oxygen. In nonathletes, these would appear as symptoms of heart disease; in endurance-trained athletes these features are accepted as nonthreatening adaptations, collectively known as *athlete's heart*.

Although these changes are a reflection of fitness, they are poor predictors of athletic performance. A larger stroke volume, for example, is an indication of a strong, trained heart, but the measured milliliters of blood pumped per minute cannot be used like the percentage of VO_2max to anticipate success in an event or to prescribe specific changes in training. Similarly, the slow resting heartbeat of an athlete, or *bradycar-*

dia, reflects cardiac enlargement, particularly hypertrophy of the left ventricle, but in exertion, endurance athletes have a peak heart rate that is not substantially different from normal individuals (between 180 and 200 beats per minute in young, healthy adults).

One provocative idea that has been suggested recently is that bradycardia by itself might produce a traininglike adaptation in the heart, stimulating hypertrophy to pump more blood to compenstate for the low number of contractions. This theory is the reverse of the accepted explanation of athlete's heart, but it leads to the interesting possibility that the major training effect on the heart occurs while athletes are at rest, rather than during exercise.

THE CARDIOVASCULAR HAZARDS OF EXERCISE

The major cause of sudden, nontraumatic death in the adult population of the Western hemisphere is atherosclerotic-related heart attacks. Autopsies show that in a majority of these deaths, 75 percent of the passageways of all three coronary arteries are clogged with atherosclerotic plaque, the fatty deposits that accumulate on the interior of blood vessels.

The tragedy of coronary heart disease is that most of the deaths from it are thought to be preventable. Coronary heart disease can begin at a young age, during the progessive buildup of fibrotic, lipid-filled plaque in the walls of major arteries, which may not lead to functional blockage until decades later. Current research suggests that the lipid content of the blood is related to the consumption of animal fats, particularly cholesterol and triglycerides, and that regular exercise increases the number of *high-density lipoproteins*, which contain an enzyme that collects cholesterol and removes it from the body—an effect that also occurs with strength training (see Chapter 5). It is because both diet and exercise can be controlled by the individual that atherosclerosis is considered preventable. Moreover, control of other risk factors, such as blood pressure and cigarette smoking, also helps to protect against coronary heart disease.

The frightening aspect of coronary heart disease is that there may be no warning signs prior to a fatal heart attack. And people who feel healthy are much less likely to have medical checkups than those plagued by symptoms. According to Brown University's Paul D. Thompson, an authority on the cardiovascular hazards of exercise, the instantaneous nature of many coronary heart disease deaths suggests that cardiac arrhythmias were the immediate cause.

The most dangerous type of arrhythmia is *ventricular fibrillation*, during which steady contraction of the ventricles is interrupted by chaotic electrical discharges, which fail to produce any synchronized contractions. Loss of effective cardiac output for three to four minutes causes irreversible brain damage; any longer and death results. This is called "sudden," in contrast to cardiac arrest, which is caused by the slow oxygen starvation of the heart muscles during exertion if the coronary arteries are blocked. The agonizing pain of this type of heart attack will usually prompt the victim to seek medical help before massive muscle fiber death, fibrillation, or other complications finally stop the heart.

Thompson has found that among the many cardiovascular changes that occur during exercise, the heart is made more susceptible to arrhythmias, including ventricular fibrillation, thereby increasing the risk of sudden death in individuals with coronary heart disease. He is quick to note, however, that "there is little risk of ventricular fibrillation in normal hearts during exercise, but the combination of ischemia [the lack or blockage of blood flow] and exercise does increase the risk of ventricular fibrillation."

Because pathological symptoms can increase during physical exertion, cardiologists have devised the *exercise stress test* to detect coronary heart disease in athletes and nonathletes alike. A treadmill in a heart clinic is the most common device for stress testing, but bicycle ergometers, wheelchair ergometers, and a simple bench step can also be used. The variables measured as the individual exercises include heart rate, blood pressure, oxygen consumption, ventilation rate, blood lactate level, perceived exertion or pain—all of which are correlated to EKG readings. Today, sports physicians advise that anyone over thirty-five, especially those at high risk of coronary heart disease (indicated by family history, high blood pressure, excessive weight, or cigarette smoking), take the stress test before embarking on a strenuous physical fitness program.[3]

For those who do not have coronary heart disease, the ghost of young Pheidippides can still cause anxiety.

The occurrence of sudden death during or immediately after exercise does not prove that exercise itself caused the fatal event. In fact, one study estimated that by *chance alone*, between five and fifteen deaths per year could occur among runners in the United States. Chance could also account for 104 deaths occurring within two hours of running.

Concerned that the reports of the dangers of strenuous exercise might frighten people away from endurance training, Larry W. Gibbons, a physician at the Institute for Aerobics Research in Dallas, conducted a survey of the cardiovascular health of 2,935 adults, age thirteen to seventy-six, who used an urban health and fitness club. During the 65-month survey period, the participants in Gibbons's study logged a total of 374,798 hours of exercise in activities such as tennis, basketball, handball, and racketball, including over 1,691,000 miles of running.

During the entire survey period there were only two cardiac events and no deaths. The first complication occurred in a sixty-one-year-old executive who entered a 3.2-kilometer competitive race, although he had not been exercising regularly. He collapsed with ventricular fibrillation but was successfully revived. The second event occurred in a thirty-five-year-old man who ran 4 kilometers following a stressful meeting, although he had not been exercising regularly; he took a cold shower and suffered an acute myocardial infarction, a heart attack caused by a sudden insufficiency of blood in the myocardium. Both men survived their heart attacks and were exercising regularly at the end of the study.

After applying statistical analysis to his data, Gibbons concluded that exercising for thirty minutes, three times per week for a year (the American College of Sports Medicine guidelines for the minimum amount of exercise needed to produce any measurable training effect) would produce a *maximum* risk estimate of 0.002 to 0.027 cardiac events per year for men and 0.005 to 0.05 events for women. In simple English this means there's a risk of between two to five heart attacks for every 100 years' worth of exercise. And that's the maximum risk; the actual risk is likely to be substantially lower.[4]

For the time being, the final word in the debate on whether vigorous physical exercise protects against or provokes sudden cardiac death is from a study by David S. Siscovick, a physician at the University of North Carolina. For the first time, in one study, he appears to have resolved the apparent contradiction of sudden death in those who are trying to obtain immunity to coronary heart disease through exercise. At the center of this study were 133 men, all of whom had their first heart attack without any prior symptoms of coronary heart disease. Some were sedentary and some exercised at various levels of intensity. Siscovick found that the risk of cardiac arrest increased during exercise for those who habitually exercised, but was even greater for those with low levels of regular exercise. However, among those who habitually exercised at any level, the *overall* risk of cardiac arrest—both during and not during exercise—was only 40 percent that of sedentary individuals.

There is certainly a small risk inherent in endurance training, especially for the nonathlete who's just starting to get into shape, that undetected diseases or anatomical abnormalities will fatally manifest themselves during vigorous physical exertion. But, as Siscovick shows, *the risk of not exercising is far greater.*

Physiologist Ernst Jokl once observed, "If a person died during exercise, he did not die from exercise."

CARBOHYDRATE LOADING

Despite the critical role of the lungs, heart, and circulatory system in prolonged aerobic exercise, it is the supply of glycogen that sets the limits in endurance activity. Glycogen is the ready-to-use sugar found in the liver and throughout the muscles.

Exercise requiring the steady expenditure of 20 kilocalories per minute or more for periods greater than 90 minutes will deplete the normal supply of stored glycogen and cause a pronounced sense of fatigue, known to some endurance athletes as "the wall."

The mode of aerobic metabolism required in most sports burns both glycogen and fats to produce ATP (adenosine triphosphate) for muscle contraction (see Chapter 2). If the duration of exercise crosses the threshold of glycogen depletion, the oxidation of fats increases, but the power output falls. For reasons that are not fully understood, fats alone cannot match the efficiency of glycogen, and it is believed that the presence of muscle glycogen is essential to maintaining intense levels of exercise.

In an average 150-pound man, the total carbohydrate reserve before exercise is about 400 kilocalories of glycogen in muscles, 200 kilocalories of glycogen in the liver, and 40 kilocalories of glucose in the blood. Since blood glucose is essential to maintaining the integrity of the nervous system, the body hoards it until all other fuels have been exhausted. This leaves a carbohydrate balance of 600 kilocalories, which, if burned at the rate of 20 kilocalories per minute, would provide only 25 percent of the energy needed for a 2,400-kilocalorie marathon. Body fat or triglyceride supply, on the other hand, contains over 100,000 kilocalories, enough for 90 to 100 hours of exertion at the same rate. The oxidation of fats alone can get the marathoner to the finish line, but he'd come in behind an otherwise equal competitor who had a greater supply of glycogen.

To prolong exercise intensity at levels over 20 kilocalories per minute, athletes must develop strategies for glycogen sparing in order to stretch the supply as much as possible. This is facilitated, in part, by endurance training. Muscles respond to overload by increasing the mitochondrial content of slow-twitch fibers, thus increasing the quantity of stored glycogen and the enzymes needed to make glycogen, and enhancing the fibers' capacity to burn fats. The normal level of muscle glycogen can be raised by about 30 percent by training-induced adaptations, but training along with a dietary manipulation known as *carbohydrate loading* can more than double the supply of this vital fuel.

Dieticians spend a considerable amount of time and energy weaning athletes from a multitude of inadequate and potentially dangerous fad diets, sold as the secret formula to superhuman strength and endurance (a partial list appears in *Fig. 5.4*). Although most athletes require only a balanced diet with a sufficient supply of calories to support their daily activities, carbohydrate loading is a recognized technique for boosting the supply of glycogen prior to long endurance events. Tests have shown that carbohydrate loading prolongs the *time to fatigue* in marathon or cross-country running, cycling, swimming, and in events that combine these activities, such as the triathlon.

Contrary to locker room hearsay, carbohydrate depletion and loading does not increase speed or strength, and the evidence is at best equivocal that this technique adds glycogen to the body's normal stores for use in short-term aerobic exercise such as basketball or even middle-distance running. It has no use in noncontinuous, anaerobic activities such as football. Moreover, after a decade of experience with carbohydrate loading, it has been found that the practice does not work for everyone.

Carbohydrate depletion and loading works due to the increased production of the enzyme that synthesizes glycogen in muscles when supplies are low. In this way, athletes can stimulate the activity of this enzyme through rigorous exercise on an extremely low-carbohydrate diet. Once the process of glycogen synthesis is in high gear, the athlete rests or reduces exercise to a minimum and consumes a high-carbohydrate diet to overstock the glycogen supply. This is possible because the synthesis of glycogen in the "starving" muscles increases in proportion to the dietary intake of carbohydrates, and because the feedback mechanism that resets glycogen synthesis back to normal levels is sluggish.

The classic Scandinavian technique of carbohydrate loading is based on a study in 1967 in which needle biopsies of active muscles measured glycogen levels in relation to diet and exercise. The results found that three days of intense exercise to exhaustion on a diet of only 10 percent carbohydrates, followed by three days of rest on a ninety percent carbohydrate diet, would double or triple glycogen levels on the seventh day— ideally, the day of the competition.

In recent years, modified regimens have been recommended to avoid some of the problems associated with this technique. Although these modified techniques do not produce the same increases in glycogen, they are easier to follow. Diets containing less that 10 percent and greater than 90 percent carbohydrates, as advocated by the classic plan, are not practical, and during both extremes there is a potential for nutritional deficiencies. Moreover, the carbohydrate-depletion phase can produce hypoglycemia, or low blood sugar, and diminish exercise capacity. Several physicians have warned that hypoglycemia has induced grand mal convulsions in otherwise healthy athletes during intense exercise, and that carbohydrate loading has been linked to arrhythmias and heart attacks in runners with coronary heart disease. The more extreme the dietary technique, the greater the need for supervision or medical consultation.

Experiments to test simpler methods of stockpiling muscle glycogen, using glucose and glycerol feedings before prolonged exercise, have met with little success. There has been some headway using high liquid carbohydrate supplements to avoid the digestion problems and bulk of the classic plan during the loading phase. One of these, Gatorlode-280 has been popular with some athletes. First introduced in 1981, this apple-flavored commercial drink mix provides 280 calories and 70 grams of carbohydrates in a 12-ounce serving. It is also fortified with 30 percent of the USRDA of vitamins C and B_2, which may enhance the metabolism of carbohydrates. Clinical studies using muscle biopsies have found that levels of muscle glycogen increase twice as much with Gatorlode-280 than with the traditional pasta and rice in 50 and 90 percent carbohyrate diets.

Caffeine, the stimulant found in coffee, tea, soft drinks, and several brands of chocolate and aspirin, has been shown to enhance endurance when taken alone or as an adjunct to carbohydrate feedings before exercise. Despite the scientific literature that supports the efficacy of caffeine in enhancing endurance, its use has not been banned by amateur or professional sports organizations as a doping substance. (See list of these drugs in *Fig. 5.5.*)

Prior to its use as a glycogen-sparing agent, caffeine was known to stimulate the nervous system, increase heart rate, and raise basal metabolism. About 90 milligrams of caffeine is found in a cup of brewed coffee; over-the-counter capsules contain up to 225 milligrams each. After oral ingestion, caffeine is rapidly and completely absorbed from the intestinal tract and reaches a maximum level in the blood between 30 and 120 minutes after ingestion. The fatal oral dose in an adult male is about 10 grams.

In 1978, David Costill reported that two to three cups of coffee, about 250 milligrams of caffeine, taken one to two hours before exercise produced a 20 percent delay in the amount of time it takes to get tired. Costill and other researchers believe caffeine accelerates the release of body fats into the blood as free fatty acids, elevating fat oxidation by as much as thirty percent and sparing the use of glycogen. In muscles, caffeine may indirectly slow the breakdown of glycogen and allow more fat to be produced for energy.

In subsequent studies, trained cyclists performed 7 percent more work in two hours with caffeine compared to a placebo, and cross-country skiers completed a 23-kilometer race 2 to 3 percent faster with caffeine. In both of these studies, the competitors chose to exercise at higher than their normal intensities with caffeine, possibly reflecting its stimulant effect. Although caffeine use has been reported by football players and weight lifters, the evidence suggests that significant improvements in performance occur only in endurance sports.

The apparent effectiveness of simple ergogenic aids such as caffeine and carbohydrate loading has sparked the invention and marketing of "natural" and "organic" sports supplements by creative entrepreneurs. The endless quest for a winning edge often seems to impair the good sense of enthusiastic athletes, making them easy prey for charlatans. At the irrational extreme is the "natural loading diet," advocated by Roy Bruder, a psychobiologist and owner of a natural food store in Kailua, Hawaii. As a substitute for the classic carbohydrate loading regimen, this plan calls for small amounts of raw or lightly cooked vegetables to be consumed during the depletion phase; a diet of 90 percent fruit for the loading phase, "with some whole-grain bread if you have an uncontrollable craving for something other than fruit"; and finally, on the day of competition, "a thorough enema first thing in the morning," with nothing but fruit juice for a pre-event meal.

It's worrying to imagine how many earnest marathon runners have discovered "Nature's carbo-loading secrets," but I doubt strongly if the diet has been used by the editors of *Runner's World*, where it first appeared in print.

OVERTRAINING IN DISTANCE RUNNERS

Overtraining, or overuse, injuries occur due to a gradual breakdown in the muscles, bones, and connective tissues in a manner analogous to metallic stress fractures. Structural failure occurs when the human locomotor system receives more stress than the tissues can tolerate. Injuries begin to occur when stress load outstrips the rate at which tissues can make compensatory changes. In endurance training, the internal metabolic processes can also become overloaded to the point where they start to fail. This can lead to such symptoms as a loss of body weight, an increase in resting heart rate, a loss of appetite or anorexia, insomnia, and depression. Chronic fatigue can also lead to a loss of motivation in athletes.

Since endurance training often involves running to exhaustion, the locomotor system can give out before the internal metabolic functions show any sign of failure. Typical overtraining ailments of this nature include stress fractures in bones, skin abrasions and blisters, joint injuries, muscle tears, tendon and ligament strains, and inflammations.

From the perspective of a sports physician, distance runners are a unique group to study. The extremely high mileage they log in training and competition magnifies the effects of disorders and abnormalities like no other aerobic sport. Every time a runner takes a step, he loads his striking foot with up to three times his body weight. An equal *ground reaction force* is transmitted up through the soft tissues and bones of his foot to the ankle, leg, knee, thigh, hip, and lower back. With every stride the energy of impact is dissipated by the shoe and the deformation of these tissues, according to each individual's running technique. In distance running there are about 300 impacts per kilometer, over 12,000 in a single marathon.

Since running is not a contact sport, all injuries arise from the foot-shoe-surface interface and are mediated by training errors, abnormal anatomy, shoe design, and surface hardness. A survey of 180 injured runners by Stanley L. James, an orthopedic surgeon attached to the University of Oregon, found that 60 percent of the ailments were associated with training errors, and *excessive mileage* accounted for 29 percent of those errors. It's interesting to note that the average weekly distance for this group was just under 50 miles, and the highest was 160 miles/week. These findings are paralleled by a separate study, which found that the risk of injury in runners increases with weekly mileage.[5]

The diagnosis and treatment of these injuries often require considerable detective work. The key, especially in overtraining injuries, is the ability to accurately dissect a runner's training routine, identify the errors in his technique, assess the structural qualities of the shoes, and spot anomalies in his bone structure from hip down. This last variable is particularly challenging because very few factors of a runner's anatomy necessarily correlate with any specific injury.

When a podiatrist or orthopedic surgeon examines a runner's foot, he knows there is an ideal position in which the bones and joints will move with optimal efficiency. Efficient movements minimize stress loads to every part of the anatomy. This ideal or *neutral position* of the foot occurs when the toes are lined up on a plane perpendicular to the vertical axis of the tibia, talus, and calcaneus *(see Fig. 9.3)*.

In the presence of congenital or training-induced abnormalities, repeated stress will cause the bones to shift away from the neutral position, forcing the bones and joints to work at inefficient angles and to place unusual loads on tendons, ligaments, and the cartilage that covers joint surfaces. Before long, the athlete's running time is down, followed by pain in the heel or ankle, leg (shin splints), knee, or hip.

Pronation, a bowed heel-foot alignment, is a shift away from the neutral position; it has been linked to many disorders, particularly Achilles' tendon pain, shin splints, and a degenerative softening of knee cartilage known as chondromalacia (see "Knee Injuries" in Chapter 10). To prevent pronation from causing further damage, a popular remedy is use of an orthopedic wedge, or *orthotics*, between the foot and the shoe to return the alignment to the neutral position.

The design of shoes in all endurance sports is essential to the prevention of injury. Gideon Ariel, the biomechanist who invented the computerized exercise machine, has also revolutionized the design and testing of athletic shoes. Unlike researchers who test shoes with mechanical feet, impactors, and

FIGURE 9.3

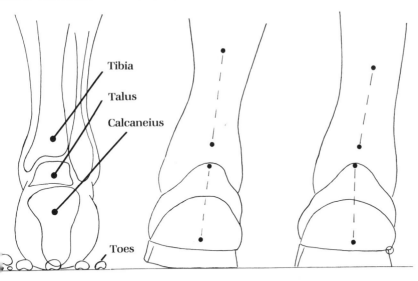

Labels: Tibia, Talus, Calcaneius, Toes

Anatomy of a human foot. When a podiatrist examines a run-ner's foot, he looks for the ideal position in which the bones and joints will move with optimal efficiency. The ideal or neutral po-sition, shown at left, occurs when the bones of the toes are lined up on a plane perpendicular to the vertical axis of the tibia, talus, and calcaneus. Pronation is a shift away from the neutral posi-tion, far right, which in excess can cause shin splints, Achilles' tendon pain, and knee injury. The runner's foot, center, has a normal alignment even though the running motion tips the foot inward.

The shoes of a runner can help stabilize the foot. Tests by the Nike athletic wear company have experimented with heel height and flare, the angle between the heel and shoe.

stretching equipment, Ariel believes that shoe performance cannot be thoroughly assessed without considering "the ath-lete in the shoe."

He began studying runners using high-speed films in con-junction with force platforms. With this equipment Ariel tested thirty-five different running shoes in 1975 and discovered that human factors were not taken into consideration in the design of athletic shoes. He found that many of the shoe characteris-tics were the exact opposite of what runners needed. Shock absorption, for example, was almost negligible in some shoes,

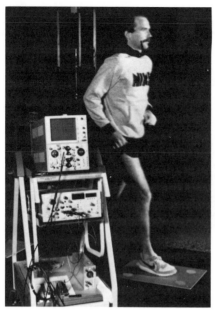

The ground reaction force and other forces involved in running can be measured on synthetic runways lined with force platforms. These platforms are so sensitive they can pick up data on how the foot-shoe-ground interface changes over a span of milliseconds. A distinct "force signature" for each type of running, from sprint starts to jogging, can be observed on an oscilloscope and chart graphs, shown to the left of the runner. (Photo by Dennis Waters/Oak Street Studio, Exeter, NH. Courtesy of Nike, Inc.)

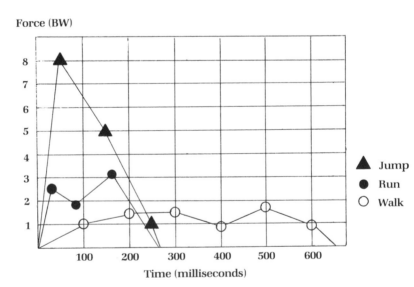

Force platforms measure the ground reaction force and center-of-pressure patterns in running or jumping. The computer recordings (above) show the marked difference between force at time of impact for a typical athlete jumping, running, and walking.

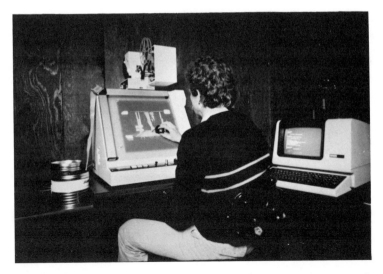

*High-speed motion picture films of athletes in motion can be
analyzed frame by frame with a special viewer, shown here. The
16-mm film is loaded into an overhead projector, shown on top
of the viewing screen, and run frame by frame, or fast forward,
or reverse with the controls at the foot of the screen. Analysis
can be made by hand or the image digitized and fed into a computer, shown at right. Here gait and foot-strike problems are being
studied by a scientist at the Nike Sport Research Laboratory.* (Photo
by Dennis Waters/Oak Street Studio, Exeter, NH. Courtesy of Nike,
Inc.)

and in others there was too much shock absorption at the wrong
area of foot-surface contact.

Much to the distress of sports shoes manufacturers, Ariel
published his findings with the conclusion that "at the present
time there are no shoes available which consider the athlete in
the shoe. In fact, some of the shoes may contribute to the injury risk factor."

In response to Ariel's research, as well as to the increasing
size, competitiveness, and sophistication of the market, and the
annual ranking of the top twenty-five shoes in the widely read
magazine *Runner's World,* manufacturers began to incorporate
shoe safety, efficiency, and performance with the biomechanics of the human foot in different types of running. Today, runners can select from over 200 models of shoes from thirty-five
makers, most of which have been designed and tested with the
athlete in the shoe, as well as by mechanically flexing, pound-

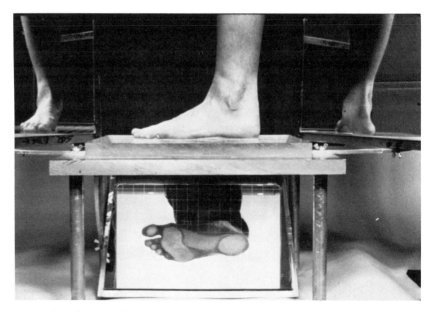

The shape and structure, or morphology, of a runner's foot can be studied using a system of mirrors that allows observation and photography from several angles simultaneously. Foot morphology studies are useful in football, basketball, soccer, and all running events. (Note slight pronation and compare with Fig. 9.3.) (Photo by Dennis Waters/Oak Street Studio, Exeter, NH. Courtesy of Nike, Inc.)

ing, dropping, ripping, sawing, and sanding it to simulate road wear.

At the Nike Sport Research Center in Exeter, New Hampshire, designers have been focusing on methods to improve rearfoot control to minimize pronation in distance running. In one recent study, the Nike engineers examined the effect of heel height, heel flare, and midsole hardness of thirty pairs of shoes on pronation (see Fig. 9.3). They used ten seasoned distance runners, who averaged between 30 to 75 miles per week, filming them from behind (200 frames/second) as they ran on a treadmill at 12.5 feet/second. The films were digitized and fed into a computer for comparison. They found that shoes with soft midsoles allowed more maximum pronation than shoes with either medium or hard midsoles; shoes with 0 degree heel flair allowed more pronation than either 15- or 30-degree flairs; and heel height had no effect on pronation or rear-foot movement.

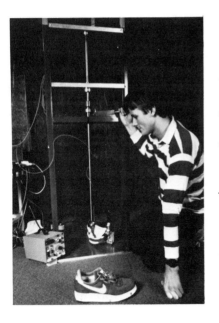

Shoe impact testing is common today for almost every type of athletic activity. As the graph on page 228 shows, each type of activity generates varying degrees of ground reaction force, from eight times the body weight in jumping to just over double the body weight for normal walking. Here a weighted shaft, instrumented and connected to a computer, is dropped onto the midsole of a shoe to collect data about its cushioning properties. (Photo by Dennis Waters/Oak Street Studio, Exeter, NH. Courtesy of Nike, Inc.)

The details of this and similar studies were integrated, fed into a computer, and are being used to design the next generation of athletic shoes.

The future of shoe design and testing is being shaped by the revolution in microelectronics. At the U.S. Olympic Training Center in Colorado Springs, the staff of the biomechanics lab is experimenting with miniature *electrodynogram sensors* to collect precise data on the forces inside the shoes of elite runners. Seven very thin, one-centimeter square (1.6-square-inch) transducers are attached to the soles of each foot, acting like separate miniature force platforms. Umbilical wires from the transducers run up the legs of the athlete to a lightweight data collection pack worn on the waist. Force data can be collected for 5-second intervals on both feet simultaneously. At the end of a run, the data is dumped from the waist pack into a microcomputer for analysis and display.

Charles Dillman, director of the biomechanics lab, believes the electrodynogram will eventually provide data more accurate than that presently collected with treadmills and pressure platforms, because measurements can be made in actual field conditions.

On another front, Gideon Ariel is designing what might be

the world's first computerized footwear: a running shoe with a microchip buried in its sole. Like the electrodynogram sensors, this chip will operate as a pressure and load gauge, recording foot impact and stride length. At the end of a training run, the athlete would remove the sensor and plug it into his home computer for an analysis of his gait, speed, distance, calories expended, and even the amount of body weight he lost. Perhaps most important, the chip has the capacity to alert the runner when he is exceeding the parameters of his training program and thus prevent overtraining injuries. If it can be programmed with the athlete's physiological profile, the intelligent shoe could warn him of impending heat stroke or even cardiac arrest.

Things might have turned out differently for Pheidippides if only he had been wearing a pair of Ariel's computerized running shoes.

TEN

SOCCER

A Game of Knees

The coach of the Santos Football Club was more than a little skeptical when Valdemar de Brito, a former Brazilian soccer star, told him of a young boy he thought should try out for the team. Considering that the candidate in question had never played in a junior division league, in fact had no experience other than rough-and-tumble sandlot ball, and was only *fifteen years old*, it's a wonder the management of one of the top professional clubs in South America didn't sack de Brito on the spot.

Yet, to the surprise of everyone, the boy got his chance, ran circles around players who were ten years older, secured a berth on the Santos's starting lineup in the 1957 season, and was elected to join the Brazilian national team in the same year. The meteoric rise of Edson Arantes do Nascimento was unprecedented in the world of soccer, or any other professional sport. In 1958, the seventeen-year-old star scored 87 goals in professional competitions, a performance record that bought him a plane ticket to Sweden with the national team to play in the quadrennial World Cup.

After sustaining a knee injury in one of the early international play-offs, do Nascimento had been forced to sit on the bench until Brazil reached the quarterfinals against Wales. Out on the pitch again, in front of a large foreign audience, he displayed dazzling legwork and popped a ball into the Welsh goal, giving the Brazilians a 1–0 victory and a shot to play France in the semifinals. He started to attract international recognition in this next round as he dribbled the ball with ease through two and sometimes three French defenders, scoring 4 goals in the

5–2 game. Sportswriters mobbed the team after the match to find out more about the sensational young player. Do Nascimento's long name was easily misspelled and mispronounced by the scribes, but they all picked up on his nickname, which within a few days would be a household word. Pelé.

On the morning of the final it was raining in Stockholm, but 60,000 Swedish fans—confident that their country's team would clinch the Cup—packed into a stadium built to hold 50,000. Dressed in wildly colored patriotic costumes, they cheered whenever their team had possession of the ball and went berserk when they took a 1–0 lead, rocking the arena with the bombilation of thousands of horns and noisemakers. Then Pelé turned the game around.

The critical play developed as Pelé stood at a distance in front of the Swedish goal, with his back to goalie Bjorn Svensson. He received a long, high pass, which he deftly trapped with his chest, letting the ball roll down his left foot. Before the checkered sphere could touch the ground, he gave it a kick, flipping it over his shoulder. Then he pivoted around while the ball was still in the air, faced the goal, swung his right foot back and blasted the ball as it came down. Svensson stood frozen in shock as the ball rocketed past him into the net.

The stadium fell silent for a moment. Even the happy Brazilians couldn't believe their eyes. Then the *Swedish fans* rose from their seats and a new sound began to fill the arena, a chant that soon developed its own cadence, a spontaneous emotional accolade transcending all allegiance to team or country. As it swelled it became clear they were crying, "Pelé, Pelé, Pelé!"

Svensson also joined in the cheering, remarking later, "I have never seen anything like that before, and I doubt I'll ever see a goal scored like that again." It was a statement echoed by many people who believe that goal was the most spectacular ever scored in a World Cup title match, which Brazil won, thanks largely to two goals by Pelé.

Over the next twelve years, playing for Santos and the Brazilian national team, Pelé would win two more World Cup titles and set an all-time career record of 1,220 goals. In 1959, the Brazilian government declared Pelé "a national asset, a national treasure," making it illegal for him to be bought by any foreign team, no matter how lucrative the offer (a decree that was overlooked when Pelé decided to play for the New York Cosmos in 1971). His international fame grew to such proportions that, while on tour in Africa, his presence brought a hiatus in the war between Nigeria and Biafra, so fans from both sides could see him play.

At one point in his career, Pelé was taken to Rio de Janeiro by Hilton Gosling, the physician attached to the Brazilian national team, where he was probed and tested at three universities in an attempt to discover the source of his genius. The scientists announced he had a very high level of endurance, peripheral vision 25 percent greater than other athletes, a reaction time a half a second faster than nonathletes, and his IQ was said to be among the top ten percent in Brazil. If accurate, these sketchy details portray a man of extraordinary dimension. Unfortunately, the actual scores of these tests were not released, either because of a misplaced concern for Pelé's privacy or for reasons of national security.

Perhaps a better measure of his genius was displayed when Pelé got together with New York Jets quarterback Joe Namath to endorse a commercial product. He was fascinated and delighted by the shape of the American football Namath was holding and borrowed it, then began bouncing it off his head as he often did with a soccer ball in practice. In this simple bit of mischief, the physical wit revealed his spontaneous capacity to mix diverse elements, come up with something new, and immediately incorporate it into his repertoire of motor skills.

The mystery of Pelé is how he acquired those motor skills so early in life. According to his family, at the age of five he was constantly kicking a big sock stuffed with rags around the streets of his home town, as he couldn't afford a soccer ball. He never went beyond the fifth grade. Neither did he have a mentor in the game. Indeed, he seems to be the perfect paradigm for those who believe "athletes are born, not made." To these notions, Pelé replies, "I don't believe there is such a thing as a 'born' soccer player. Perhaps you are born with certain skills and talents, but quite frankly it seems impossible to me that one is actually born to be an ace soccer player."

It's too bad that the young Pelé wasn't studied with modern biomechanical techniques. The early test results that showed he had a large aerobic capacity and good peripheral vision should have held little surprise; it should have also been ob-vious just watching him on the field that his reaction time, flexibility, and coordination were also above normal. Pelé could control the ball using almost any part of his body, and his foot-work was particularly mesmerizing, but a biomechanical analy-sis would likely reveal that the real magic came from his knees.

THE KNEE—ANATOMY OF THE KICKING JOINT

Science writer William F. Allman once wrote, "If God had in-tended for us to become athletes, he would not have given us knees," a clear reference to the high rate of injury in this vul-nerable joint. Despite its maligned reputation, the architecture of the knee is a marvel of evolutionary engineering, a perfect tradeoff between stability and mobility. The thumb or shoulder will pop out of its socket if forced, but the only way to dislo-cate a knee is to break the bone. As the principal weight-bear-ing joint in the leg, stability in the knee is essential for effective locomotion. One knee alone can support the entire weight of the body in motion, as its companion disengages to dribble or kick. Anyone who has seen Pelé flip over on his back, kick the ball in the air, reverse somersault, bounce up from the ground, pivot on one foot, and sprint off in the opposite direction has witnessed a complete display of the knee's range of motion. Even in less talented players, a knee can bend 150 degrees, swing from side to side, and even twist on itself while sustaining loads up to five times the normal body weight.

Studies have shown that when a player kicks a ball toward the goal, its flight path is determined by its initial launch angle, launch velocity, and the aerodynamic characteristics of the ball, factors that operate identically to those in basketball (see Chapter 2). The difference, of course, is that the soccer ball is launched by a foot.

The earliest studies of the biomechanics of kicking found that the launch angle of the ball was a function of the path of the foot during impact with the ball, and the launch velocity was primarily a function of the angular velocity of the knee. More recent studies have amended this to include other variables, such as the position on the ball where the foot strikes relative to its vertical and horizontal axes, imparting the same spin mechanics seen in basketball and baseball. The angle of foot on impact, the angular velocity of the thigh, and the linear (forward) velocity of the body are now also considered major contributors to the momentum imparted to the ball. (The sum of these factors is listed in *Fig. 10.1.*)

Pelé never studied biomechanics, but his experience gave him some natural insights laboratory studies may have overlooked. In his recent book on soccer techniques, *Learning Soccer with Pelé*, the master says, "The leg that does the kicking is less important than your supporting leg, which allows the other one to swing at a right angle. For example, if your foot of your support leg is behind the ball, the ball will tend to rise. . . . When, by mistake, the support foot is in front of the ball, the power of the shot will be reduced and the ball will probably hit the ground and ricochet." The optimal position for the supporting foot is next to the ball, or just slightly behind the ball, so that the swinging leg is almost parallel to the supporting leg at the moment of impact, providing a low, knee-high trajectory at maximum velocity.

In some ways this is analogous to the position of a golfer's feet relative to the tee in the downswing of a long drive, where optimal support of the body enables the pendulumlike swing of arms and club to attain maximum velocity at the lowest point in the swing—which should coincide with the placement of the ball (see Chapter 8). In kicking, the leg also resembles the same double-pendulum motion, reaching the highest speed at the lowest point on the downswing, at a position near the supporting foot.

Efficiency of motion often eludes biomechanical analysis because the segments of the body that contribute to overall efficiency may not be directly involved in the motion itself. Efficiency is the ratio between the energy expended in a movement and the total work done in that movement. An expert and novice soccer player, both equipped with the same biological equipment, can both expend 1 kilocalorie of energy kicking a ball at a target 15 feet away, but the expert obtains a launch velocity of 65 feet/second, and the novice only 55 feet/second. The expert has done more work with the same energy, and his higher efficiency stems from better technique.

A study of soccer players at the University of Tokyo, con-

FIGURE 10.1

Effects of the Angle and Velocity of Body Segments on the Flight of a Kicked Ball*

	Player One	*Player Two*	*Player Three*
Body velocity (feet/second)	10.2	8.5	12.6
Thigh velocity (degrees/second)	1.9	3.7	1.5
Knee velocity (degrees/second)	2008.1	1788.6	1532.2
Foot velocity (feet/second)	77.9	76.7	76.5
*BALL VELOCITY (feet/second)***	82.0	89.2	89.0
Foot inclination (degrees)	34.0	31.0	33.9
Foot path angle (degrees)	11.0	6.1	7.2
*BALL LAUNCH ANGLE (degrees)****	24.7	17.7	25.1

Quick knees are the principal force behind the speed of a kicked ball. An early study of three highly skilled football players in Australia shows that the launch angle of any ball kicked off the ground depends on the path and inclination of the striking foot, and the ball's launch speed is determined primarily by the angular velocity of knee extension. Foot path is the angle between the ground and forward motion of the striking foot; foot inclination is the angle between a plane perpendicular to the ground and a plane running between ankle and toes. Knee velocity is measured at the point (or frame in the high-speed films) that coincides with maximum foot velocity just before impact with the ball. When motions of all the body segments above the foot are added together, they do not equal the final foot velocity, and there is considerable variation in this anomaly between players. This error suggests there are other factors being overlooked in the mechanics of a kicked ball, but those listed above still remain the principal predictors of a ball's speed and trajectory.

*Source: M. B. Macmillan (1975, p. 52), in bibliography.
**Ball Velocity is the result of the factors above it.
***Ball Launch Angle is the result of the factors above it.

ducted by biomechanist T. Z. Asami, found that not only could skilled players kick the ball faster than unskilled players using the same amount of energy, but that the accuracy of the kick, as measured by bull's-eye target scores 15 feet from the players, was highest in any player kicking the ball at about 80 percent of his maximum foot velocity. From this Asami concluded that when the highest efficiency was attained in a kick, the direction of the kick was also the most accurate. In other words, the higher the efficiency, the more accurate the kick.

One link between speed and accuracy in a kicking motion is the knee. When it's not bearing the weight of the body, this joint possesses a higher degree of stability because its natural two-dimensional hinge motion is no longer compromised by the torque forces of the upper body rotating against the immobile foot planted on the ground. Instead of negotiating the three-dimensional twists, sways, and wobbles imposed on it by five times the body's weight, the knee only has to control the freely suspended leg and foot, which on the average-size athlete weigh only 4 to 5 pounds (2.9 percent of total body weight). Since the same muscles and ligaments that stabilize the knee also power and control the leg motions in a kick, maximum foot velocity and foot-path accuracy are obtained in one simple mechanical function—knee extension.

Maximum efficiency in the extension, or forward thrust, of the knee occurs when the straight hinge action is unimpaired by side-to-side wobbling. This lateral motion is contained by ligaments that circle the joint, particularly by two collateral ligaments on either side of the knee. In a healthy knee, stability is augmented by the smooth, shiny cartilage that lines the surface of the bones. Roughly speaking, the knee can be visualized as a round ball lying on a flat table, where any disturbance to the ball's stability will make it roll; cartilage acts as a gasket or ring of packing material that surrounds the ball, or rounded stump of the femur, restricting its range of motion. Additional support and stability is provided by the quadriceps, the muscle group on the top of the thigh, which contracts to extend the leg. The most important muscle of this group is the vastus medialis, located along the inner thigh, which keeps the patella, or kneecap, in place.

Strength training and conditioning of the leg muscles and connective tissue increase stability of the knee; kicking exercises in the field or with a Cybex or computerized weight machine will increase the rate and force of muscle contraction—all of which will improve efficiency.

Future advances in kicking performance will stem from investigations into the role of torso leverage on knee velocity, the placement of the supporting foot relative to the ball, the interaction of the ball and foot at impact, and the role of the quadriceps in knee extension.

According to Tzu C. Huang, a mechanical engineer at the University of Wisconsin, the angular acceleration of the knee reaches a maximum shortly after the time when the muscles of the thigh reverse the motion of the leg from flexion to extension. Huang believes the quadriceps, which play a central role in achieving the acceleration in knee extension, must also be involved in slowing knee flexion prior to pushing the knee forward. This is a phenomenon similar to the movement in a golfer at the height of the backswing—the takeaway loop—where the muscles that slow the backswing are also those that start the downswing. This means that the backward rotation of the leg of a kicker during knee flexion provides an inertial load acting against the quadriceps. It's possible that this loading, like stretching an elastic band, may provide some of the initial angular impulse in the forward motion of the kick. If true, there may be an optimal degree of knee flexion to obtain maximum velocity during extension, and once identified, it can be used as an important tool in coaching.

KNEE INJURIES

In their private moments together before facing the press, Pelé and Joe Namath joked about knees. The Brazilian's had bothered him since the 1958 World Cup play-offs, when he was benched until the quarterfinals against Wales. In the 1962 World Cup play-offs he was forced to sit out a match against Hungary (which Brazil lost) because of a knee sprain he'd gotten in a grueling game against Bulgaria days before; then he forced himself to play against Portugal and was later escorted from the field in pain. The agony came and went until he retired.

Compared to Namath, however, Pelé's knees were in perfect condition. When Sonny Werblin, president of the New York Jets, was building his franchise, he said he was looking for a quarterback "who could do more than just play." Werblin watched Namath play for the University of Alabama in the 1965 Orange Bowl where, despite pain from the first of his knee injuries, the young quarterback threw precision passes that almost defeated the favored Texas team. Werblin later said, "I don't know how to define a star, but I knew Joe had what it takes when he limped off the bench that night and 72,000 people moved to the edge of their seats."

Namath's knees dominated his life and prematurely terminated what might have been a very long, brilliant career in professional football. Just before he started playing for the Jets, doctors found that a large pad of cartilage (medial meniscus) had shredded and rolled back into a tight wad between the femur and tibia in his right knee. During the operation to remove the damaged cartilage, doctors saw that a key ligament had been stretched out of shape and had to be plicated, or pleated, with sutures. More trouble followed.

"The knee is the most poorly constructed joint in the body," reports James A. Nichols, director of the Institute for Sports Medicine at New York's Lenox Hill Hospital and the surgeon who looked after Namath's knees.

Gerald A. M. Finerman, an orthopedic surgeon at the UCLA School of Medicine, says, "The knee has a ligament system so placed that it allows for complete stability. . . . It's quite brilliant."

And a third opinion: "It's not that the knee is necessarily flawed in design, it's that people abuse it and tax the joint in ways it was never intended," says Stanley James, a consulting orthopedic surgeon at Nike's Athletics West track club, who has attended the joints of such world-class runners as Joan Benoit and Mary Decker.

Who's right?

It appears that, to an extent, they all are. The knee is an efficient, stable joint that provides a wide range of motion and mobility for walking, running, climbing, and jumping. Its critical role in basic locomotion suggests that the design of the knee has worked well since man's forebearers fell from the trees over a million years ago. As basic survival prior to the automobile depended on a durable set of legs, it is inconceivable that the present rate of knee injury has persisted over the millennia. Activities such as football, basketball, marathon running, and soccer were simply not included in the original design specifications for the knee. The millions of joggers and recreational athletes, many of whom are out of shape or abuse their bodies by overtraining (see Chapter 9), give rise to an inflated rate of knee injury, which almost certainly wouldn't exist otherwise.

Soccer's worldwide popularity—there are an estimated 22 million players—has caused a global epidemic of knee injuries. In Europe alone, soccer is responsible for over 50 percent of all sports injuries, and one survey found that of *all* injuries treated in European hospitals, including nonsport injuries, soccer-related knee injuries accounted for up to 2 percent. If this phenomenal incidence of human suffering were caused by a contagious disease, Europe would be living in a state of panic.[1]

Jan Ekstrand, a surgeon at the University Hospital in Linkoping, Sweden, studied injuries in a senior soccer division of twelve teams over one year, beginning in January 1981. During this period, 124 out of 180 players incurred 256 injuries, 20 percent of which were located in the knee, the most common site of injury. Ekstrand categorized all the soccer injuries as either minor, moderate, or major. Of the major injuries, knee ligament sprains were the most frequent (32 percent). Of the traumatic knee injuries, 61 percent occurred during collision with another player and 31 percent were caused by overtraining.

About a dozen surveys on soccer injuries in Europe have been published since 1965, and despite variations in the rate of injury, most agree on the knee's peculiar vulnerability. Ekstrand's study is unique, however, in that he also compared the rate of injury to the training and success of individual teams. He found a direct correlation between a team's success, measured by the number of goals scored, and hours of training. As a whole, teams that had accumulated over 1,400 man-hours of practice scored more than twenty goals in the season, which seems like good common sense. What doesn't make sense—especially in light of the fact that 31 percent of the injuries were attributed to overtraining—is that the number of injuries *decreased* as practice hours rose from 1,400 to 1,800. Ekstrand explains that the decrease in injuries with training is due primarily to a drop in traumatic injury; the rate of overuse injuries apparently remained constant regardless of hours practiced.

There may be a second explanation worth considering: overtraining injuries should not necessarily increase in relation to increases in exercise. *Overtraining occurs when the rate of stress exceeds the rate of adaptation.* As the athletes in Ekstrand's study were all in a senior soccer division, it is fair to assume that training was supervised, stress loads were applied in acceptable increments, and the players' tolerance to increasing hours of practice grew as their bodies became more conditioned.

In the knee, overtraining occurs when the stress load exceeds the ability of the connective tissue to adapt. A similar phenomenon occurs in tennis elbow, where microtears of the tendons surrounding the joint accrue faster than the body can heal properly, leading to inflammation and pain. The knee is more complex, bears more weight, and more can go wrong.

One of the most common knee injuries is a torn *meniscus*, one of two C-shaped disks of cartilage tucked between the femur and tibia, which helps to distribute the load evenly across the surface of the joint and also acts as a shock absorber. Repairs to a torn meniscus account for about 90 percent of all knee surgery. Problems arise if a loose piece of the meniscus becomes trapped in another area of the joint, eating away at the healthy cartilage, impairing movement, and often causing excrutiating pain. The outer third of a healthy meniscus has an active blood supply, which allows it to grow new tissue in response to wear and tear, an adaptation similar to work calluses on hands. But this process is slower than the rapid adaptations seen in muscles. Although the quadriceps and hamstring in the thigh may seem to be gaining strength through training, connective tissue around the knee does not respond as quickly, and overtraining can literally grind these tissues down to the bone.

Another common injury from overtraining is a ligament tear, although this can occur in highly conditioned athletes from a traumatic injury, such as a fall or collision with another player. When torn, the collateral ligaments, which keep the knee from bending sideways, heal quickly. The two cruciate ligaments, which cross each other inside the knee joint, are difficult to repair once torn.

Injuries to the knee are further complicated by the reaction of the *synovium*, or protective lining of the joint, which lubricates the knee by secreting a fluid with a viscosity just higher than that of cooking oil. In the presence of a loose shred of meniscus, an inflamed ligament, or just as the result of a traumatic blow to the knee, the synovium will produce an excess amount of lubricant as a defensive reaction, causing stiffness and swelling in the joint, commonly known as water on the knee.

The potential for overtraining, which can lead to these injuries, is high in soccer, especially during preseason practice, when the body hasn't fully adapted to the rigor of constant running, jumping, kicking, and otherwise overloading the knee. According to Ekstrand, a soccer player takes about 15,000 steps during a game, roughly equivalent to running a marathon.

Any athletic activity involving prolonged stress on the knees can lead to an overtraining injury. Distance runners seem to be most vulnerable and, in addition to the maladies described for soccer players, can experience an inflammation of the patella tendon and acquire a condition known as *chrondromalacia*, where the underside of the kneecap is so worn that it begins to resemble shredded crabmeat. The abrupt twisting stops in basketball can completely rupture the patella tendon, requiring surgery and long, tedious hours of therapy. Tennis players often rip their meniscus. Skiers can tear knee ligaments as easily as they can snap a bone.

Fortunately, advances in orthopedic surgery have kept pace with the explosion of knee injuries and today it's possible to send a player back out to the pitch, whereas only a decade ago he might have had to sit on the sick bench for months. The first practical breakthrough was *arthrography*, an X-ray technique developed in the mid-1960s. A special dye is injected into the knee, clearly highlighting all the tissues, thus making a diagnosis easier. Then came *ligament reconstruction*, a process by which tendons are transplanted from other parts of the body and sewn into the knee to increase stability.

Arthroscopy, introduced a decade ago, allows surgeons to peek inside the knee using a small fiber-optic light and lens system, so that the architecture of the knee can be inspected and repaired without slicing the entire joint open. More than any other orthopedic advance to date, the arthroscope has accelerated the rate at which athletes can return to the field. Joan Benoit is a well-known example. In April 1984, after sustaining an injury to her right knee that caused pain that even rest would not cure, and facing the Olympic marathon trials in May, she went to see Stanley James, orthopedic surgeon of the Athletics West track club. He used arthroscopic surgery on her knee—a technique he compares to "building a ship in a bottle"—and snipped off a cluster of collagen fibers in the front of her knee that seemed to be causing the problem. *Seventeen days later* she won the U.S. Olympic marathon trial with a time of 2:31:04, and in August won the first Olympic women's marathon ever held.

Although traumatic injuries to the knee are unpredictable and difficult to prevent, injuries from overtraining are generally considered 100 percent preventable. Jan Ekstrand, the orthopedic surgeon who authored the studies on the incidence of soccer injuries, devised an injury-prevention program that he tested in a random trial, using twelve Swedish soccer teams. Half of them were put on the program, the other half served as controls. The test group used a special twenty-minute warmup session before every practice or game, during which calisthenics were replaced by ten minutes of relaxed ball passing and ten minutes of stretching and flexibility exercises. Each practice session was followed by a five-minute cool-down period of jogging and stretching. Players with knee instabilities were excluded from play, and those with prior ankle injuries were taped, even if they no longer had any symptoms. Finally, all players were issued plastic shin guards, which extended from the top of their shoes to just below the bottom of their knees.

As a result, the injuries to the test teams were 75 percent lower than to the control groups. In addition, the most common types of soccer injuries, sprains and strains of the knee and ankle, were significantly reduced. Studies such as this, which show that stretching and other passive warmup techniques are effective in preventing injuries, help to underscore the need to incorporate these techniques into athletic training. Despite this evidence, cold showers, calisthenics, sprint drills, and shots on goal remain the predominant method of warming up for soccer practice.

Overtraining in soccer, as in other sports, can be avoided by carefully orchestrating the stress loads applied to various anatomical structures of the body, which do not all adapt at the same rate. The relatively rapid response of skeletal muscles to strength or endurance training, for example, is not mirrored in the connective tissue of the knee. Although a 6 percent increase in leg strength may be obtained after several weeks of intensive training due to hypertrophy of the muscle fibers, the ligaments in an adult knee do not respond in kind and are *just* capable of stretching six percent of their length in a year. If they are forcibly and suddenly stretched to this length or beyond by the newly acquired power in the leg muscles, they will snap.

Gradually increasing the stress loads placed on the knee, or any other joint, is the only known way to maximize the training effects of exercise and also prevent injuries. Just before practice, stretching and flexibility exercises prepare muscles and joints for the higher levels of stress to follow. Warmup exercises prepare tissues for change, actually raising their temperature, making them more malleable. During practice, increases in exercise intensity and duration must not outstrip the body's ability to adapt.

An estimated 20 percent of all novice runners have knee problems severe enough to require a doctor's attention within the first three months of training because they're imposing loads faster than the tissues can respond. Over 30 percent of all joggers—and there are 10 to 15 million of them in the United States—suffer from an overtraining syndrome known as runner's knee. These injuries may cost the health-care system a billion dollars every year and exact an unfathomable cost in pain and suffering—and they are largely preventable.

Of the patients seen by Stanley James, the orthopedic surgeon who operated on Joan Benoit, 60 percent come to him with injuries from such training errors as excessive mileage, a rapid increase in exercise intensity, or a sudden change in an athlete's training program. "The body is a tremendously adaptable mechanism, but it takes time to accommodate stress," says James. "Unfortunately, most people are not willing to give the body time to adapt."

AGING AND ATHLETIC PERFORMANCE

In the first fifty years of World Cup competition, Brazil was the only nation to win the trophy three times, an accomplishment that must be credited heavily to the presence of Pelé. Then, in 1982, the Italian national team—the Azzuri—equaled this feat in Madrid with a decisive 3–1 victory over West Germany in the final match.

Italy possessed no Pelés, although twenty-five-year-old Paulo Rossi proved to have a deadly foot. For twenty years their game has been primarily defensive, a stark contrast to Brazil's aggressive and constantly innovative offensive style. However, if there was a single hero on the Azzuri team it would be goalkeeper Dino Zoff, the much-admired team captain. During the play-offs he was a decisive factor in coordinating the tactics of the Italian defenders, and when the ball slipped through, his awesome gymnastics in front of the goal constantly frustrated the challangers' shots.

Aside from his remarkable talents on the pitch, Zoff is best known for his longevity. In 1982, at age forty, he was the oldest player to ever appear in a World Cup final, his hundred and eighth international game. His professional career began in 1961. Ten years later he joined Juventus, a perennial power in the Italian league, where for a seven-year stretch he kept substitute goalies sitting on the bench—not once during his reign did any of them play one minute for Juventus. At one point, he set a division record of 1,145 minutes in the goal without allowing a single ball into the net.

Unlike older American baseball heroes Pete Rose or Carl Yastrzemski, Zoff has never touched a weight-lifting machine, nor does he follow a strict diet, as does forty-nine-year-old discus thrower Al Oerter. Yet his skills never seemed to wane with the passing years. Today Zoff is the deputy director of the Italian Football Commission, a position he accepted after retiring in 1982.

In soccer the better goaltenders are, on average, much older than players in active field positions. On the professional level, a goalie enhances his physical performance with a long memory, which comes with age, of the feints and shots opposing players have used in the past. In 1958, the Swedish goalie Bjorn Svensson was caught with his pants down when Pelé pulled his trick shot in the World Cup final, but if he had to face Pelé again it's unlikely he'd be fooled twice.

The goal mouth measures 8 yards wide by 8 feet high, a large area to protect from balls being shot from 20 to 50 feet away, traveling at speeds of up to 90 feet per second and swerving with the unpredictability of a knuckle ball. At this velocity, a ball shot from 20 feet takes 0.22 second to reach the net—in which time the keeper must somehow propel his body over 4 or even 8 yards to intercept the ball. This split-second timing leaves little margin for error. The old goalie's ability to anticipate a shot is worth much more than the faster reflexes of the young rookie.

The tradeoff between the experience of age and the vitality of youth only works in certain positions in a limited number of sports. Successful athletes over thirty are usually found in events that demand explosive strength and precise motor skills, but do not require a high aerobic capacity (although 80-year-old marathon runners do occasionally cross the finish line ahead of competitors half their age). Discus thrower Al Oerter, who won the last of four Olympic gold medals in 1968 at the age of thirty-two and almost made it to the 1980 and 1984 Games, is a classic example. So is Yankee knuckle-ball pitcher Phil Niekro. At forty-six, he's the oldest pitcher in the major leagues, out-hurling players young enough to be his children. As of 1984, he had won 268 games, lost 230, and struck out 2,912 batters in 4,619 innings. Only eight other pitchers in history have struck out more batters.

Dino Zoff's retirement came as a surprise to many because his age had not affected his performance, and after the 1982 victory he vigorously denied having any plans to quit, saying, "Other players have gone on longer than I." Insiders insinuated that Zoff capitalized on his World Cup notoriety and accepted the prestigious post on the Football Commission before his fame faded, swapping a few more years in the goal for long-term job security.

Whether or not this is true, the gossip highlights the abbreviated duration of peak-performance years in competitive athletics. In professional sports, an aging star may have a well-preserved body not significantly different from that of teammates a few years younger, but when it's time to renew his contract the telltale deterioration in performance will put him on the unemployment line. In amateur sports, the Olympic hopefuls caught in the 1980 boycott of the Moscow Games were distraught, not over ideological objections to Jimmy Carter's decision, but because in the four years until the Los Angeles Games most of them would be past their prime. Four crucial years.

The perception that the glory dies before the man can have a profound psychological effect on any athlete who's worried about age—even adolescent gymnasts. Former baseball slugger Mickey Mantle, now employed by a chemical company, has a recurrent dream that he's stuck in a taxi trying to get to Yankee Stadium. Once he arrives the young security guard doesn't recognize the champion and won't let him inside. Locked out, Mantle finds a hole in the fence just big enough to look through and sees his friends Whitey and Yogi and Casey getting ready to play. Suddenly, over the public address system he hears, "And now batting . . . number seven . . . Mic-key Man-tle!" Then he wakes up, palms sweaty.

A. E. Housman's tribute "To an Athlete Dying Young" includes the lines "And early though the laurel grows/It withers quicker than the rose." It's sadly ironic that our athletic heroes, whose vitality and daring often seem to mock death, are touched so young by the process of aging. But there's justice. This outrage of mortality is somewhat balanced by the certain knowledge that many of the effects and diseases of aging are reduced or eliminated through lifelong athletic endeavor.

If Dino Zoff's present desk job reduces the time he previously spent in active exercise, the effects of his twenty-two-year career will begin to vanish. All the hard-earned physiological adaptations will be thrown into reverse: muscles will shrink, aerobic capacity will decline, reflexes will fail. These effects do not happen simply because he is now forty-three years old; they are the result of *hypokinesis*, the disuse of vital functions, which accompanies a sedentary life-style. It would have occurred if he had become inactive at thirty or even twenty. The symptoms of disuse and aging are so similar that it's tempting, but incorrect, to think they are the same phenomenon. Is there *any* link? Does disuse accelerate aging? Or does aging amplify the effects of disuse?

The language of gerontology, the study of aging, can be confusing, and the perplexity of terms used to describe "getting old" reflects the present uncertainty about the biological process of aging, especially as it relates to exercise, training effects, and performance. Most researchers are in agreement about the general effects of aging easiest to observe in the general population: as time passes for any individual the risk of death increases. In addition, as public health has improved in the last 300 years, the life expectancy has increased. Today the average life expectancy is about 85 years. The maximum life span, however, has remained at about 110 years for the past three centuries, in spite of tremendous advances in medicine.

Many believe that the maximum life span, which has remained constant for so long regardless of nurture, is an absolute limit imposed on the individual by something resembling a genetic clock. Place a culture of bacteria in a petri dish, give it the best possible conditions in which to thrive, and each individual bacterium will divide and multiply—and then the process suddenly stops. Depending on species, there appears to be an absolute limit on the number of cell divisions. Most human cell cultures divide fifty times, then die. Identical twins tend to die within two to four years of each other; fraternal twins within eight to ten years.

If we assume for a moment that we could clone a hundred people from the same genetic material—basically making a hundred identical twins—and we knew from prior experiments that under ideal conditions they had a maximum life span of 100 years, then we could draw a straight line from the day of birth to the day of death a century later and this would describe the *rate of aging*. In this hypothetical situation, the clones would age at the rate of 1 percent per year. As they approached their maximum life span we would expect aberrations in their genetic material to produce defects in their anatomy and physiology. For example, their bones would lose their minerals, connective tissue would lose its elasticity, fluids would seep from tissues like the lens of the eye impairing vision, muscle fibers in the heart would contract with less force, and cardiac output would fall. These inevitable defects could be generalized as the *effects of aging*, and in the ideal environment they would culminate in death in the hundredth year, give or take four years to allow for the random expression of aberrant genetic material among individuals in our group.

However, if we took the clones out of the ideal environment and scattered them around the globe, the results of the exper-

iment would be entirely different. Exposure to natural radia-
tion, mutagenic chemicals, and viruses would randomly dis-
rupt their genetic material and it would appear as if the effects
of aging had started prematurely. Our group would also be exposed to environmental factors that had no direct effect on their
genetic processes—variations in diet, traumatic injury, bacte-
rial infection—but still appeared to hasten the onset of the effects of aging. By the end of the experiment, few if any of the
clones would live to be 100. On the average, most would live to
about 85, conforming to the life expectancy of the general population. In other words, the rate of aging would be accelerated
by environmental factors.

Back in the real world, there is considerable disagreement
among gerontologists about the relative contributions of genetic versus environmental factors on the effects of aging and
the rate at which they appear, but all agree that the process of
aging is affected by both. The real controversy doesn't begin,
however, until the sports scientist gets involved.

In Belgium, at the University of Liege, physiologist Vassilis
Klissouras studied twenty-three identical and sixteen fraternal
twins (who share only 50 percent of the same genes), ranging
in age from nine to fifty-two years, to see what intrapair differences might exist in functional adaptation to athletic training—where adaptation is considered an expression of the genes
and training a factor of the environment. He measured VO_2max,
EKG, heart volume, maximum heart rate, maximum muscular
force, and even nerve conduction velocities. Some of the twins
had been separated for many years and had led different lives;
others had lived together since birth.

In all the variables measured, except VO_2max, Klissouras found
nothing but diversity among intrapair adaptations to exercise,
suggesting that physiological changes in the body are pro-
foundly affected by training even in individuals who have
identical genes. The exception was VO_2max, which showed remarkable intrapair similarities among identical twins but not
among fraternal twins, suggesting that oxygen uptake may be
influenced primarily by hereditary factors.

In one intriguing case, forty-nine-year-old fraternal twins had
a different VO_2max despite similar life-styles: one had an oxygen uptake of 32 milliliters per kilogram per minute (ml/kg-min)

251

and the other 45 ml/kg-min. They had lived together all their lives, had the same profession, and had both played competitive soccer from early childhood until they were twenty-two. What happened to these men? Why weren't their maximum oxygen uptake levels higher and why were they so different?

The phenomenal aerobic demands of playing soccer for over a decade require much more oxygen than their test levels indicate, implying that they once had a higher aerobic capacity, but they lost it when they became inactive. Assuming that VO_2max is strongly influenced by the genes, Klissouras concluded that the reversal of their training-induced adaptations was also controlled by their genes. In other words, without continuous stimulation of sufficient magnitude from training the level of oxygen uptake in an individual reverts to a baseline set by heredity; in this case, the baseline was different because the two subjects were fraternal twins.

Out in the general population, surveys have also found that inactivity produces changes in the body that appear to be almost identical to the effects of aging. Similarly, clinical studies of sedentary *or* elderly individuals who are put on an exercise program have found there to be a rapid improvement in physiological functions and a reduction of the apparent effects of aging.

At present, the cutting edge of this research is the new science of space medicine, which has gathered a tremendous amount of information of the effects of physical activity on healthy, conditioned astronauts, and correlated it to the effects of aging. The large number of across-the-board similarities between the effects of aging, life in the confines of space, and earthside inactivity must be more than coincidence. It remains unknown, however, how these three states of being affect each other.

At present the only certainty is that endurance training, and to a much lesser extent, strength training, reverses the majority of the degenerative effects associated with hypokinesis and many of the effects associated with aging. One study, for example, looked at middle-aged, sedentary midwestern males and found that a vigorous conditioning program can recapture *forty years'* *worth* of VO_2max. A study at the University of Toronto found that men and women, age sixty to eighty-three, can improve their VO$_2$max by 24 percent in only seven weeks of endurance training. A similar study found a 40 percent increase in seventy-year-olds with three months of training. At the University of Southern California, physiologist Herbert deVries found that 112 males, ages fifty-two to eighty-seven, who participated in jogging, stretching, or swimming for only one hour, three times a week, under supervision, experienced an improvement in oxygen transport capacity, as well as improvements in work capacity and blood pressure. Exercise has also been shown to improve the mineral content in the bones of the elderly, even at age eighty. Training will also improve the range of motion in the shoulder by 10 percent and in the ankle by 50 percent after twelve weeks.

Evidence of this nature continues to mount. Of course, no reputable gerontologist has claimed that physical inactivity is the cause of aging, nor that athletic endeavor is a cure for aging, but nearly all agree that training is capable of retarding or reversing the *effects* of aging. If nothing else, this research clearly shows that there is a method to at least improve the quality of life for sedentary and elderly individuals.

Although this is good news for gerontologists, the social implications may be even more profound.

In 1985, approximately 50 percent of the U.S. population was over fifty years old. Soon the "baby boom" of the 1950s will become a senior citizen explosion—and the socioeconomic consequences could be devastating. Over the next three decades the nation's economic base will come to depend more and more on the production of a dwindling number of young, healthy people in the work force, who will also be required to divert their limited resources to the care of a predominantly elderly society. What will become of national defense, health care, Social Security, welfare? At no other time in Western civilization has there been such a disproportionate demographic shift.

There is no miracle drug in sight that can restore forty years of VO$_2$max, nor is there ever likely to be, but this astonishing achievement now appears obtainable with exercise alone. Who would have suspected that scientists working with athletes over the past twenty years, looking for new ways to shave a few seconds off the mile run, or looking for methods to keep a thirty-year-old athlete in his prime, would stumble upon such a simple and effective remedy for the effects of aging?

Today, individuals may elect a life-style that will diminish the rate of aging. Tomorrow, well, tomorrow we may have to endure fifty-year-old Olympic hopefuls complaining that the latest boycott deprives them of performing just when they were at their peak.

ELEVEN

EXTREME ENVIRONMENTS

From Chomolungma to Death Valley

In late 1977, a group of Austrian alpine climbers announced that they had assembled a team to scale Everest. Ordinarily, this wouldn't have caused much of a stir, as sixty-five men, two women, and one seventeen-year-old boy had already stood upon the roof of the world. If anything, the Austrian expedition sounded a little flaky: plans for the adventure included live television broadcasts from the summit, a hang-glider flight from 24,000 feet, and a final ascent by two men without the use of supplemental oxygen.

The Austrians' announcement would have passed unnoticed but for the words "without oxygen," which evoked memories for some physiologists of the days when men argued that Everest could be scaled "with lungs alone." That notion was buried when Edmund Hillary, with tanks and mask, made it to the top in 1953, but the plans of the young Austrians made more than a few old-timers wonder if it was still possible.

Certainly the human body has the capacity to adapt to the thin air of high altitudes, an observation first recorded by Jose de Acosta, a priest and chronicler attached to the Spanish conquest of Peru in the 1530s. In his report on the Incas, de Acosta pointed out that Spaniards accustomed to life at sea level became strangely ill if they ascended directly to the mountain homes of the Indians, but those who had meandered through the plains of intermediate altitude seldom displayed any symptoms. Although the physiological mechanisms causing this malady remained a mystery for centuries, the Spaniards soon concluded that the body could adapt to high altitudes given enough time, but if their lust for gold, glory, and exotic women exceeded their caution, then the alien "mountain sickness" would strike, sometimes with deadly results.

Today millions of people live in oxygen-impoverished environments and lead active, healthy lives, performing the same forms of work and exercise as at sea level. The fact that the 1968 Olympic Games were staged successfully in Mexico City, at an altitude of 7,350 feet, demonstrated that athletic performance is not adversely affected at this height—indeed, the reduced air resistance and gravity may have contributed to several world records.

Mexico City and Denver, Colorado (5,400 feet), are considered to lie within an altitude range that requires only minimal adaptation, but the summit of Mount Everest (29,028 feet) is considered an *extreme environment*, where external stress is generally beyond the ability of the body to adapt, no matter how long it's given to acclimate. The extremes of high and low temperature, high and low air pressure, are fascinating natural laboratories for the sports scientist. It's not that a large number of athletic events are conducted in these conditions, but that competitions in more hospitable climes often simulate or approach these extremes.

Extreme environments also pose a more fundamental interest for sports scientists, who are constantly looking for ways to translate the adaptive responses of the human body to new performance records. Can training in simulated tropic conditions help the urban marathoner ward off heart stroke—or even improve his time in the heat? Can high-altitude training increase oxygen transport in a manner analogous to blood doping (see Chapter 2,) to enhance endurance at sea level?

Conventional athletic training obtains specific adaptations by overloading the body with measured doses of stress, carefully designed around the physical demands of a sport. Environmental physiologists are not constrained by these practical considerations. When they apply themselves to sports research, they will expose any willing athlete to extreme environmental conditions, often simulated in the lab, monitoring every vital sign, taking dozens of tissue samples, observing the volunteer's behavior around the clock—hoping to net a new and unexpected adaptation.

EXPOSURE TO ALTITUDE

In the same year Father de Acosta was filing his report on the effects of altitude on the health of his *conquistadores*, a Spanish priest of the Jesuit mission to Akbar, the Mongol emperor of Hindustan, published the first known map of the Himalayas. "Peak XV," known to the natives as Chomolungma, or Goddess Mother of the World, held no interest for the West until Andrew Waugh, the surveyor general of India, suspected that this noble peak was one of the highest in the world. After carefully considering the protocol of tradition, he decided to name it "Mount Everest" to commemorate his predecessor, Sir George Everest. The Royal Geographic Society in Britain agreed it was an excellent choice and made the new name official on world maps in 1866.

Of course, the Goddess Mother had been explored by Sherpas, Tamangs, and other Tibetan tribes centuries before British colonial rule put Everest on the map, but not a scrap of native folklore alludes to any ancient hero who had scaled the summit. The mountain had remained inviolate from the day it emerged from the collision of continents until the first half of the twentieth century.

In 1922, a British assault pushed beyond the 25,000-foot mark, using oxygen for the first time. This early equipment was awkward and heavy, prompting some climbers to question its necessity. The oxygen debate continued into 1924, when E. F. Norton led a British expedition to Everest, taking oxygen along, but hoping not to use it.

At 25,000 feet, Norton began to feel the deleterious effects the thin air had on human behavior. The simplest tasks seemed to require phenomenal energy, and a lethargy pervaded his team. It took Norton four hours to convince his usually reliable Sherpa porters to agree to ascend just another 2,000 feet—and in return he promised they could quit and return to base camp. Once that had been accomplished, he reported, "We no longer had any porters to stimulate, and this was fortunate, for as you near 27,000 feet you have no great surplus of determination."

At 27,500 feet, Norton started seeing double, his resting pulse had jumped twenty beats per minute, his extremities felt very cold despite "perfect weather," and mental confusion often made him think he was slipping. As the cost of exertion became too dear, he turned back at 28,126 feet, resigned to letting the men with the oxygen flasks make the next assault. They went up, with less than 1,000 feet to the top, but never returned.

Even after Edmund Hillary made the first successful ascent in 1953 using oxygen, Norton remained convinced that a fit man could make the summit without masks and tanks. Physiologists, who now had a good idea about the energy requirements of exercise and the amount of oxygen needed to produce that energy, came to disagree with Norton. The air on Everest was too thin to support the metabolism of an active climber. Some believed there wasn't enough oxygen to support basal metabolism. Although the amount of oxygen in the atmosphere remains at a constant 21 percent up to an altitude of 350,000 feet, the air is compressed by the arms of the earth's gravitational field, resulting in a larger number of gaseous molecules—hence higher pressure—at sea level and fewer molecules of oxygen at higher altitudes. Everest was deemed beyond the pale.

Then, as now, the effects of hypoxia—oxygen insufficiency—are relative to the body's ability to adapt. As de Acosta noted, slow ascent to 18,000 feet can be accomplished with little discomfort, aside from an occasional shortness of breath, a temporarily diminished work or exercise capacity, and an irregular breathing pattern at night, called Cheyne-Stokes syndrome. If ascent is too rapid, hypoxia will bring on symptoms of *acute mountain sickness*, often within two hours of changing elevations. Acute mountain sickness usually starts around 10,000 feet, but can vary among individuals from 6,000 to 15,000 feet. The illness arises from the chemical imbalances caused by the lack of oxygen, especially an increase in water in the brain and cerebrospinal fluid, and symptoms usually include headache, insomnia, loss of appetite, vomiting, tachycardia (rapid heart action), and breathing disturbances. As the body adapts, the symptoms subside, usually within two to three days. In rare cases, however, pulmonary edema (waterlogged lungs) or cerebral edema can occur, and both are life-threatening if the victim is not moved quickly to lower altitudes.

Mountain climbing would be a physically exhausting activity even at sea level. At 20,000 feet, with up to thirty pounds of equipment and clothing, it's a wonder it's possible at all. Although the body adapts by improving oxygen transport, the climber must also make compromises with nature. If he is to avoid exhaustion or hypoxia at 20,000 feet, he must cut his work load in half; if he was capable of eight hours of climbing at 10,000 feet, he must reduce this to about four hours of active climbing. This is usually accomplished by establishing an ascent cadence, climbing for five or ten steps and resting for an equal amount of time. A sea-level athlete might be tempted to push himself to provoke further adaptation, but neither prolonged exposure nor greater exertion at 20,000 feet has ever led to improved levels of acclimation. In fact, adaptation to altitude levels off at 18,000 feet—11,000 feet below the summit of Everest.

All things considered, it would appear that Norton was wrong—lungs alone are not enough. Yet he came within a thousand feet of his goal.

Reinhold Messner and Peter Habeler, the two Austrian climbers who proposed to make it to the top without oxygen, had of course studied all the problems and were aware that expert opinion was decidedly against them. Messner was a very accomplished climber who had two Himalayan expeditions under his belt; in one of them he conquered Hidden Peak without using fixed ropes, high camps, or oxygen. "By fair means" was Messner's philosophical approach to Everest, but in truth that would only be possible if all the experts had made a basic miscalculation somewhere.

Certainly, the thirty-three-year-old Messner was in good condition to take advantage of any oversight. He had been clocked climbing 1,000 meters (3,281 feet) vertically in thirty-four minutes, work that required about 4 liters of oxygen per minute.[1] Assuming this is 75 to 80 percent of his VO_2max, then 100 percent VO_2max would be about 70 milliliters of oxygen delivered to every kilogram of tissue per minute, which represents a high level of fitness at sea level. Of course, at 29,000 feet, maximum oxygen consumption falls off sharply (see Fig. 11.1). If Messner's hearty lungs could continue to deliver, say, 70 per-

FIGURE 11.1

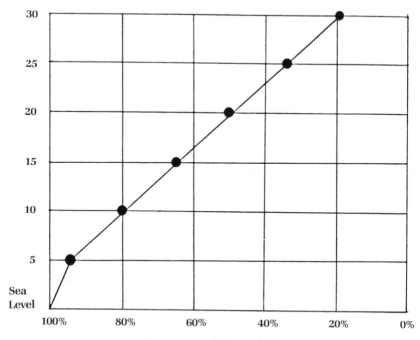

Feet (Thousands)

Percentage of Normal VO₂ max

Reinhold Messner's greatest challenge in his bid to climb Mount Everest "with lungs alone" was that the body's ability to consume oxygen declines rapidly with altitude. This is shown in the graph above. If Messner's maximum aerobic capacity, known to be about 70 ml/kg-min, could work at 70 percent VO₂max throughout his climb, his body would receive only 11 ml/kg-min at the summit. This is enough to support a casual walk on a sunny beach, but hardly enough for climbing the world's tallest mountain.

cent VO₂max throughout his climb, then a rough calculation predicts that at the summit he'd receive only 11 milliliters of oxygen per kilogram per minute, perhaps enough to support a casual stroll on a sunny beach, but hardly enough for climbing the peak of the world's tallest mountain, with temperatures in the range of minus 40 degrees Celsius.

On the other hand, these figures suggest it was at least theoretically possible for Messner to survive at the summit and move around cautiously if he could get there, whereas a less fit climber with a VO_2max of 60 ml/kg-min, even working at 75 percent capacity, could deliver only about 9 ml/kg-min at the summit, enough to maintain basal metabolism at home in bed.

Messner's hunch that there had been a miscalculation somewhere was right in one respect. In 1978 no one had ever taken a measurement of the air pressure at the summit, and if they had it would have been known that it was substantially higher than predicted by standard International Altimeter Calibrations, the method of barometric readings by which aircraft deduce their altitude. In 1981, a scientific expedition to Everest found the pressure at the summit close to 250 millimeters of mercury (the same yardstick used in domestic barometers), whereas the predicted pressure was 235 millimeters of mercury, giving the summit a "physiological altitude" about 1,500 feet lower than its surveyed value. The reason for the higher readings on Everest is that barometric pressure 4 to 16 kilometers above sea level fluctuates with latitude, due to the large, cold mass of air in the stratosphere above the equator, squashing the air below. At 28 degrees North latitude, Everest climbers actually enjoy more oxygen than they would on mountains farther to the north due to this equatorial bulge in the atmosphere.

In planning their ascent without oxygen the Austrians must have also anticipated, or at least hoped for, marginal errors in actual oxygen transport in the blood beyond those predicted by theory. Though the extent of altitude-induced adaptation is fairly established, the net physiological benefits are difficult to quantify because there are so many different—and apparently contrary—changes occurring in the body of a lowlander placed at an extreme altitude.

The first and simplest reaction of the body to the shortage of oxygen is to increase the rate of ventilation to compensate for the "shortage of breath." This brings the level of oxygen back to normal, but as the production of carbon dioxide in the body has remained constant, the faster breathing flushes more carbon dioxide out than oxygen coming in. This results in a drastic imbalance in the acidity of the blood; the tissues become alkaline and normal biochemical processes are disrupted. After two to three days, the body manufactures less sodium bicarbonate, which neutralizes body acids, so the problem of excessive alkalinity passes. Sodium bicarbonate, however, is used to mop up many acids, including lactic acid, which forms as a waste product of anaerobic metabolism (see Chapter 2) and is linked to fatigue. Thus, in the presence of reduced sodium bicarbonate, a climber must rely more on aerobic metabolism to avoid the early onset of fatigue, but the Catch-22 is less oxygen to support aerobic metabolism.

After a few days at a new altitude, the higher rate of ventilation returns to normal levels as the number of red blood cells increases. Within hours of oxygen deprivation, the effects of hypoxia stimulate bone marrow to produce more red blood cells, which can increase by about 25 percent in only a few days. In a simpler world we would be able to predict exactly how much more oxygen was being carried in the blood. Normally, each gram of hemoglobin can transport 1.33 milliliters of oxygen; at sea level a healthy man has 15 grams of hemoglobin in every 100 milliliters of blood, and after acclimation his hemoglobin will increase to 20 grams. But at high altitudes, the atmospheric pressure is lower outside as well as inside the lungs, so that the partial pressure systems that coax oxygen into the lung's blood vessels are not as effective. Due to this low pressure, hemoglobin is only saturated with a fraction of the oxygen found at sea level.

Red blood cells make a second adaptation to altitude that further complicates the estimate of how much oxygen is actually being delivered. In response to the stress of hypoxia, the billions of new red blood cells are manufactured with a higher concentration of a chemical—2,3-diphosphoglycerate—that *decreases* the affinity of hemoglobin for oxygen. At first this seems to make no sense. We'd expect the legions of new red blood cells would be equipped to grab more oxygen as they passed through the lungs, not less. It turns out the reason for increasing the dissociation factor between oxygen and hemoglobin is an attempt to make it easier for oxygen to detach from the hemoglobin when it arrives in the tissues. The loss of oxygen accumulated in the lungs due to the decreased affinity of hemoglobin is compensated by the increased number of red blood cells. But, as all these factors must vary from individual to individual at different altitudes (or levels of hypoxia), it is difficult to put an exact number on the net improvement in oxygen transport caused by the multiple adaptations.

The increase in red blood cells is also accompanied by an inexplicable drop in blood plasma, the fluid medium that contains and moves the solid particles, collectively known as the hematocrit. As plasma declines in proportion to the hematocrit, the viscosity of the blood goes up. As recently as 1978, the Austrian expedition scientists believed that when the hematocrit exceeded 50 to 60 percent, the blood would become too thick to circulate through the microscopic capillaries supplying vital tissues. According to this theory, if climbers removed some of their blood and replaced it with plasma or some other neutral fluid, the alleged viscosity problem would clear up and oxygen transport would be improved.

When the Austrians had reached 15,000 feet, two physicians on the team experimented with this theory on themselves, removing a whisky bottle full of whole blood from each other. Almost immediately their acclimated bodies became acutely hypoxic and they were confined to their beds, breathing emergency oxygen until they had readjusted to altitude. Disappointingly few physiological measurements were made during the Austrian expedition, but following this near disaster, hematocrit counts were occasionally recorded. They soon discovered that it never exceeded 60 percent unless a climber became extremely dehydrated, so that the theoretical viscosity problem could be prevented if an adequate fluid intake was maintained. Subsequent research has found that the effects of blood viscosity are mediated by the muscle tone of the blood vessels, and animal experiments found no impairment of oxygen delivery to active muscles when the hematocrit was artificially raised as high as 70 percent.

When Messner and Habeler set out toward the summit, the first team of four Austrians had already reached the top and returned using oxygen. In camp, feelings were divided on whether the risk of an assault without oxygen would be too great. The doctors warned of brain hemorrhage or convulsions, but Messner, who had earlier refused to let the physicians draw any of his blood, did not have great faith in expert opinion, although he was worried by the experience of one of the mountaineers in the first assault. At 28,000 feet this Austrian had tried climbing for a while without oxygen and said, "It took all my strength . . . simply to thrust out my chest to take in air." He also reported such profound mental confusion—"as if in a trance, I thought I was floating above the ground"—that he considered a final ascent without oxygen impossible.

Nevertheless, Messner and Habeler proceeded, hoping to make it as far as possible, but taking two small bottles of oxygen with them for emergencies. At their last camp, at 28,000 feet, the going was as tough as predicted. They woke often in the middle of the night gasping for breath. At 28,500 feet, wading through knee-deep snow, they collapsed after every few steps. Talking required too much effort and they used sign language: Habeler pointing down, Messner shaking his head, pointing up. And then a sudden storm hit them.

The struggle to make the last 100 yards is described graphically by Messner in his book *Everest.* "Peter Habeler and I dragged ourselves on all fours along the summit ridge in a snowstorm. We could only manage five meter stages before collapsing in the snow, gasping for breath for a full five minutes or more. This was the only way we could compensate for the lack of oxygen and muster sufficient strength to continue. The last hundred meters of height took us more than an hour to climb."

Once at the top, Habeler was beset with cramps and, fearing something worse, immediately began to retrace his steps. Messner stayed to take photographs, but his degree of mental confusion was apparent: at one point he took fresh film from his pocket to load into the camera, but threw it over the mountain instead; he laid down to catch his breath and suddenly thought he had been there for hours. It is truly remarkable that he made it off the summit in this condition unassisted, especially over the treacherous stretch known as the Hillary step.

The success of Messner and Habeler made headlines around the world and prompted curious physiologists to try to figure out how it had been accomplished and how close the Austrians had come to disaster.

A group of American "climbing scientists" headed by John West, a physician and physiologist at the University of California, organized an expedition to Everest in 1981 to investigate Messner's feat and learn more about the adaptations of the human body to high altitude. Known as the American Medical Research Expedition to Everest (AMREE), the fourteen scientists and six highly experienced Himalayan climbers established a rigid, prefabricated laboratory at base camp (17,700 feet), and minilabs in shelters in high camps at 20,700 feet and 26,400 feet. From the first day of operation they monitored blood chemistry, lung gases, VO_2, EKG, and sleeping EEG in all participants when possible, including a few samples taken at the summit.

Blood samples taken at the summit yielded some interesting clues about the biological activity inside the bodies of Messner and Habeler as they struggled in the thin air. Although the AMREE climbers all used oxygen, experiments indicated that acute hypoxia threatened the tissues of the Austrians, despite their high degree of fitness and acclimation. As they hyperventilated, often for a few minutes between every few steps, the carbon dioxide was rapidly flushed out of their bodies and must have caused extreme alkalosis—much higher than West had ever anticipated. At about 17,500 feet, there is no further improvement in the removal of sodium bicarbonate from the body, and as the Austrians pushed themselves higher, panting and gasping, they threw the acid balance of their blood and tissues completely off the scale. That neither climber experienced serious discomfort other than cramps and confusion is difficult to understand in light of the impairments in their body chemistry.

After reviewing all the data, West believes that Messner and Habeler must have had a maximum oxygen consumption that provided them with little more than the requirements of basal metabolism. That, coupled with the failure of Norton's oxygenless assault and the anecdotes of the Austrian climbers, led West to conclude that altitudes of about 29,000 feet must be near the limits of human tolerance. If Everest was another 1,000 feet higher (said to be geologically possible) or another 20 degrees to the north of the equator, Messner and Habeler may never have reached the top.

West also conducted experiments to see how oxygen deprivation might affect the brain. The AMREE climbers were given neuropsychological tests before, during, and after the expedition, measuring the functions of memory and coordination. The test results indicated a significant decline in verbal learning and short-term memory while subjects were living at altitude, but their scores return to pre-expedition levels within a year. The most significant abnormality to emerge was a reduction in the "finger-tapping speed test." Here the subject depresses a simple lever with one finger as rapidly as possible over a period of ten seconds. Of the sixteen scientists tested, fifteen showed continued impairment after the expedition, and thirteen members still had the abnormality one year later. West says this type of impairment has been found in other altitude studies, but the cause is not clear. It could be related to brain dysfunction, possibly permanent, caused by prolonged and severe hypoxia—although the AMREE scientists all used oxygen whenever it was needed.

If this test does indicate brain damage from oxygen insufficiency at high altitude, the effects on behavior and motor performance do not seem to be profound in seasoned climbers, some of whom have spent decades crawling on the mountains of the world, a pastime that requires exceptional motor skills and mental stability if one is to survive.

On the other hand, maybe Reinhold Messner *did* acquire a little brain damage during the Austrian expedition: he repeated the experiment in 1980 with a *solo ascent* to the roof of the world.

EXPOSURE TO EXTREME TEMPERATURES

The ability of human beings to survive almost anywhere on the surface of the earth is due to the fact they are *homeotherms*, maintaining a relatively constant body temperature with a wide range of physiological mechanisms. The capacity to function more or less independently of the environment's temperature, augmented by intelligence, is a principal reason man has become the dominant species on the planet. Animals such as reptiles and insects are *poikilotherms*—their body temperature fluctuates with the environment—and they live at the mercy of the elements.

Despite the body's homeothermic properties, the temperature of the environment has a profound effect on athletic performance. The extremes of hot and cold weather impair exercise capacity and with prolonged exposure have killed many athletes. "Hot" and "cold" are, of course, merely the subjective perceptions of physical temperature, or the measure of heat. At absolute zero (− 273.16 degrees Celsius), any substance has absolutely no molecular movement, or no heat. Any energy applied will increase molecular motion, making the material warmer.

In the human body, which lives and dies by the dance of molecules within its trillions of cells, too little heat brings the biochemical economy to a standstill, too much heat increases the kinetic movement of molecules to the point at which they break away from the chemical bonds that hold them to other molecules, and cell structure deteriorates. Thus, at body temperatures above 44 degrees Celsius, nerve cells begin to denature, and heat stroke, brain damage, and death will follow, unless temperature is rapidly reduced. At body temperatures below 32 degrees Celsius body metabolism is greatly reduced, and cardiac arrhythmias, coma, and death follow unless temperature is raised.

The body adapts to extreme temperatures as it does to other forms of environmental stress, but as yet, sports scientists have found no practical applications that can be used to enhance performance, although many interesting possibilities suggest themselves.

In cold environments, acclimation is characterized by a slower onset of shivering. Of course the body has to be exposed to the cold to adapt; living in heated buildings, using heated transportation, and wearing layers of clothing will not produce any physiological response. (There are cases, in fact, of overdressed people living in cold environments who have suffered heat stroke.) The reason behind the delayed shivering is not understood, although many physiologists believe it results from an alternative method of heat generation (nonshivering thermogenesis). If this method of heat production can be isolated and controlled, it might lead to an energy-sparing strategy in competitive winter sports. Shivering is the result of muscle contraction, which can increase basal metabolic rate by three to five times, using substantial amounts of glycogen. For an endurance athlete who carbohydrate loaded (see Chapter 9) and began shivering prior to the beginning of exercise, the extra stores of glycogen would be depleted at a faster rate, reducing his competitive edge.

The primary adjustment to the cold by the circulation is vascular resistance, causing a reduction in blood flow to the skin. Ironically, a second characteristic of acclimation to the cold is the maintenance of the temperature of the hands and feet after weeks of exposure. How this is done without recruiting an increased blood flow to the surface of the extremities is unknown. It has been suggested that the body selectively inhibits vascular restriction in the hands and feet of cold-acclimated individuals; others think it may be a form of chemical thermogenesis.

Several studies have shown that improved physical fitness brought about by intense endurance training improves the body's tolerance to the cold, with average skin temperatures warmer by 1 degree Celsius and extremity temperatures warmer by 5 degrees Celsius, compared to temperatures before training. Core temperatures in trained subjects did not change, nor did contraction speed or force in muscles (which is known to decline with temperature).

The body's circulatory response to heat is the reverse of its response to cold. The vessels dilate to enhance the conduction of excessive heat in the core of the body to the skin, where it can be released into the air. This is facilitated by a 10 to 15 percent increase in blood plasma volume within five days of exposure. There is also an increase in sweat capacity, from 1.5 liters per hour to 4 liters per hour.

The dangers of excessive heat buildup in the body are known to most athletes: dehydration can seriously impair performance, and continued exertion after dehydration can lead to heat cramps in the skeletal muscle, weakness and low blood pressure associated with heat exhaustion, and collapse seen in heat stroke. Heat acclimation significantly delays the onset of these systems by increasing the capacity to remove heat from the body, but researchers believed, for many years, that acclimation could only occur in warm weather environments.

According to Carl V. Gisolfi, a physiologist at the University of Iowa, heat acclimation can be obtained by training in a cool environment. His research is based on an original but controversial study that found that competitive distance runners performed as fully heat-acclimatized men during *winter months* if they participated in only 85 minutes of moderate exercise in 23 degree Celsius dry heat. This suggested that physical training in a cool environment "preacclimated" the runners for their summer events, a finding thought to be absurd by many exercise physiologists.

Gisolfi recently conducted a study that supports this idea and seems to have silenced the critics. He obtained a 50 percent improvement in heat tolerance from eight weeks of moderate training on a treadmill, working out for 100 minutes a day in a temperature of 27 degrees Celsius temperature. These adjustments were found to occur in both men and women and were unrelated to their aerobic capacity or other traditional yardsticks of athletic performance. The key to an improvement in thermal tolerance with training in a cool environment, says Gisolfi, is to maintain an elevated internal body terperature through exercise for a sufficient period of time to produce an adaptive response.

Even acclimated athletes run the risk of dehydration if they don't replace the fluid lost through sweating—and the rate of loss can be surprisingly high. One study of marathon runners found that the average loss of fluid ranged from 1.5 to 3 liters per hour. Dehydration is defined as the loss of body fluid in excess of 1 percent (700 milliliters) or more, and these figures represent losses of 2 to 4 percent within the first hour of the race. Without replacing these losses, after two hours between 4 and 8 percent deficits would occur.

The effects of dehydration begin with thirst (1 percent deficit), discomfort, irritability, and impaired performance (5 percent). More dangerous symptoms follow: difficulty in swallowing (7 percent), difficulty walking and moving (10 percent), delerium and shriveled skin (15 percent), skin cracking and bleeding (20 percent). This last is the maximum tolerance point before death. In conditions of extreme heat or exercise, dehydration beyond 10 percent usually leads to heat exhaustion and heat stroke. If the victim is not rested, cooled, and rehydrated, the heat will kill him before dehydration does.

What should an athlete drink to rapidly replace fluid losses during exercise? The answer to this question depends on who is asked. Physiologists are almost unanimous in their belief that water is best because it contains no additives to slow its exit from the stomach to the intestines, where it's absorbed into the bloodstream. Some athletes, however prefer sweetened or fla-vored sports drinks to water. The manufacturers of sports drinks, a $75 million a year market in America, claim their products are even better than water. The maker of one "thirst quencher" said its product got into the bloodstream "twelve times faster than water." Many sports drinks are advertized as "isotonic," having the same solid-to-liquid ratio as natural body fluids, which allegedly accelerates the rate of absorption.

These claims became too hard to swallow for Edward F. Coyle, an exercise physiologist at the University of Arizona, who con-ducted clinical trials on three popular sports drinks and water to determine their gastric emptying rates. After fasting for twelve hours, twelve volunteers were given 400 milliliters of the var-ious drinks. After fifteen minutes, the contents of their stom-achs were evacuated with a tube. As expected, water left the stomach faster than any of the other drinks, and those drinks with low sugar content were close behind. The sports drink with the slowest gastric emptying time, 35 percent slower than any of the other drinks, was Gatorade, with 4.5 grams of carbohy-drates per 100 milliliters of fluid. This confirmed findings of other studies, which indicated that sugars in sports drinks are the primary factor in determining the rate of emptying; a carbo-hydrate content in excess of 2.5 grams/100 milliliters appears to be the threshold at which fluids are retained in the stom-ach.

The mechanism that retards gastric emptying in high-car-bohydrate drinks is a receptor in the duodenum, the first part of the small intestine, which responds to the osmotic pressure created by solutions flowing through it from the stomach. Con-trary to popular belief, exercise has no significant effect on gas-tric emptying rates.

Sugars are added to most sports drinks (see Fig. 11.2) to im-prove taste. But some advertisements would have athletes be-lieve the carbohydrate content gives them a quick energy boost. In fact, sugars entering the bloodstream just prior to and dur-ing exercise can have the opposite effect, triggering the release of insulin and the rapid onset of fatigue (see Chapter 5).

FIGURE 11.2
Contents of Selected Sports Drinks*

Drink	Carbohydrates	Sodium	Potassium
	(grams per 8-ounce serving)		
Apple juice	30	trace	248
Coca-Cola	24	20	trace
Energade	30	106	31
Gatorade	12	115	23
Orange juice	29	2	500
V-8 juice	11	738	unknown
MAXIMUM CONCENTRATION	6	.055	.046

Too many nutrients can spoil the drink. That's the message from the American College of Sports Medicine (1975), which has published guidelines for the maximum concentration of carbohydrates and electrolytes in sports drinks, based on clinical studies that have measured the rate at which popular drinks are absorbed into the bloodstream. Although proper nutrition is essential to peak athletic performance, a high concentration of some nutrients in sports drinks may impair an athlete's ability to replace fluids during exercise lost through sweating. Water is the best drink for rehydration, but sports drinks can be used if diluted to conform with the ACSM guidelines.

*Source: adapted from Beckwith (1981), in bibliography.

Similarly, too many electrolytes can spoil a sports drink. Although some drinks claim to be isotonic, because potassium, sodium, and various chloride salts have been added, many are actually *hypertonic*—compared to the ratio of solids to fluid in the blood, they contain too many electrolytes. When these drinks are ingested they draw body fluids into the stomach to help dilute them, decreasing fluid supply in the blood, which defeats the purpose of fast rehydration during exercise. The dilution process also delays gastric emptying.

Diluting sports drinks with three to five parts of water will reduce excessive electrolytes and carbohydrates without totally destroying palatability. If an athlete refuses to dilute his drink or drink plain water, however, physiologists say the commercial sports drinks are still better than risking dehydration by drinking nothing at all.

THE FRONTIER: CHRONOBIOLOGY

Time is a critical factor in all biological activity and a measure of performance in many sports, yet it is seldom considered a component of the environment, like temperature and pressure, to which the body adapts. Although time is not a form of external stress, time-related functions in the environment—such as the variations in daylight with latitude, seasons, and the revolution of the earth—trigger profound biological responses in the body. Body temperature, metabolic rate, levels of alertness, arousal, sexual activity, and other functions have all been found to vary with time.

As some biological activities are inherently discontinuous, like eating and sleeping (although it may appear that some people indulge continuously in either), physiologists believe an internal regulating mechanism evolved to optimize these activities to time-related cues in the environment. Nocturnal predators, for example, are at their physiological peak during the evening; hibernating species experience a drastic reduction in metabolism during winter months. These are alternations in function prompted by an internal biological clock that sets itself according to sensory input from the environment.

Human beings who use rapid air transportation and live in steady-state climate-controlled buildings can easily confuse their internal clocks. When American athletes travel to South Korea for the 1988 Olympics, they will pass through at least eleven time zones; without time to adjust to these changes, jet lag will destory their chances of success. Similarly, amateur athletes who have daytime jobs and train at night in indoor gyms may not perform up to their nighttime peaks. The understanding of these time-related problems is essential to ensure that athletes perform their best, but the real promise of *chronobiology*, the study of biological functions in relation to time, lies in the ability to manipulate the body's biological clock in ways that might enhance performance.

At Harvard Medical School, chronobiologist Charles Czeisler is investigating the effects of time on the biological clocks of selected athletes, in a study sponsored by the U.S. Olympic Committee. At one time, the biological clock was an abstract idea, presumed to exist in the brain, but its location defied detection. Today, Czeisler and other researchers believe the clock is a pinhead-size cluster of only 10,000 neurons in the brain. Called the *chiasmatic nucleus*, it controls many physiological cycles, including the release of key hormones.

National champion body builder Larry Bernstein spent some time in Czeisler's Neuroendocrinology Laboratory, staying awake for forty-eight to seventy-two hours at a stretch, sitting in a computerized exercise chair, working out once every four hours. Every twenty minutes, samples were taken from his saliva and blood, once every three hours from urine, and continuous monitoring checked temperature, body motion, and EKG. The windowless lab was kept at a constant level of illumination, since changes in lighting alter the amount of hormones released in the body. Long after Bernstein left the lab, Czeisler and his staff analyzed the samples, looking for billionth-of-a-gram changes in hormones, correlating them to changes in temperature, exercise, and actual time of day.

Using this data from Bernstein and other athletes who come to his lab, Czeisler can track the twenty-four-hour cycles of biological activity, or *circadian rhythms*, in his athletes, plotting how they begin to deviate in the artificial environment without sleep. Many athletes and their coaches say that adequate sleep is essential for peak performance, although there is very little known about the physiological and psychological effects of sleep loss on athletic activity. Sleep is one of the key components in the study of circadian rhythms, an activity most people have always assumed involves healing and growth. Recent evidence suggests the contrary and raises interesting questions about why people sleep, whether there is an absolute need for sleep, and how this passive period might be manipulated to benefit performance.

According to J. A. Horne, a prominent sleep researcher at the University of Loughborough in England, the popular belief that sleep is essential to growth and repair of the body's tissues is based on studies finding that certain anabolic or tissue-building hormones, such as human growth hormone (see Chapter 5), are released in greater quantities during sleep. Horne points out that the breakdown of tissues, or catabolism, and assembly of tissues, or anabolism, is a continuous activity that takes place twenty-four hours a day. There is no substantial scientific evidence that anabolism is increased during sleep, says Horne; in fact, it appears that anabolic activity is geared more to the supply of nutrients than rest. One study has found that after eating, the manufacture of proteins throughout the body increases, whereas "fasting" after dinner—which happens during sleep—causes a 27 percent reduction in anabolism and a 35 percent increase in catabolism. This trend peaked about five to seven hours after the last meal (in this study, 2:00 A.M.), and continued through the night until after breakfast. Refeeding, not wakefulness, reestablished the daytime pattern of anabolism.

Dozens of studies have shown that when volunteers are subject to eight to eleven days without sleep, there is no failure in the body's ability to repair and grow new tissue, as long as sufficient nutrients are supplied. This also translates to the capacity to perform exercise or do work. Studies involving three to five days of sleep deprivation found absolutely no effects on strength or endurance and no alternations of heart rate or VO_2 uptake. There have been many similar studies to support these findings.

On the other hand, everyone knows from experience that sleep is essential; in scientific studies it is difficult to keep most people awake for more than ten days without drugs. Sleep seems essential to the brain, but it is not known why. After only a few days of sleep deprivation, most subjects become irritable and suspicious, speech becomes slurred, and there is abnormal EEG activity in epileptics; but the lack of sleep does not induce psychotic states described in popular films and literature. According to Horne, the cerebrum, the upper portion of the brain, appears to be functionally disconnected from the lower parts of the brain and the rest of the body during sleep.

In discovering that sleep plays no significant role in physiological functions, chronobiologists gain considerable scope in designing alternative sleep strategies around biological cycles that do affect physical performance. One of these cycles is known as the *diurnal rhythm*, distinct morning and evening patterns of activity, marked by peaks of body temperature and motor skill efficiency over the day, as well as peaks in the subjective perception of fatigue and arousal. Unlike circadian rhythms, which seem to affect almost everyone, diurnal rhythms vary considerably among individuals and affect performance in various sports differently, opening the possibility of custom-made training schedules.

In a recent study comparing the diurnal performance of golfers to water polo players, no differences could be found among low-performing athletes; but in the high-performing group, golfers showed consistently higher morning scores, and the water polo players were better in the evening, suggesting optimal times of day for playing these two sports. A study of aerobic capacity in which athletes cycled to exhaustion at 95 percent VO_2max on stationary bicycle ergometers found that although there was no significant effect of time of day on *perceived* exertion, their exercise tolerance time and total work done did peak at 10:00 P.M. Of course, studies like these need considerable substantiation before practical changes can be made in scheduling sports activities, but they do suggest that coaches and trainers need to reassess the traditional training schedule of "early to bed, early to rise," and that some athletes may consistently underperform because arbitrary schedules are imposed on their natural diurnal and circadian rhythms.

Research in chronobiology has also exposed spurious notions such as "biorhythms" as having no basis in reality. Serious inquiries about biorhythms from elite athletes, particularly in track and field, prompted researchers to take a careful look. The theory is that human behavior is influenced by three cycles, beginning at the moment of birth and continuing throughout life with fixed periods. The physical cycle is said to affect characteristics such as strength and endurance, the emotional cycle affects judgment and moods, and the mental cycle affects intelligence and concentration. The great appeal of biorhythms is their simplicity; they offer a plan anyone can follow to maximize performance. However, innumerable studies have found absolutely no correlation between biorhythms and athletic performance; those who advocate biorhythms have never had a study published in peer-reviewed scientific literature.

"The future is wide open," says Charles Czeisler, "but we don't want to get into a situation like biorhythms, making assumptions and predictions based on little evidence. At present we don't know where this research will lead. Certainly it should prove helpful . . . [to] athletes with practical problems such as jumping time zones. Meanwhile, we'll keep taking measurements, sifting through the data and hope to find a basis for reliable environmental scheduling."

TWELVE

THE FUTURE OF ATHLETIC PERFORMANCE

Human athletic activity spans an enormous range, from the 50-meter sprint finished in seconds to bicycling odysseys covering thousands of miles and months of time. Each event requires different skills and different levels of strength or endurance, yet quite remarkably, among *all* events there is a steady progression of new records set over time, a progression that seems relentless.

In the past century, the men's long jump record has increased by about 66 percent, the distance of the shot put by 100 percent, and the ski jump by a phenomenal 700 percent.

The rate of acceleration for footracing over all distances has averaged about 2.5 feet per minute per year. On an annual basis, this rate of growth may seem like a crawl, but measured over the past 100 years, it represents a staggering improvement.

Can these records continue to grow indefinitely, and if not, when and where will they begin to taper off?

Despite evidence that structured athletic events have been held for thousands of years, from the Uto-Aztecan Indians of Mexico to the ancient Greeks, accurate written measurements of performance were first recorded in England only in the mid-nineteenth century. If the progression of records is plotted from this point in time, all growth trends can be represented by upward swinging, parabolic curves, which have known mathematical characteristics that can be extrapolated, or projected into the future.

It is this apparently smooth and orderly progression of records over the past century that makes predictions of short-term performance quite reliable. Tests of the reliability of the extrapolations were conducted by several analysts for the Tokyo and Los Angeles Olympics with a high degree of success. Of course, actual performances never precisely fit the extrapolated curves, which only reflect general trends. In the last century, for example, the distance for the men's long jump has improved from 19 feet 5 inches to 29 feet 2.5 inches; but the smoothness of improvement is apparent only over time. Close examination shows there were long periods of little or no change between 1901–21, 1935–60, and recently between 1968–85, contrasted by sudden advances in 1872, 1896, 1900, 1935, 1964, and 1968.

Although over the long run, world records in all events appear to be eroding at an astonishingly steady rate, most analysts believe the parabolic curves cannot continue to climb indefinitely—the curves must begin to flatten, or exhibit *asymptotic deflection,* sooner or later.

At Massey University in New Zealand, biophysicist Trevor Kitson has tinkered with the growth curves of athletic records to see when a leveling off could be anticipated. He began by finding the average annual growth in the time it took to run the mile, marking records as of January 1 every year, from 1914 to 1984. The resulting curve predicted that the mile will be run in just under 3:45 in 1987 and just under 3:30 by 2023. When Kitson followed the projected curve all the way to end of the time axis, he predicted that on August 1, 2528, the mile will ultimately be run in *no time at all.* Even with the bizarre physics of Einstein, it's difficult to imagine how this could be accomplished, and if it could, Kitson predicts it would be "a feat which will presumably ruin athletics as a spectator sport."

Kitson then looked at the changing records for the mile over the last thirty years, instead of the last seventy, and found that the current world record of 3:47.33 is likely to stand until 1987. Then the curve begins to flatten dramatically, suggesting that the "ultimate mile" will be run near the turn of the century in 3:46.66. This prediction, however, based solely on the extrapolation of past records, stands in sharp contrast to other predictions for the mile, which use the progression of world records

FIGURE 12.1
Men's Track Records for the 100-Meter, Mile, and Marathon Races

Year	100 Meters	1 Mile	Marathon
1925	10.37	4:10.4	2:29:01
1950	10.10	4:01.4	2:25:39
1975	9.95	3:49.4	2:08:33
1985	9.93	3:46.3	2:08:13
2000	9.74	3:44	2:04:20
2025	9.65	3:40	2:04:10
2050	9.50	3:35	2:04:00
"Ultimate"	9.00	3:00	1:37:30

Will sports decline as athletes approach their "ultimate" limits? For the first 100 years of accurate athletic records, made possible because of the introduction of precise chronometers, such as the stopwatch in the mid-nineteenth century, growth trends maintained a steady rate of improvement. In recent years, however, analysts such as Kitson (1984) have detected a flattening of the upward curves, suggesting that man is beginning to reach his ultimate level of athletic performance, at least as it is conceived today. Predictions beyond 1985 are made both upon the extrapolation of existing trends and anticipated improvements in technology, training, and various physiological and biomechanical factors. The "ultimate" performance values were calculated by Rumball (1970) based on a coefficient of fatigue for various distances, which he believed at the time would occur around 2075, but given the more recent predictions of several other authors, would more likely occur between 2100 and 2175. See Jokl (1984), Lloyd (1982), Ryder (1976), and Wilkinson (1982) in the bibliography for information behind the predictions listed above.

only as a starting point to map the physiological growth of champions (see Fig. 12.1).

An alternative approach for charting the future of athletic performance is based on calculations of the maximal amount of energy an "ideal athlete" can generate in a given event. Factors involved in such calculations include the energy required to move the body over the required distance, the energy needed to overcome air resistance (which changes with altitude), the extra power needed if a footrace is held on a circular track, and the energy gained from the elastic properties of modern running surfaces. These and other considerations produce a mathematical expression of when the ideal athlete will literally run out of energy, a *coefficient of fatigue*, for various times and distances.

Another approach is to find the theoretical biomechanical limitations of limb movement—the absolute top speed at which muscles can contract and move an arm or leg over a given range of motion. This method is used in short, explosive events where a coefficient of fatigue has little application. In the 100-meter sprint, for example, one study found that the knee appears to limit the rate of energy with which the legs can move, setting a ceiling on stride frequency, and thus speed.

Regardless of the method used to predict the future of performance in any event, all present techniques lead to a flattening of the century-old growth curves, and ultimately to what some call the "absolute limits" of athletic performance. But the notion of absolute limits has always provoked some controversy.

The conventional school of thought holds that despite the ongoing breakthroughs in training and technology, man will reach his ultimate level of performance in all events within the next 100 to 125 years. As this level is approached, many futurists predict that new sports will arise, as well as new methods of measuring existing events—for instance, races will be clocked in increasingly smaller fractions of a second.

A more optimistic, but unorthodox view is that there are no limits to athletic performance. Certainly, at first glance, this seems no more than wishful thinking, but the idea deserves some exploration.

Reinhold Messner climbed to the top of Everest without oxygen, but if the mountain had been another 1,000 or 3,000 feet higher, would he have made it? Obviously, somewhere between the peak of Everest and the hard vacuum of space there is an absolute limit for maintaining metabolism in the thin air. Similarly, the laws of physics suggest there is a ceiling on how far a quarterback can throw a spiral, or how many pounds a weight lifter can press. But these limits are hard to pinpoint due to the incredible adaptability of the human body. Whenever someone makes such a prediction, even when it's based on the most ingenious calculations, they are courting embarrassment. One need only remember how Roger Bannister broke the "insuperable" four-minute mile. Athletes can frustrate and confuse scientists, especially when it comes to predictions of performance, and there is a pleasant justice in this.

One of the best cases in which the experts were caught unprepared for a spectacular athletic feat, was the still-standing 1968 record long jump by Bob Beamon at the Olympic Games in Mexico City. At that time, the officials used an optical measuring device that could slide down a rail 28 feet in length. No one thought anyone would jump beyond this range; the previous gold medal winner in 1964 hit 26 feet 5 inches.

Beamon, who had no full-time coach, had nearly fouled out in the qualifying rounds, and had engaged in sexual intercourse the night before, did not feel confident. But when it was his turn, he stood on the runway motionless for twenty seconds, then sprinted forward and leapt 29 feet 2.5 inches—a jump hailed as one of the greatest athletic achievements of all time.

Because the jump was longer than the measuring rail, Beamon didn't realize what he had done. The officials had to roll out an old fashion tape to measure the distance. When Beamon finally learned of the extraordinary record he had just set, his legs gave out and he sank to the ground in a cataplectic seizure, overcome with tears and nausea.

Beamon's jump prompted University of Kentucky physiologist Ernst Jokl to develop a new concept in sports science, the *mutation performance.* "If you follow sports records, you know the rate of improvement is fairly constant, but in the case of Beamon, the magnitude of improvement had no precedent," observed Jokl. "In biology we talk about the appearance of new structures that do not have any precedent and we call them mutations. Beamon's long jump is what I call a 'mutation performance' because it has no precedent. In sports as in biology, new phenomena will arise unexpectedly, shatter our perception of what is normal, and constantly surprise us about the ability of the human body to adapt and excel."

Predictions of athletic performance do not allow for the "Beamon effect." Indeed, all predictions of future performance are based on the human body as it is known today, as if it were a static, inanimate mechanical device—and this may be a greatly

281

flawed perception. In some respects, sports science has proceeded to a point analogous to physics prior to Einstein: New-
tonian mechanics was a useful tool for understanding and predicting local physical events, like the apple falling from a tree,
but anomalies in the orbit of Mercury or the behavior of suba-
tomic particles eludes classic mechanics. Today, as classic biological principles such as oxygen debt and the constancy of
muscle fiber type are challenged by observations and tests of
athletes, there is a need for an imaginative reassessment of the
human body.

Until quite recently, blood flowing through the body was
treated as if it had the physical properties of a fluid like water
and tissues were treated as solids obeying Hooke's classic laws
of elasticity—approaches now known to be wrong as biologists
continue to gather new data on the mechanical properties of
biological tissues. Cartilage, for example, is now seen as a two-
phase material—acting as *both* a solid and a liquid—which helps
to explain and understand its simultaneous mechanical and
lubricative behavior. Thus, descriptions of blood or cartilage
based on earlier models fail to accurately predict their behavior in the extremes of human exertion.

Living materials possess a property that has no counterpart
in the inanimate world. Unlike all of the materials studied by
engineers, the sports scientist must consider the capability of
living tissues to grow, to resorb, and to adapt to stress. Living
tissues defy predictability because they can change dimension
and sometimes alter their mechanical properties. But perhaps
most important, organisms evolve from generation to generation.

Unless these dynamic qualities of the human body are considered, predictions of "ultimate performance" will necessarily
fall short of the mark. The rate of evolution, in particular, can
dramatically alter the expectations of human potential only 50
or 100 years from now.

The most significant difference between today's athlete and
the athlete of only a half century ago is physical stature. Today's champions are taller and heavier than those of the 1920s
and 1930s. Although there have been no significant functional
or geometric changes in the human body in recent history, the

size of muscles has grown in proportion to the height of athletes. The ratio of cross-sectional area of all skeletal muscles to their length is 1.13 to 1. As brute strength, disregarding motor recruitment patterns (see "Strength Training" in Chapter 1), is set at about 100 pounds per square inch of cross-sectional area, a few inches in overall height can double muscle strength. The average athlete who is 6 percent taller than his counterpart in 1925 possesses 13 percent more muscle strength. In fact, studies have shown that the maximal work output of the average athlete today is over 20 percent higher than forty years ago.

In addition, increases in body mass correspond to increases in endurance, as the number of mitochondria and red blood cells, blood volume, and heart and lung size have also increased proportionately. Thus Jokl has found that today's athletes have a 13 percent higher rate of oxygen uptake than those of forty years ago.

Of course, the increase in stature does not necessarily confer advantages in all sports. In gymnastics, for example, smaller may still be better, as the increase in muscle mass is offset by increases in body weight. In a simple chin-up, a taller athlete's arms must lift a bigger body. In such sports as basketball or football increases in stature have obvious benefits. One study has found that in the past thirty years, there has been a 10 percent increase in weight and a 6 percent increase in the speed of the 40-yard dash in the average NFL player (although some of the increase in speed must be attributed to the faster artificial turf).

In terms of stature alone, there can be little doubt that we are witnessing a relatively rapid evolution of the human body over a very short period of time. Some biological changes take many thousands of years. To grasp the magnitude of the change in stature, one need only take average-size high school students to a museum and see that the boys couldn't possibly fit into armor made for adult medieval knights or the girls into most eighteenth-century wedding dresses.

The rapid advance in technology is another reason why it is difficult to set an upper limit on athletic performance.

From one point of view, the sports scientist should really be called a sports engineer, as engineering is the art and science concerned with the practical application of scientific knowledge in the design, construction, and operation of something, in this case, the human body.

With the recent explosion of genetic engineering and bionics, the terms "design" and "construction" may have real application to the athlete in the next few decades. At present, athletes may compete with artificial joints and blood vessels. Why not synthetic muscles? Today, there is no artificial substitute for human skeletal muscle, although a team of researchers at MIT, headed by biophysicist Toyoichi Tanaka, are creating gels that, when placed in an electric field, can rapidly shrink down between one-third and one-hundredth of their original size. The gels are now being tested at tensile strengths seen in human muscle. Imagine if Tanaka can create an artificial muscle with just twice the strength of human muscle, which can be transplanted and used in competition.

Research on artificial blood that can transport more oxygen than human blood has been under way for over a decade. If it works, it will be a breakthrough in medicine, and it will revolutionize endurance events.

RNA, the chemical messenger for the DNA blueprint in every living cell, has been extracted from the cells of trained animals and successfully injected into untrained animals, which then display many of the same motor skills, even though they had never been exposed to the task or maze of the trained donors. A mind-boggling concept.

The possibilities of enhancing athletic performance are unfolding at a pace with developments in training and technology. When these advances are coupled with the increasing number of competitors, the increasing body size of athletes, and the more effective means of profiling and selecting potential champions, there can be no doubt that the so-called "absolute limits" will recede before the press of human growth and ingenuity.

Yet, over and above these physical considerations, the essential attributes of the champions who will assault the performance records during the next century may be qualities we can't quantify. The peculiar eccentricities of John McEnroe, the daring of Reinhold Messner on Everest, the special hunger of Arnold Palmer at Cherry Hills, the courage of Jacques Plante in returning to the ice minutes after seven stitches were added to the 200 previously sewn into his face—this may be the true essence of championship material.

Maximum performance is not something the sports scientist can *give* to an athlete. It must come from within. A championship performance is essentially a solo venture, an experiment conducted by the individual, melding body and spirit, stretching his limits, redefining himself, and essentially redefining our perception of the capabilities and potential of man. His only barriers are his imagination and his determination.

The future of mankind is wide open, and at the cutting edge is the athlete. No one knows more than he that man is a marvel of the universe. He has no limits.

His destiny, as ours, is expressed by Shakespeare's Julius Caesar: "Now bid me run, and I will strive with things impossible."

APPENDIX

Metric Conversions

DISTANCE

1 millimeter = 0.039 inches
1 centimeter = 0.392 inches
1 meter = 3.281 feet
1 kilometer = 0.621 miles

MASS

1 gram = 0.035 ounces
1 kilogram = 2.204 pounds

VOLUME

1 milliliter = 0.03 fluid ounces
1 liter = 1.06 quarts or 2.1 pints

SPEED

1 meter per second = 3.281 feet/second or 2.237 miles per hour
1 mile per hour = 1.467 feet/second or 0.447 meters/second
1 foot per second = 0.682 miles per hour or 0.305 meters/second

FORCE

1 Newton = 0.22 pounds
1 kilopond = 9.8 Newtons

WORK AND ENERGY

1 Joule = 1 watt-second
1 Newton-meter = 1 Joule
1 kilopond-meter = 9.807 Joules
1 foot-pound = 1.356 Joules
1 Calorie = 4.18 Joules

POWER

1 watt = 44.2 foot-pounds/minute
1 horsepower = 745 watts or 33,000 foot-pounds/minute
1 kilopond-meter/minute = 0.163 watts

TEMPERATURE

1 degree Celsius = 9/5° Fahrenheit
1 degree Fahrenheit = 5/9° Celsius

CHAPTER NOTES

(Note: *Authors and titles referred to in these notes can be found in the bibliography.*)

ONE: FOOTBALL

1. Intensity and repetition are terms used in strength training to denote the load a muscle is required to resist or move so many times before resting. Manipulation of load intensity versus the number of repetitions produces a variety of adaptations in muscles, discussed in Chapter 5.

2. Avid football fans who have followed John Riggins; observed his ball handling, timing, agility and heart; and wondered why he has not accumulated the yardage of Franco Harris or Walter Payton may want to read the principal study on which this idea is based. See Hickson (1980) in bibliography.

3. This hypothetical situation would occur only as a result of a head-on collision; an oblique collision could have ended many ways. If McNeal had the position, opportunity, and speed presented in this scenario, it's most likely Riggins would have seen him and either slanted toward the sideline or cut across the grain toward the center, forcing the cornerback to attack from a greater angle to Riggins's line of motion. Drawing an oblique tackle may be an instinctive move, but it's also good physics: the sum of momenta of the two players remains constant, but as the ball carrier increases the tackler's angle of incidence, the resultant vectors of collision buy the rusher more yardage. See Hay (1978, pp. 14–44) for a concise overview of linear kinematics in sports and Brancazio (1984, pp. 202–44) for an easy course in the mathematics of sports collisions.

4. The National Operating Committee on Standards for Athletic Equipment (NOCSAE) was formed in 1969 for the purpose of making competitive sports as free from injury as possible through protective equipment standards. As of 1983, the fatalities in football have decreased by about 50 percent since NOCSAE has been in operation. See Hodgson (1975) for a typical NOCSAE report on helmet testing.

5. Donzis's timidity is understandable, but during the 1920s, a traveling salesman known as Foulproof Taylor peddled protective cups for boxers and spectators after fights at fairs and carnivals. With a hand on each hip and legs spread wide, he'd invite the toughest guy in the crowd to punch him below the belt. And if interest lagged, Foulproof allowed spectators to belt him with a baseball bat. For more on protective cups, see "Fear of Injury" in Chapter 3.

TWO: BASKETBALL

1. The idea of raising the basket is not new. It was first suggested in 1932 by Kansas coach Phog Allen, and an NBA scout, Pete Newell, the former coach at the University of California, experimented with 12-foot baskets with some success. Newell reported that the higher baskets neutralized the taller players and made the game much faster.

2. This problem is more than academic whimsy. The U.S. Department of Defense has been unable to produce a system of comparable complexity to control a modern type of battleship gatling gun that can track and hit high-speed, sea-skimming missiles such as the Exocet. Similar problems arise in the design of tracking and control systems for the so-called "Star Wars" space-based antimissile defense system, where a tight laser beam or stream of sub-atomic particles must be held onto a missile flying over 1,000 miles away, long enough to penetrate the booster's outer skin and damage internal components.

3. If the ball is dropped into the hoop from directly above—an entry angle of 90 degrees—it has an 18-inch-diameter circular opening through which it can pass. Approaches from smaller angles present the ball with a smaller opening. The minimum entry angle for a swish is just under 33 degrees, presenting a rim 9.71 inches in diameter, the same size as the ball.

THREE: ICE HOCKEY

1. A classic example of this occurred at the Pro Indoor Tennis tournament in Philadelphia on January 25, 1985, when John McEnroe was trailing challenger Miloslav Mercir of Czechoslovakia in the second set by 5–1. McEnroe suddenly pulled a temper tantrum, protesting a call and kicking a television camera he said was too close to him. This display distracted Mercir, whose game suddenly fell apart. He lost the set and the match, prompting the Czech to remark, "I was bothered by his protesting, and that lost my concentration." However, the effects of McEnroe's temper vary considerably among players. In fact, surveys of the star's performance have found that he loses more games after a tantrum, often to inferior players he has beat in the past. (See Chapter 7.)

FOUR: BOXING

1. Instead of putting further restrictions on the boxer, the state of New Jersey passed legislation in January 1985 that increased the role of the ring physician, who can now inspect gloves before and after a fight, and more important, he can stop a fight at any time, regardless of the judgment of the referee. New Jersey law also states that three knockdowns will automatically end a fight, and the referee can give a standing 8-count to call a technical knockout.

2. A Newton is a standard unit of force that measures an acceleration of 1 meter (3.281 feet) per second squared to a mass of 1 kilogram (2.2 pounds). Or, more appropriately, one Newton is roughly equivalent to the force exerted by the weight of a large apple. Thus, the impact of a 3,000-Newton punch can be imagined as catching the weight of 3,000 apples on the chin.

290

CHAPTER NOTES

3. There is one other study, but it remains unpublished and relatively unknown which found that three times as many "injuries" occurred in boxers who did not wear headgear as in those who did. Until the protocols of the study and such terms as "injuries" can be assessed, it's difficult to know how to interpret this data. See Estwanik (1984).

FIVE: STRENGTH TRAINING

1. There is considerable overlap in the use of many terms in sports science. Ariel calls this technique variable resistance exercise, others call it variable strength training. Strength training, the term used throughout this volume, is also known as weight training or resistance training. It's common for many people to use the terms exercise and training interchangeably. Here, strength training is used to describe training that increases strength, in contrast to endurance training, which increases aerobic capacity in such athletes as distance runners (see Chapter 9). The term "exercise" will be used throughout the text to denote any form of physical activity that contributes to or maintains a level of strength or endurance; "training" will be used for exercise that overloads the body enough to *increase* levels of strength or endurance. "Practice" refers to the repetition of a physical activity to acquire, maintain, or fine tune a motor skill, like shooting a basketball. (See Chapter 8.)

2. A study of football players at Syracuse University may have found clues to the problem of how much protein or how many calories active athletes should consume. The average daily caloric intake of these players was a staggering 5,270 kilocalories, and average protein intake was about 200 grams. The athletes all maintained their normal weight despite the hefty intake in this unsupervised diet. In the off season, intake declined naturally. The message of this study seems to be to let athletes eat until sated, as long as the diet is balanced and there is no excessive weight gain.

3. During the 90 degree heat of the 1960 Rome Olympics, Knut Jensen, a prominent member of the Danish cycling team, appeared to faint in the middle of the 100 kilometer race, fall from his bike, then died on the way to the hospital. The reasons for his death came out slowly. At first officials said he had collapsed from sunstroke and suffered a fractured skull in the fall. An autopsy later determined that Jensen had taken (some say he was given) a large dose of Ronicol, a blood circulation stimulant. This drug, in combination with strenuous exertion in hot weather, may have precipitated or mimicked the symptoms of sunstroke. Jensen was the first athlete to die in Olympic competition since the 1912 marathon, and the drug connection prompted the International Cycling Federation to become the first amateur governing body to introduce doping controls.

SIX: BASEBALL

1. Aerodynamic factors over which the pitcher has no control, but which will slightly affect the flight of the ball, include air temperature, air pressure, and humidity. Drag *decreases* as temperature rises, pressure falls, and humidity rises. This last factor may seem wrong, because in terms of our

291

senses, humid days seem "heavy"; but in fact, in damp air, oxygen and nitrogen molecules are replaced by *lighter* water molecules.

2. The number 500 degrees per second may seem confusing, since there are only 360 degrees in a circle. What this refers to is the angular distance covered if the ball had traveled at the same speed for a whole second. An entire pitch takes under a half second, and the angular distances involved in batting are covered in milliseconds. The unit of one second of time is used as a constant value to facilitate comparisons.

SEVEN: TENNIS

1. Bernhang also found that good players had only a short period of maximal grip pressure, which coincided with impact with the ball, whereas the poor players frequently began the stroke with maximal grip pressure and maintained this grip throughout the stroke. Unfortunately, grip data were not collated to see if there was any relation between grip firmness, playing ability, and tennis elbow.

EIGHT: GOLF

1. Just after the 1972 World Series at the Firestone Country Club, Jack Nicklaus was told by a scientist that centrifugal force was so great in the downswing that by the time the club head was parallel to the hips, a golfer's problem was not to accelerate the club more, but simply to go along with it as long as he didn't brake the forward momentum. Nicklaus replied that he felt he did accelerate the club all the way through in a full shot. The scientist said this *feeling* was correct; if a golfer doesn't feel he's accelerating, then there's a possibility he may be holding back on the shaft. This anecdote may explain the discrepancy between what the pros preach and practice. Today, Nicklaus is one of the authors who does not advocate wrist pressure; he advises novices to let the centrifugal force of the club unlock the wrists spontaneously. See Nicklaus (1974).

2. The launch speed for Palmer's 346-yarder was obtained from a formula the Dunlap Sports Company developed from experience with their driving machines. For an initial velocity of v (in feet/second), the carry plus run in yards equals 5/4 v - 27. For golfers who wish to compute carry only, in case of a high chip landing on a soft green, the formula is yards = 3/2 v-105. The velocity of Palmer's club head just prior to impact (213 feet/second) was obtained by solving for V, where launch speed = mass of the club head (M) times V times (1 + the ball's COR)/M + the mass of the ball (m). Using both these formulas, golfers can calculate and compare club speed and ball speed from shot to shot, using different clubs and balls.

NINE: ENDURANCE TRAINING

1. There is some controversy among historians about the true identity of the Greek messenger who ran from Marathon to Athens. All sources agree Pheidippides (or Philippides) ran to Sparta and back, seeking military aid to repulse the Persians, but many scholars believe that another, unknown messenger ran from Marathon to Athens. There is also uncertainty about what

killed the original marathoner. Sudden death in the first three minutes after strenuous exercise may be caused by dramatic fluctuations in body chemistry, where the levels of adrenaline and norepinephrine, two hormones that stimulate heartbeat, can jump up to ten times their resting norm. In abnormal or diseased hearts, this can lead to irregular contractions and cardiac arrest. Physicians say it's better to wind down slowly than to stop exercise abruptly, hence the cool-down period following aerobic exercise. Other possible causes of Pheidippides's death include cardiac ischemia, aortic aneurism, a cerebrovascular stroke, or heat stroke coincident with the end of his run.

2. Accurate reporting of this study should include the fact that there was a significant decrease in the time these athletes completed their 10-kilometer run toward the end of the experiment. This decline in performance, despite increases in oxygen uptake, was attributed to the intensity of training in the experiment, where tissue damage and carbohydrate depletion in the muscles did not have time to recover due to the repeated overload. This has implications for assessing the threshold between optimal training and overtraining. In addition, Mikesell suggests that the chronic fatigue produced in this experiment caused a deterioration in motivation among the runners. For more on linear increases in VO$_2$max, see Hickson (1977).

3. We can be sure that Jim Fixx, who was a strong advocate of fitness programs, would want it to be known that reports immediately after his death indicated he did not have a regular physician, he had not taken a stress test, had not even gone to a doctor for a routine checkup as a family member had urged him to do, even though he had once been overweight and a smoker, and his father had had a heart attack at the age of thirty-five and died of a second at forty-three. Physicians generally agree that individuals as young as thirty-five should consult with their doctor before they start any form of endurance training.

4. For the sake of clarity, Gibbons's data have been abbreviated. The 374,798 hours of exercise is a collective figure referring to man-hours. The risk estimates apply to man-years, so that two to five heart attacks per 100 years of exercise means 100 years of exercise time put in by the total exercise population under consideration. If a million Americans exercise for one hour per day, that's slightly over 100 years of exercise time (874,000 hours) per day.

5. In fact, not all running injuries are a result of the foot-shoe-surface interface. One study found that 4 percent of distance runners had been bitten by dogs, 0.2 percent hit by bicycles, 0.6 percent hit by motor vehicles, and an unbelievable 7 percent were hit by a thrown object, including cans, bottles, ice, liquids, and even in one case a rock-filled bag. (It often seems that some researchers gather data useful only for chapter notes.) See Koplan (1982).

TEN: SOCCER

1. American researchers claim that the risk of injury in football is five times higher than soccer in the United States. Nevertheless, the rate of knee injury in both contact and noncontact sports in America is as high as that caused by soccer in Europe. A study of 1,877 football injuries by Culpepper (1983),

cited in Chapter 1, found that the most common site of injury was the knee (22 percent). A study of 1,819 running injuries by Clement (1981), cited in Chapter 9, found that 42 percent were knee injuries.

ELEVEN: EXTREME ENVIRONMENTS

1. According to J. R. Sutton (1983, p. 428), Messner's 1,000-meter climb in thirty-four minutes represents a power output of 1,800 kilopond/minute, which equals 17,640 Joules of energy or 4.2 kilocalories/minute. This seems low relative to the energy requirements of other athletic activities, in which case the estimates of Messner's VO_2 would have to be revised upward.

BIBLIOGRAPHY

INTRODUCTION: SELECTED READINGS

Bannister, R. *The Four-Minute Mile*. New York: Dodd, Mead, 1981.

Brancazio, P. J. *Sportscience: Physical Laws and Optimum Performance*. New York: Simon & Schuster, 1984.

Brooks, G. A. *Exercise Physiology: Human Bioenergetics and Its Applications*. New York: John Wiley, 1984.

Bunn, J. W. *The Scientific Principles of Coaching*. Englewood Cliffs, NJ: Prentice-Hall, 1972.

Garfield, C. A. *Peak Performance; Mental Training Techniques of the World's Greatest Athletes*. Los Angeles: Jeremy Tarcher, 1984.

Hay, J. G. *The Biomechanics of Sports Techniques*. Englewood Cliffs, NJ: Prentice-Hall, 1978.

Jerome, J. *The Sweet Spot in Time*. New York: Summit Books, 1980.

Jokl, E. *The Physiological Basis of Athletic Records*. Springfield, IL: Charles Thomas, 1968.

Leonard, G. *The Ultimate Athlete*. New York: Viking Press, 1979.

Michener, J. *Sports in America*. New York: Random House, 1976.

Northrip, J. W. *Introduction to Biomechanical Analysis of Sport*. Dubuque, IA: William C. Brown, 1976.

Plagenhoef, S. *Patterns of Human Motion*. Englewood Cliffs, NJ: Prentice-Hall, 1971.

Schrier, E. W. *Newton at Bat*. New York: Charles Scribners, 1984.

Shephard, R. J. *The Fit Athlete*. London: Oxford University Press, 1978.

Thomas, V. *Science and Sport*. Boston: Little, Brown, 1970.

Tricker, R.A.R. *The Science of Movement*. New York: American Elsevier, 1967.

Wells, K. F. *Kinesiology: Scientific Basis of Human Motion*. Philadelphia: W. B. Saunders, 1976.

Winter, D. A. *Biomechanics of Human Movement*. New York: John Wiley, 1979.

Young, J. Z. *An Introduction to the Study of Man*. London: Oxford University Press, 1971.

ONE: FOOTBALL

Albright, J. P. "Nonfatal cervical spine injuries in football." *JAMA* 236 (1978): 1243.

Arnold, J. A. "New football rules and athletic injuries." *J Ark Med Soc* 74 (1977): 163–65.

Blyth, C. S. "When and where players get hurt." *Phys Sports Med* 2 (1974): 45–52.

Brancazio, P. J. *SportScience*. New York: Simon & Schuster, 1984.

Cain, T. E. "Use of the air-inflated jacket in football." *Am J Sports Med* 9 (1981): 240–43.

Carter, D. R. "Biomechanics of hyperextension injuries to the cervical spine in football." *Am J Sports Med* 8 (1980): 302–9.

Compton, M. "Sideline computing in the NFL." *Personal Computing,* January 1984, pp. 29–32.

Costello, F. "Using weight training and plyometrics to increase explosive power for football." *NSCA Journal,* April–May 1984, pp. 22–24.

Culpepper, M. I. "High school football injuries in Birmingham, Alabama." *So Med J* 76 (1983): 873–78.

Eskow, D. "Dressed to kill." *Pop Mech,* October 1983, pp. 89–92, 175–76.

Funk, F. F. "Injuries of the cervical spine in football." *Clin Orthop* 109 (1975): 50–58.

Gerberich, S. G. "Concussion incidences and severity in secondary school varsity football players." *Am J Pub Health* 73 (1983): 1370–75.

Gollnick, P. D. "The muscle fiber composition of skeletal muscle as a predictor of athletic success." *Am J Sports Med* 12 (1984): 212–17.

Gonyea, W. J. "Role of exercise in inducing increases in skeletal muscle fiber number." *J Appl Physiol* 48 (1980): 421–26.

Hay, J. G. *The Biomechanics of Sports Techniques.* Englewood Cliffs, NJ: Prentice-Hall, 1978.

Hickson, R. C. "Interference of strength development by simultaneously training for strength and endurance." *Eur J Appl Physiol* 45 (1980): 255–63.

Hodgson, V. R. "National Operating Committee on Standards for Athletic Equipment football helmet certification program." *Med Sci Sports* 7 (1975): 225–32.

Holland, R. G. "Speed training." *Athl J,* February 1984, pp. 50–51.

Kindel, S. "Plugged-in pigskin." *Forbes,* November 1982, pp. 39–40.

Lipschutz, N. "Equipment proposals reduce sports injuries." *Industrial Design,* January–February 1980, pp. 12–13.

Lyons, R. S. "Coaching by computer." *Saturday Evening Post,* September 1983, pp. 64, 104.

Myers, E. "Playing by the system." *Datamation,* March 1983, pp. 63–74.

Norman, R. W. "Biomechanical evaluations of sports protective equipment." *Exerc Sport Sci Rev* 11 (1983): 232–74.

Ostler, S. "The stronger I get, the meaner I feel." *Sports Fitness* 1 (1985): 39–43, 118.

Radford, P. "The nature and nurture of a sprinter." *New Scientist,* 2 August 1984, pp. 13–15.

Reid, S. E. "Brain tolerance to impact in football." *Surg Gyn Obs* 133 (1971): 929–36.

Stanitski, C. L. "Synthetic turf and grass: a comparative study." *J Sports Med* 2 (1974): 22–26.

Stingley, D. *Happy to Be Alive.* New York: Beaufort Books, 1983.

Sullivan, G. *The Great Running Backs.* New York: Putnam, 1972.

Torg, J. S. "Effect of shoe type and cleat length on incidence and severity of injuries among high school football players." *Res Q* 42 (1971): 203–11.

BIBLIOGRAPHY

———. "Severe and catastrophic neck injuries resulting from tackle football." *College Health* 25 (1977): 224–26.

Virgin, H. "Cineradiographic study of football helmets and the cervical spine." *Am J Sports Med* 8 (1980): 310–17.

Williams, K. R. "A model for the calculation of mechanical power during running." *J Biomech* 16 (1983), 115–28.

TWO: BASKETBALL

Bannister, R. G "The effects on respiration and performance during exercise of adding O_2 to the inspired air." *J Physiol* 125 (1954): 118–21.

Bizzi, E. "The coordination of eye-head movements." *Sci Am,* October 1974, pp. 100–106.

Blakeslee, T. R. *The Right Brain.* New York: Anchor Press, 1980.

Brancazio, P. J. "Comments on 'Kinematics of the free throw in basketball.'" *Am J Phys* 50 (1982): 944–46.

———. "Physics of basketball." *Am J Phys* 49 (1981): 356–65.

———. "The science of basketball shooting," in *SportScience.* New York: Simon & Schuster, 1984, pp. 306–14.

Brooks, G. A. "Metabolic response to exercise," in *Exercise Physiology.* New York: John Wiley, 1984, pp. 189–219.

———. "Temperature, skeletal muscle mitochrondrial function and oxygen debt." *Am J Physiol* 220 (1971): 1053–59.

Busk, J. "EEG correlates of visual-motor practice in man." *Electroenceph Clin Neurophysiol* 38 (1975): 415–22.

Cousey, B. *Basketball Concepts and Techniques.* Boston: Allyn & Bacon, 1983.

Davies, K.J.A. "Biochemical adaptation of mitochondria." *Arch Biochem Biophys* 209 (1981): 539–54.

Dolson, F. "Chamberlain pours in 100." *Philadelphia Inquirer,* 3 March 1962.

Dreher, H. "Wilt Chamberlain's 100-point game," in *Great Sport Thrills.* New Jersey: Watermill Press, 1981.

Ekblom, B. "Central circulation during exercise after venesection and reinfusion of red blood cells." *J Appl Physiol* 40 (1974): 379–83.

———. "Response to exercise after blood loss and reinfusion." *J Appl Physiol* 33 (1972): 175–80.

Evarts, E. V. "Brain mechanisms of movement." *Sci Am,* September 1979, pp. 164–79.

Henry, F. M. "Increased response latency for complicated movements and a 'memory drum' theory of neuromotor reaction." *Res Q* 31 (1960): 448–58.

Hermansen, L. "Anaerobic energy release." *Med Sci Sports* 1 (1969): 32–38.

Holloszy, J. O. "Effects of exercise on mitochondrial oxygen uptake and respiratory enzyme activity in skeletal muscle." *J Biol Chem* 242 (1967): 2278–82.

Holzman, R. *A View from the Bench.* New York: W. W. Norton, 1980.

Isaacs, L. D. "Relationship between depth perception and basketball shooting over a competitive season." *Percept Motor Skills* 53 (1981): 554.

STRETCHING THE LIMITS

McArdle, W. D. "Aerobic capacity, heart rate and estimated energy cost during competitive basketball." *Res Q* 42 (1971): 178–86.

Mizusawa, K. "Comparative studies of color fields, visual acuity fields, and movement perception limits among varsity athletes and non-varsity groups." *Percept Motor Skills* 56 (1983): 887–92.

Rebert, C. S. "Differential hemispheric activation during complex visuomotor performance." *Electroenceph Clin Neurophysiol* 44 (1978): 724–34.

Regan, D. "The visual perception of motion in depth." *Sci Am*, July 1979, pp. 136–51.

Rostaing, B. "Triumphs tainted with blood." *Sports Illustrated,* 21 January 1985, pp. 12–21.

Russell, B. *Second Wind.* New York: Random House, 1979.

Scharf, S. M. "Second wind during inspiratory loading." *Med Sci Sports Exerc* 16 (1984): 87–91.

Schnabel, A. "Assessment of anaerobic capacity in runners." *Eur J Appl Physiol* 52 (1983): 42–46.

Suinn, R. M. "Behavior rehearsal training for ski racers." *Behavior Therapy* 3 (1972): 519–20.

———. "Psychology for Olympic champions." *Psychol Today,* July 1976, pp. 38–42.

———. "Removing emotional obstacles to learning and performance by visuomotor behavior rehearsal." *Behavior Therapy* 3 (1972): 308–10.

Tan, A. "Kinematics of the free throw in basketball." *Am J Phys* 49 (1981): 542–44.

Thirer, J. "Effects of abusive spectator behavior on performance of home and visiting intercollegiate basketball teams." *Percept Motor Skills* 48 (1979): 1047–53.

Torrey, L. "How science creates winners." *Science Digest* 92 (1984): 33–40.

Toyoshima, S. "Effects of initial ball velocity and angle of projection on accuracy in basketball shooting," in A. Morecki, ed., *Biomechanics VII-B.* Baltimore: University Park Press, 1981.

Waitley, D. E. "Sports psychology and the elite athlete." *Clin Sports Med* 2 (1983): 87–99.

Wurtz, R. H. "Brain mechanisms of visual attention." *Sci Am*, June 1982, pp. 124–35.

THREE: ICE HOCKEY

Alexander, J. F. "Comparison of the ice hockey wrist and slap shots for speed and accuracy." *Res Q* 34 (1963): 259–65.

Anderson, D. "The mask that changed hockey's face." *Sport*, November 1980, pp. 73–75.

Dillman, C. J. "Speed capabilities of ice hockey players." Unpublished U.S. Olympic Committee research paper, 1984.

Dore, R. "Dynamometric analysis of different hockey shots," in P. V. Komi, ed., *Biomechanics V-B.* Baltimore: University Park Press, 1976, pp. 277–85.

BIBLIOGRAPHY

Emmert, W. "The slap shot: strength and conditioning program for hockey at Boston College." *NSCA Journal*, April–May 1984, pp. 4–6, 68.

Frayne, T. "The school of hard knocks returns." *Macleans*, 21 March 1983, p. 36.

Fussman, C. "Protecting your privates." *Esquire*, November 1982, pp. 21–22.

Gitler, I. *Blood on the Ice*. Chicago: Henry Regnery, 1974.

Goldstein, J. H. "Sports violence." *Nat Forum* 62 (1982): 9–11.

Green, H. "Time-motion and physiological assessments of ice hockey performance." *J Appl Physiol* 40 (1976): 159–63.

Hayes, D. "Injuries and protective equipment in hockey." Proceedings of the 18th Conference on the Medical Aspects of Sport, 1977, pp. 46–51.

———. "A mechanical analysis of the hockey slap shot." *J Can Assoc Health Phys Ed Rec* 31 (1965): 17–26.

Horn, J. C. "Sir Lancelot of the rink: the ritual of hockey fights." *Psychol Today*, February 1981, pp. 15–16.

Kelly, B. R. "Personality dimensions of aggression: its relationship to time and place of action in ice hockey." *Human Relations* 32 (1979): 219–25.

Kiester, E. "The uses of anger." *Psychol Today*, July 1984, p. 26.

Landers, D. M. "The arousal-performance relationship." *Res Q Exerc Sport* 51 (1980), 77–90.

Levine, D. "Gretzky: way ahead of the game." *Sport*, May 1984, pp. 39–41.

Martens, R. "Arousal and motor performance." *Exerc Sport Sci Rev* 2 (1974): 155–89.

McCarthy, J. F. "Aggression, performance variables, and anger self-report in ice hockey players." *J Psychol 99 (1978): 97–101.*

Mikita, S. *Inside Hockey*. Chicago: Henry Regnery, 1971.

Minkoff, J. "Evaluating parameters of a professional hockey team." *Am J Sports Med* 10 (1982): 285–92.

Norman, R. W. "Relative impact-attenuating properties of face masks of ice hockey goaltenders," in E. Asmussen, ed., *Biomechanics IV* Baltimore: University Park Press, 1974.

Percival, L. *The Hockey Handbook*. Toronto: Copp Clark, 1961.

Power, C. "Cashing in on heavy checking," *Psychol Today*, November 1979, p. 39.

Roy, B. "Biomechanical features of different starting positions and skating strides in ice hockey," in E. Asmussen, ed., *Biomechanics VI-B* Baltimore: University Park Press, 1978, pp. 137–41.

———. "Kinematics of slap shot in ice hockey as executed by players of different age classifications," in P. V. Komi, ed., *Biomechanics V-B*. Baltimore: University Park Press, 1976, pp. 286–90.

Russell, G. W. "Crowd size and competitive aspects of aggression in ice hockey: an archival study." *Human Relations* 29 (8)(1976): 723–35.

Smith, M. D. "Hockey violence: a test of the violent subculture hypothesis." *Social Problems* 27 (1979): 235–47.

Tator, C. H. "National survey of spinal injuries in hockey players." *Can Med Assoc J* 130 (1984): 875–80.

———. "Spinal injuries due to hockey." *Can J Neurol Sci* 11 (1984): 34–41.

Therrien, R. G. "Mechanics applications to sports equipment: protective helmets, hockey sticks, and jogging shoes," in D. N. Ghista, ed., *Human Body Dynamics*. Oxford, Clarendon Press, 1982.

Widmeyer, W. N. "Aggression in professional ice hockey: a strategy for success or a reaction to failure?" *J Psychol* 117 (1984): 77–84.

Wilson, K. "Facial injuries in hockey players." *Minn Med* 60 (1977): 13–24.

Zimmer, J. "Courting the gods of sport: athletes use of superstition." *Psychol Today*, July 1984, pp. 36–40.

FOUR: BOXING

Annas, G. J. "Boxing: atavistic spectacle or artistic sport?" *Am J Pub Health* 73 (1983): 811–12.

Battalia, J. E. "Brain injury in boxing." *JAMA* 249 (1983): 254–57.

———. "Physician contends young boxers risk brain damage." *Am Fam Phys*, February 1982, p. 129.

Brayne, C.E.G. "Blood creatine kinase isoenzyme in boxers," *Lancet*, 11 December 1982, pp. 1308–09.

Carr, D. B. "Physical conditioning facilitates the exercise-induced secretion of beta-endorphin and beta-lipotropin in women." *New Eng J Med* 305 (1981): 560–63.

Casson, I. R. "Brain damage in modern boxers." *JAMA* 251 (1984): 2663–67.

Colt, E.W.D. "The effect of running on plasma b-endorphin." *Life Sci* 28 (1981): 1637–40.

Davis, G. C. "Endorphins and pain." *Psychiat Clin N Am* 6 (1983): 473–87.

Estwanik, J. J. "Amateur boxing injuries at the 1981 and 1982 USA/ABF national championships." *Physician and Sportsmedicine* 12 (1984): 123–28.

Fraioli, F. "Physical exercise stimulates marked concomitant release of b-endorphin and ACTH in peripheral blood in man." *Experientia* 36 (1980): 987–89.

Joch, W. "Biomechanical analysis of punching in boxing," in A. Morecki, ed., *Biomechanics VII-B* Baltimore: University Park Press, 1981, pp. 343–49.

Johnson, J. "Peak accelerations of the head experienced in boxing." *Med Biol Eng*, May 1975, pp. 396–404.

Johnson, W. "Human body mechanics in some sports and games," in D. N. Ghista, ed., *Human Body Dynamics*. Oxford: Clarendon Press, 1982.

Jokl, E. *The Medical Aspects of Boxing*. Pretoria: Smith & Smith, 1941.

Kaste, M. "Is chronic brain damage in boxing a hazard of the past?" *Lancet*, 27 November 1982, pp. 1186–88.

Koob, G. F. "Opiate-like stimulant properties of endorphins," in R. Collu, ed., *Brain Neurotransmitters and Hormones*. New York: Raven Press, 1982.

Lampert, P. W. "Morphological changes in brains of boxers." *JAMA* 251 (1984): pp. 2676–79.

Landis, D. "Boxing: five training ingredients." *NSCA Journal*, April–May 1984, pp. 26–30.

Levin, D. C. "The runner's high: fact or fiction?" *JAMA* 248 (1982): 24.

BIBLIOGRAPHY

Lundberg, G. D. "Boxing should be banned in civilized countries." *Jama* 251 (1984): 2696–98.

Moore, M. "The challenge of boxing: bringing safety into the ring." *Phys Sportsmed* 8 (1980): 101–5.

Roberts, A. H. *Brain Damage in Boxers*. London: Pittman Publishing, 1969.

Ross, R. J. "Boxers: computed tomography, EEG, and neurological evaluation." *JAMA* 249 (1983): 211–13.

Schmid, L. "Experience with headgear in boxing." *J Sports Med & Phys Fit* 3 (1968): 171–75.

Shaffer, T. E. "Participating in boxing among children and young adults." *Pediatrics* 74 (1984): 311–12.

Stoler, P. "Ali fights a new round." *Time*, 1 October 1984, p. 60.

Timperley, W. R. "Banning boxing." *Brit Med J* 285 (1982): 289.

FIVE: STRENGTH TRAINING

Anderson, I. "Goodbye steroids, hello growth hormone." *New Scientist*, 17 November 1983, p. 478.

Basmajian, J. V. *Muscles Alive: Their Functions Revealed by Electromyography*. Baltimore: Williams & Watkins, 1967.

Beckett, A. H. "Use and abuse of drugs in sports." *J Biosoc Sci Suppl* 7 (1981): 163–70.

Bedgood, B. L. "Nutrition knowledge of high school athletic coaches in Texas." *J Am Dietet Assoc*, December 1983, pp. 672–77.

Beecher, H. K. "Amphetamine sulfate and athletic performance." *JAMA* 170 (1959): 102–17.

Chandler, J. V. "The effect of amphetamines on selected physiological components related to athletic success." *Med Sci Sports Exerc* 12 (1980): 65–69.

Cox, R. J. "Myoelectric and force feedback in the facilitation of isometric strength training." *Psychophysiol* 20 (1983): 35–43.

Didinger, R. "U.S. medal candidate Guy Carlton." *Philadelphia Daily News*, 5 July 1984, pp. 90–91.

Ekholm, J. "Load on knee joint structures and muscular activity during lifting." *Scand J Rehab Med* 16 (1984): 1–19.

Fleck, S. J. "Types of strength training." *Orthop Clin N Am* 14 (1983): 449–58.

Garhammer, J. "Power production by Olympic weightlifters." *Med Sci Sports Exerc* 12 (1980): 54–60.

Goldberg, L. "Changes in lipid and lipoprotein levels after weight training." *JAMA* 252 (1984): 504–6.

Hakkinen, K. "Alterations of mechanical characteristics of human skeletal muscle during strength training." *Eur J Appl Physiol* 50 (1983): 161–72.

Hatfield, M. "Bigger, faster, stronger: the legacy of squats." *Sports Fitness* 1 (1985): 17–19.

Hill, J. A. "The athletic polydrug phenomenon." *Am J Sports Med* 11 (1983): 269–71.

Hurley, B. F. "High-density-lipoprotein cholesterol in bodybuilders v. powerlifters." *JAMA* 252 (1984): 507–13.

Ikai, M. "Some factors modifying the expression of human strength." *J Appl Physiol* 16 (1961): 157–63.

Kamen, G. "Strength recovery patterns following exercise with an imposed myotatic stretch." *Arch Phys Med Rehabil* 65 (1984): 178–81.

Kulund, D. N. "Warm-up, strength and power." *Orthop Clin N Am* 14 (1983): 427–48.

Lamb, D. R. "Anabolic steroids in athletics: how well do they work and how dangerous are they?" *Am J Sports Med* 12 (1984): 31–38.

Lasagna, L. "Breakfast of champions." *The Sciences*, March–April 1984, pp. 61–62.

Looney, D. S. "A test with nothing but tough questions." *Sports Illustrated*, 9 August 1982, pp. 24–29.

Mandell, A. "The Sunday syndrome." Proceedings of the National Amphetamine Conference, San Francisco, California, 1978.

Marshall, E. "Drugging of football players curbed by central monitoring plan." *Science* 203 (1979): 626–28.

Massey, B. H. "Effects of high frequency electrical stimulation on the size and strength of skeletal muscles." *J Sports Med Phys Fit* 5 (1965): 136–44.

McCutcheon, M. L. "The athlete's diet: a current view." *J Fam Pract* 16 (1983): 529–34.

Mole, P. "Adaptations in muscle to exercise." *J Clin Invest* 50 (1971): 2323–30.

Murray, T. H. "The coercive power of drugs in sports." *The Hastings Center Report*, August 1983, pp. 24–30.

Percy, E. C. "Erogogenic aids in athletes." *Med Sci Sports* 10 (1978): 298–303.

Porcello, L.A.P. (1984), "A practical guide to fad diets," *Clin Sports Med.*, 3(3): 723–729.

Rozenek, R. "Protein metabolism related to athletes." *NSCA Journal*, April–May 1984, pp. 42–45, 62.

Sale, D. G. "Neuromuscular function in weight trainers." *Experimental Neurol* 82 (1983): 521–31.

Sanford, T. L. "The effects of electrical stimulation of normal quadriceps on strength and girth." *Med Sci Sports Exerc* 14 (1982): 194–97.

Short, S. H. "Four-year study of university athletes' dietary intake." *Am Dietet Assoc* 82 (1983): 632–45.

Smith, M. J. "Muscle fiber type." *Orthop Clin N Am* 14 (1983): 403–11.

———. "Nutrition and the athlete." *Am J Sports Med* 10 (1982): 253–55.

Solberg, S. "Anabolic steroids and Norwegian weightlifters." *Brit J Sports Med* 16 (1982): 169–71.

Sperryn, P. "Drugged and victorious: doping in sport." *New Scientist* 2 August 1984, pp. 16–19.

Surburg, P. R. "Neuromuscular facilitation techniques in sportsmedicine." *Physician and Sportsmedicine* 9 (1981): 115–27.

Taylor, A. W. "The effects of faradic stimulation on skeletal muscle fiber area." *Can J Appl Sports Sci* 3 (1978): 185.

Tesch, P. A. "Muscle capillary supply and fiber type characteristics in weight and power lifters." *J Appl Physiol* 56 (1984): 35–38.

BIBLIOGRAPHY

Thomason, H. "Drugs and the athlete," in B. Davies, ed., *Science and Sporting Performance*. Oxford: Clarendon Press, 1982, pp. 100–10.

Todd, T. "He bends but he does not break [Lamar Gant]." *Sports Illustrated,* 22 October 1984, pp. 46–62.

U.S. Olympic Committee. "Drug Information for Athletes," USOC pamphlet, 1984.

Wiktorsson-Moller, M. "Effects of warm-up, massage, and stretching on range of motion and muscle strength in the lower extremity." *Am J Sports Med* 11 (1983): 249–52.

Zimmer, J. "Floppy-disk diets." *Health,* January 1984.

Zurer, P. S. "Drugs in sports." *Chem and Eng News,* 30 April 1984, pp. 69–78.

SIX: BASEBALL

Adams, G. L. "Effect of eye dominance on baseball batting." *Res Q* 36 (1965): 3–9.

Bahill, A. T. "Why can't batters keep their eyes on the ball?" *Am Sci* 72 (1984): 249–53.

Baila, D. L. "Fastball: hot or cold?" *Science World,* 16 September 1966, pp. 10–11.

Bennett, J. M. "An evaluation of major league baseball offensive performance models." *Am Statist* 37 (1983): 76–83.

Bowe, J. "Sporting goods designers cash in on aluminum's virtues." *Modern Metals,* February 1981, pp. 26–32.

Brancazio, P. J. "The hardest blow of all," *New Scientist,* 22–29 December 1983, pp. 880–83.

———. "The physics of judging a fly ball." *Physics Today,* January 1984, pp. 55–56.

———. "Science and the game of baseball," *Science Digest,* July 1984, pp. 66–69, 90.

Breen, J. L. "What makes a good hitter." *J Health Phys Ed Rec* 38 (1967): 36–39.

Briggs, L. J. "Effect of spin and speed on the lateral deflection of a baseball." *Am J Phys* 27 (1959): 589–96.

Bryant, F. O. "Dynamic and performance characteristics of baseball bats." *Res Q* 48 (1977): 505–9.

Chapman, S. "Catching a baseball." *Am J Phys* 36 (1968): 868–70.

Cook, E. *Percentage Baseball.* Cambridge, MA: MIT Press, 1966.

Edwards, D. K. "Effects of stride and position on the pitching rubber on control in baseball pitching." *Res Q* 34 (1963): 9–14.

Frohlich, C. "Aerodynamic drag crisis and its possible effect on the flight of baseball." *Am J Phys* 52 (1984): 325–34.

Grazier, J. "Science goes to bat." *Pop Mech,* May 1984, pp. 71–74, 220.

Jobe, F. W. "An EMG analysis of the shoulder in throwing and pitching." *Am J Sports Med* 11 (1983): 3–5.

Kalmer, D. "Proper pitching mechanics." *Athletic Journal,* January 1981, pp. 30–79.

Kennedy, R. "It's the apple of his eye: A's manager Steve Boros leads baseball into the computer age." *Sports Illustrated,* 6 June 1983, pp. 72–74.

Kephart, K. "Strength for baseball." *NSCA Journal,* April–May 1984, pp. 36–39.

Kirkpatrick, P. "Batting the ball." *Am J Phys* 31 (1963): 606–13.

Krane, K. S. "Probability, statistics, and the World Series of baseball." *Am J Phys* 49 (1981): 696–97.

Line, Les. "Of ashes and heros." *Audubon,* May 1983, pp. 6–8.

Lotz, R. "Aspects of traditionalism in modern sports organizations." *Soc Sci J* 19 (1982): 8–19.

Lyons, R. D. "If the ball is too fast to follow, how can anyone hit it?" *New York Times,* 12 June 1984, pp. C1–C4.

Maslow, J. E. "Baseball by computer." *Saturday Review,* 12 April 1980, pp. 42–43.

Pedegana, L. R. "The relationship of upper extremity strength to throwing speed." *Am J Sports Med* (1982): 352–54.

Poole, W. H. "The biomechanics of pitching." *Athletic Journal,* February 1984, pp. 12–14, 69.

Schadewald, R. "It's 1-2-3 strikes and yer out at the old ballistics game." *Science Digest,* September 1979, pp. 56–61.

Selin, C. "An analysis of the aerodynamics of pitched baseball." *Res Q* 30 (2)(1959): 232–40.

Tullos, H. S. "Throwing mechanism in sports." *Orthop Clin N Am* 4 (1973): 709–20.

Watts, R. G. "Aerodynamics of a knuckleball." *Am J Phys* 43 (1975): 960–63.

Weissman, S. "The microchipped diamond." *Psychol Today,* August 1983, pp. 45–51.

SEVEN: TENNIS

Andrews, J. G. "A mechanical analysis of a special class of rebound phenomena," *Med Sci Sports Exerc* 15 (1983): 256–66.

Bak, D. J. "Injected-molded frame increases racket's performance." *Design News,* 24 January 1983, p. 93.

Baker, J.A.W. "Tennis racket and ball responses during impact under clamped and freestanding conditions." *Res Q* 50 (1979): 164–70.

Bartoszynski, R. "Some remarks on strategy in playing tennis." *Behavioral Science* 26 (1981): 379–87.

Bernardo, S. "Physics of the sweet spot." *Science Digest,* May 1984, pp. 62–66, 95.

Bernhang, A. M. "The many causes of tennis elbow." *NY State J Med* 79 (1979): 1363–66.

———. "A scientific approach to tennis elbow." *Orthop Rev* 4 (1975): 35–41.

———. "Tennis elbow: a biomechanical approach." *J Sports Med* 2 (1974): 235–60.

Brattberg, G. "Acupuncture therapy for tennis elbow." *Pain* 16 (1983): 285–88.

Brody, H. "Physics of the tennis racket." *Am J Phys* 47 (1979): 482–87.

BIBLIOGRAPHY

———. "Physics of the tennis racket II: the sweet spot." *Am J Phys* 49 (1981): 816–19.

Bunn, J. W. *The Scientific Principles of Coaching.* Englewood Cliffs, NJ: Prentice-Hall, 1955.

Cleary, S. "Does string tension really matter?" *World Tennis,* December 1983, pp. 56–57.

Deford, F. "So, why can't you smile [John McEnroe]?" *Sports Illustrated,* 25 June 1984, pp. 70–84.

Elliott, B. C. "Tennis: the influence of grip tightness on reaction impulse and rebound velocity." *Med Sci Sports Exerc* 14 (1982): 348–52.

———. "Vibration and rebound velocity characteristics of conventional and oversized tennis rackets." *Res Q Exerc Sport* 51 (1980): 608–15.

Fiott, S. "Frames of reference." *World Tennis,* December 1984, pp. 20–23.

Fisher, A. "Super racket." *Pop Sci* 210 (1977): 45–46, 150.

Grabiner, M. D. "Resultant tennis ball velocity as a function of off-center impact and grip firmness." *Med Sci Sports Exerc* 15 (1983): 542–44.

Greenberg, J. "Traumatic tennis: a state of shock." *Science News* 126 (1984): 72.

Hatza, H. "Forces and duration of impact, and grip tightness during the tennis stroke." *Med Sci Sports* (1976): 88–95.

Hay, J. G. *The Biomechanics of Sports Techniques.* Englewood Cliffs, NJ: Prentice-Hall, 1978.

Kalyn, W. "Building the brave new athlete [Martina Navratilova]." *World Tennis,* April 1983, pp. 55–61, 104.

Legwold, G. "Tennis elbow: joint resolution by conservative treatment and improved technique." *Physician and Sportsmedicine* 12 (1984): 168–89.

Lendrem, D. "Should John McEnroe grunt?" *New Scientist,* 21 July 1983, pp. 188–89.

Liu, Y. K. "Mechanical analysis of racket and ball during impact." *Med Sci Sports Exerc* 15 (1983): 388–92.

McFarland, K. "Effects of hemispace on concurrent task performance." *Neuropsychologia* 20 (1982): 365–67.

Nirschl, R. P. "Conservative treatment of tennis elblow." *Physician and Sportsmedicine* 9 (1981): 43–54.

———. "Tennis elbow." *Orthop Clin N Am* 4 (1973): 787–800.

Pain, H. J. *Physics of Vibrations and Waves.* New York: John Wiley, 1968.

Priest, J. D. "Elbow injuries in sports." *Minn Med,* September 1982, pp. 543–51.

Schalen, L. "Quantification of tracking eye movements in normal subjects." *Acta Otolaryngol* 90 (1980): 404–13.

Schechter, A. "Who can see best where a tennis ball bounces on the court?" *Sports Illustrated,* 15 November 1982, pp. 34–35.

Strizak, A. M. "Hand and forearm strength and its relation to tennis." *Am J Sports Med* 11 (1983): 234–39.

Terauds, J. *Science in Racket Sports.* Del Mar, CA: Academic Publishers, 1979.

Tilden, W. T. *Tennis A to Z.* London: Victor Gollancz, 1960.

EIGHT: GOLF

Aksamit, G. "Feedback influences on the skill of putting." *Percept Motor Skills* 56 (1983): 19–22.

Alderman, R. B. "A comparative study on the effectiveness of two grips for teaching beginning golf." *Res Q* 38 (1967): 3–9.

Asanuma, H. "Cerebral cortical control of movement." *The Physiologist* 16 (1973): 143–66.

Bouisset, S. "The organization of a simple voluntary movement as analysed from its kinetic properties." *Brain Res* 71 (1974): 451–57.

Budney, D. R. "Kinetic analysis of golf swing." *Res Q* 50 (1979): 171–79.

Carlsoo, S. "A kinetic analysis of the golf swing." *J Sports Med Phys Fit* 7 (1967): 76–82.

Cochran, A. *The Search for the Perfect Swing* (the GSGB study), London: Heinemann Educational Books, 1968.

Daish, C. B. *Learn Science Through Ball Games.* New York: Sterling, 1972.

Davis, J. M. "The aerodynamics of golf balls." *J Appl Phys* 20 (1949): 821–28.

Engelhorn, R. "Motor learning and control: microcomputer applications." *J Phys Ed Rec Danc* 54 (1983): 30–32.

Erlichson, H. "Maximum projectile range with drag and lift, with particular application to golf." *Am J Phys* 51 (1983): 357–62.

Gardner, E. B. "The neuromuscular base of human movement: feedback mechanisms." *J Health Phys Ed Rec*, October 1965, pp. 61–62.

Grimsley, W. "I want that grand slam." *Saturday Evening Post*, 18 June 1960, pp. 24, 101–2.

Henderson, S. E. "Role of feedback in the development and maintenance of a complex skill." *J Exper Psychol* 3 (1977): 224–33.

Henry, F. M. "Increased response latency for complicated movements and a 'memory drum' theory of neuromotor reaction." *Res Q* 31 (1960): 448–58.

Hogan, C. A. "Your mind hits the shots." *Golf*, December 1984, pp. 46–50.

Jorgensen, T. "On the dynamics of the swing of a golf club." *Am J Phys* 38 (1970): 644–51.

Landers, D. M. "The arousal-performance relationship revisited." *ResQ Exerc Sport* 51 (1980): 77–90.

Lindsley, D. B. *Brain Function and Learning.* Los Angeles: University of California Press, 1967.

Martens, R. "Arousal and motor performance." *Exerc Sport Sci Rev* 2 (1974): 155–88.

Nagao, N. "A kinematic analysis of the golf swing by means of fast motion picture." *J Sports Med* 14 (1974): 55–62.

Nicklaus, J. *Golf My Way.* New York: Simon & Schuster, 1974.

Riedlinger, T. "Golf club firm tees off with cast stainless steel 'woods,' " *Modern Metals*, October 1982, pp. 24–25.

Schmidt, R. A. "Control processes in motor skills." *Exerc Sport Sci Rev* 4 (1976): 229–61.

———. "A schema theory of discrete motor skill learning." *Psychol Rev* 82 (1975): 225–60.

BIBLIOGRAPHY

Shea, J. B. "Motor control." *Clin Sports Med* 3 (1984): 171–83.

Simek, T. C. "Immediate auditory feedback to improve putting quickly." *Percept Motor Skills* 47 (1978): 1133–34.

Steinhaus, A. H. "Your muscles see more than your eyes," *J Health Phys Ed Rec* September 1966, pp. 38–40.

Tarler-Benlolo, L. "The role of relaxation in biofeedback training: a critical review of the literature." 85 (1978): 727–55.

Thompson, D. H. "Immediate external feedback in the learning of golf skills." *Res Q* 40 (1969): 589–94.

Vaughn, C. L. "A three-dimensional analysis of the forces and torques applied by a golfer during the downswing," in A. Morecki, ed., *Biomechanics VII-B*. Baltimore: University Park Press, 1981.

Williams, D. *The Science of the Golf Swing.* London: Pelham, 1969.

Williams, K. R. "The mechanics of foot action during the golf swing and implications for shoe design." *Med Sci Sports Exerc* 15 (1983): 247–55.

NINE: ENDURANCE TRAINING

Adner, M. M. "Elevated high-density-lipoprotein levels in marathon runners." *JAMA* 243 (1980): 534–36.

Altman, L. K. "James Fixx: the enigma of heart disease." *New York Times*, 24 July 1984.

———. "Study finds fitness doesn't insure health." *New York Times*, 16 September 1979.

Ariel, G. B. "Biomechanics of athletic shoe design," in P. V. Komi, ed., *Biomechanics V-B*. Baltimore: University Park Press, 1976.

Bassler, T. "Immunity to atherosclerosis." *Ann NY Acad Sci* 301 (1977): 579–92.

Bates, B. T. "An assessment of subject variability, subject-shoe interface, and the evaluation of running shoes using ground reaction force data." *J Biomech* 16 (1983): 181–91.

Bruce, R. A. "Exercise stress testing in evaluation of patients with ischemic heart disease." *Progr Cardiovasc Dis* 11 (1969): 371–84.

Bruder, R. "Nature's carbo-loading secrets." *Runners World*, April 1978, pp. 50–51.

Cavagna, G. A. "Mechanical work in running." *J Appl Physiol* 19 (1964): 249–56.

Clarke, T. E. "The effects of shoe design parameters on rearfoot control in running." *Med Sci Sports Exerc* 15 (1983): 376–81.

Clarkson, P. M. "High-density-lipoprotein cholesterol in young adult weightlifters, runners and untrained subjects." *Human Biol* 53 (2)(1981): 251–57.

Clement, D. B. "A survey of overuse running injuries." *Physician and Sportsmedicine* 9 (1981): 47–58.

Convertino, V. A. "Exercise training-induced hypervolemia." *J Appl Physiol* 48 (1980): 665–69.

Costill, D. L. "Carbohydrate loading without depletion." *Runners World*, August 1978, pp. 17–25.

————. "Influence of caffeine and carbohydrate feedings on endurance performance." *Med Sci Sports* 11 (1979): 6–11.

————. "Muscle glycogen utilization during prolonged exercise on successive days." *J Appl Physiol* 31 (1971): 834–38.

————. "Physiology of marathon running." *JAMA* 221 (1972): 1024–29.

————. *A Scientific Approach to Distance Running.* New York: Track & Field News Books, 1979.

Davies, K.J.A. "Biochemical adaptation of mitochondria." *Arch Biochem Biophys* 209 (1981): 539–54.

Eddy, D. O. "The effects of continuous and interval training in women and men." *Eur J Appl Physiol* 37 (1977): 83–92.

Ekblom, B. "Effect of physical training on O_2 transport in man." *Acta Physiol Scand* (suppl) *328* (1969): 5–45.

Essig, D. "Effects of caffeine ingestion on the utilization of muscle glycogen." *Int J Sports Med* 1 (1980): 89–90.

Foster, C. "Effects of pre-exercise feedings on endurance performance." *Med Sci Sports* 11 (1979): 1–5.

Gibbons, L. W. "The acute cardiac risk of strenuous exercise." *JAMA* 244 (1980): 1799–1801.

Gobel, M. F. "Predictors of coronary artery disease from exercise stress testing." *Minn Med* 64 (1981): 143–48.

Hagberg, J. M. "Faster adjustment to and recovery from submaximal exercise in the trained state." *J Appl Physiol* 48 (1980): 218–24.

Hickson, R. C. "Linear increase in aerobic power induced by a strenuous program of endurance exercise." *J Appl Physiol* 42 (1977): 372–76.

Holt, B. "Ignoring doctor's orders Rep. Byron ran for his life." *Washington Star,* 16 November 1978.

James, S. L. "Injuries to runners." *Am J Sports Med* 6 (1978): 40–50.

Konstam, M. A. "Effect of exercise on erythrocyte count and blood activity." *Circulation* 66 (1982): 638–42.

Koplan, J. P. "An epidemiological study of the benefits and risks of running." *JAMA* 248 (1982): 3118–21.

Mikesell, K. A. "Influence of intense training on aerobic power of competitive distance runners." *Med Sci Sports Exerc* 15 (1984): 371–75.

Mole, P. A. "Adaptation of muscle to exercise." *J Clin Invest* 50 (1971): 2323–30.

Moore, M. "Carbohydrate loading: eating through the wall." *Physician and Sportsmedicine.* 9 (1981): 97–103.

Paffenbarger, R. S. "Work activity and coronary heart mortality." *N Eng J Med* 292 (1975): 545–50.

Pedoe, D. T. "The way to an athlete's heart." *New Scientist,* 2 August 1984, pp. 32–33.

Phinney, S. D. "The human metabolic response to chronic ketosis without caloric restriction." *Metabolism* 32 (1983): 769–76.

Pollock, M. L. "The quantification of endurance training programs." *Exerc Sport Sci Rev* 1 (1973): 155–88.

BIBLIOGRAPHY

Schoene, R. B. "Nutrition for ultra-endurance." *Clin Sports Med* 3 (1984): 679–92.

Shapiro, L. M. "Effect of training on left ventricular structure and function: an echocardiographic study." *Br Heart J* 50 (1983): 534–39.

Sherman, W. M. "The marathon: dietary manipulation to optimize performance." *Am J Sports Med* 12 (1984): 44–51.

Siscovick, D. S. "The incidence of primary cardiac arrest following vigorous exercise." *N Eng J Med* 311 (1984): 874–77.

Thompson, P. D. "Cardiovascular hazards of physical exercise." *Exerc Sports Sci Rev* 10 (1982): 208–35.

Williams, C. "The biological basis of aptitude: the endurance runner." *J Biosoc Sci Suppl* 7 (1981): 103–12.

Williams, K. R. "A model for the calculation of mechanical power during distance running." *J Biomech* 16 (1983): 115–28.

Wyndham, C. H. "Physiological requirements for world-class performances in endurance running." *S Afr Med J* 43 (1969): 996–1002.

TEN: SOCCER

Asami, T. Z. "Energy efficiency of ball kicking," in P. V. Komi, ed., *Biomechanics V-B*. Baltimore: University Park Press, 1976.

Bortz, W. M. "Disuse and aging." *JAMA* 248 (1982): 1203–8.

Bruce, R. A. "Exercise, functional aerobic capacity, and aging." *Med Sci Sports Exerc* 16 (1984): 8–13.

Brunner, D. *Physical Activity and Aging*. Baltimore: University Park Press, 1970.

Derscheid, G. L. "Medial collateral ligament injuries in football." *Am J Sports Med* 9 (1981): 365–68.

deVries, H. A. "Physiological effects of an exercise training regimen upon men aged 52 to 88." *J Gerontol* 25 (1970): 325–36.

Ekstrand, J. "Incidence of soccer injuries and their relation to training and team success." *Am J Sports Med* 11 (1983): 63–67.

———. "Prevention of soccer injuries." *Am J Sports Med* 11 (1983): 116–20.

———. "Soccer injuries and their mechanisms: a prospective study." *Med Sci Sports Exerc* 15 (1983): 267–70.

Gifford, R. W. "Exercise programs for the elderly." *JAMA* 252 (1984): 544–46.

Hogan, D. B. "Marathoners over sixty years of age." *J Am Geriatr Soc* 32 (1984): 121–23.

Huang, T. C. "Biomechanics of kicking," in D. N. Ghista, ed., *Human Body Dynamics*. Oxford: Clarendon Press, 1982.

James, S. L. "Injuries to runners." *Am J Sports Med* 6 (1978): 40–50.

Klissouras, V. "Adaptation to maximal effort: genetics and age." *J Appl Physiol* 35 (1973): 288–93.

Langer, E. J. "Environmental determinants of memory improvement in late adulthood." *J Personal Psychol* 37 (1979): 2003–13.

Larson, R. L. "The knee," *Clin Sports Med* 4 (1985): 209–397.

Macmillan, M. B. "Determinants of the flight of the kicked ball." *Res Q* 46 (1975): 48–57.

Marcus, J. *The World of Pelé.* New York: Mason-Charter, 1976.

Moretz, J. A. "Long-term follow-up of knee injuries in high school football players." *Am J Sports Med* 12 (1984): 298–300.

Parker, J. L. "Sawdust memories." *Ultrasport* 2 (1985): 64–67.

Rand, J. A. "The role of arthroscopy in the management of knee inuries in the athlete." *Mayo Clin Proc* 59 (1984): 77–82.

Sidney, K. H. "Frequency and intensity of exercise training for the elderly subject." *Med Sci Sports* 10 (1978): 125–31.

Stoner, L. J. "Variation in movement patterns of professional soccer players when executing a long range and medium range soccer kick," in A. Morecki, ed., *Biomechanics VII-B.* Baltimore: University Park Press, 1979, pp. 337–42.

Wiktorsson, M. "Effects of warm-up, massage, and stretching on range of motion and muscle strength in the lower extremity." *Am J Sports Med* 11 (1983): 249–52.

Zernicke, R. F. "Lower extremity forces and torques during systematic variation of non-weight bearing motion." *Med Sci Sports* 10 (1978): 21–26.

ELEVEN: EXTREME ENVIRONMENTS

Beckwith, P., cited in "Too many electrolytes spoil the drink," *Science News,* 120 (1981): 104.

Colquhoun, W. P. *Biological Rhythms and Human Performance.* New York: Academic Press, 1971.

Coyle, E. F. "Gastric emptying rates for selected athletic drinks." *Res Q* 49 (1978): 119–24.

Frisancho, A. R. "Functional adaptation to high altitude hypoxia." *Science* 187 (1975): 313–19.

Gisolfi, C. V. "Relationships among training, heat acclimation, and heat tolerance in men and women." *Med Sci Sports* 11 (1979): 56–59.

Holmes, D. S. "Biorhythms: their utility for predicting post-operative recuperative time, death and athletic performance." *J Appl Psychol* 65 (1980): 233–36.

Horne, J. A. "Human sleep and tissue restitution: some qualifications and doubts." *Clin Sci* 65 (1983): 569–78.

———. "Time of day effects with standardized exercise upon subsequent sleep." *Electroenceph Clin Neurophysiol* 40 (1976): 178–84.

Horvath, S. M. "Exercise in a cold environment." *Exerc Sport Sci Rev* 9 (1981): 221–63.

Houston, C. S. *Going High: The Story of Man and Altitude.* New York: American Alpine Club, 1980.

Hultgren, H. N. "Circulatory adaptation to high altitude." *Ann Rev Med* 19 (1968): 119–51.

Jokl, E. *Exercise and Altitude.* New York: S. Karger, 1968.

Lenfant, C. "Adaptation to high altitude." *N Eng J Med* 284 (1971): 1298–1309.

Martin, B. J. "Exercise after sleep deprivation." *Med Sci Sports Exerc* 13 (1981): 220–23.

Messner, R. *Everest.* New York: Oxford University Press, 1979.

BIBLIOGRAPHY

Quigley, B. M. " 'Biorhythms' and men's track and field world records." *Med Sci Sports Exerc* 14 (1982): 303–7.

Reilly, T. "Influence of time of day on reactions to cycling at a fixed intensity." *Brit J Sports Med* 17 (1983): 128–30.

Rossi, B. "Diurnal individual differences and performance levels in some sports activities." *Percept Motor Skills* 57 (1983): 27–30.

Surman, B. S. "Beating the clock." *Technology Review* 87 (1984): 33.

Sutton, J. R. "Exercise at altitude." *Ann Rev Physiol* 45 (1983): 427–37.

———. "Thermal illness in fun running." *Am Heart J* 100 (1980): 778–81.

West, J. B. "Human physiology at extreme altitudes on Mount Everest." *Science* 223 (1984): 784–88.

White, J. "The hydration and electrolyte maintenance properties of an experimental sports drink." *Brit J Sports Med* 17 (1983): 51–58.

Winslow, R. M. "Red cell function at extreme altitude on Mount Everest." *J Appl Physiol* 56 (1984): 109–16.

Wyndham, C. H. "The physiology of exercise under heat stress." *Ann Rev Physiol* 35 (1973): 193–220.

TWELVE: THE FUTURE OF ATHLETIC PERFORMANCE

Berg, K. "Physiological and anthropometric determinants of mile run time." *J Sports Med* 20 (1980): 390–96.

Chapman, A. E. "Kinetic limitations of maximal sprinting speed." *J Biomechanics* 16 (1983): 79–83.

Epstein, S. H. "World records: any limits?" *Science '84*, April 1984, pp. 84–85.

Jokl, E. "The future of athletic records." *Track Field Q Rev* 84 (1984): 5–16.

———. *The Physiological Basis of Athletic Records*. Springfield, IL: Charles C. Thomas, 1968.

Kitson, T. "The ultimate mile." *New Scientist*, 2 August 1984, pp. 34–35.

Koppett, L. "Can technology win the game?" *New York Times*, 24 April 1978, pp. C1, C10.

Lindsey, B. I. "Sports records as biological data." *J Biol Ed* 9 (1975): 86–91.

Lloyd, B. B. "Athletic achievement: trends and limits," in B. Davies, ed., *Science and Sporting Performance*. Oxford: Clarendon Press, 1982, pp. 86–99.

———. "The champion athlete: limiting factors in record breaking." *Proc Roy Soc Med* 62 (1969): 1164–66.

———. "World running records as maximal performances." *Suppl I to Circulation Research*, vols 20 and 21, March 1967, pp. I-218, I-226.

Nelson, R. C. "Cradle-to-Olympics athletes." *Research/Penn State*, December 1983, p. 2.

Nicholas, J. A. "The value of sports profiling." *Clin Sports Med* 3 (1984): 3–10.

Phinizy, C. "The unbelievable moment [Bob Beamon]." *Sports Illustrated*, 23 December 1968, pp. 53–56, 61.

Riegel, P. S. "Athletic records and human endurance." *American Scientist* 69 (1981): 285–90.

Rumball, W. M. "Analysis of running and the prediction of ultimate performance." *Nature* 228 (1970): 184–85.

Ryder, H. W. "Future performance in footracing." *Scientific American,* June 1976, pp. 109–19.

Tanaka, K. "A multivariate analysis of the role of certain anthropometric and physiological attributes in distance running." *Ann Human Biol* 9 (1982): 473–82.

Voy, R. O. "Technology, health and human performance." *Technology Review* 87 (1984): 29–37.

INDEX

INDEX

Carlton, Guy, 120
Carr, David, 108
Casson, Ira R., 100
Cavum septi pellucidi, 100
Celtics, Boston, 46, 57
Center of percussion, tennis racket and, 170–71
Chamberlain, Wilt, 41–42
Chandler, Joseph V., 129
Chargers, San Diego, 29, 31
Cheyne-Stokes syndrome, 258
Chiasmatic neucleus, 273
Chiefs, Kansas City, 29, 31
Cholesterol, 126–27
   coronary heart disease and, 206, 217, 220
   diet and, 217
   endurance training and, 206–7
   strength training and, 207
Chrondromalacia, 226, 244
Chronobiology, 8, 272
Cinematography, high-speed, biome-chanical analysis and, 24–26, 81–82
Cineradiography, 37
Circadian rhythms, 273
Circulation, arterial, 209–10, 213. *See also* Blood flow.
Clayton, Derek, 212, 216
Cocaine, effects of, on athletic perfor-mance, 129, 135
Coe, Sebastian, 2
Coefficient of fatigue, 280
Coefficient of friction, 103
Coefficient of restitution, values for, base-ball, 155–56
   tennis ball, 173
   tennis racket, 169, 170, 174
Colburn, Kenneth, Jr., 67
Colt, Edward, 108
Computer(s)
   baseball strategy with, 139, 160–62
   football plays, designed with, 22–29
   golf, in swing analysis, 203
   running shoes and, 232
   Sportspac, 28–29
   strength training and, 118, 120–21
   tennis rackets, designed with, 175
Concentration, effects of, on athletic per-formance, 70
Concussions, levels of, 94–95
Contraction, muscular. *See* Muscle, con-traction of.
Cook, Earshaw, 158, 160

Cooper, Ken, 118
Coronary heart disease, 206, 217, 220
Cortisone, effects of, 129
Costill, David L., 211–12, 214, 224
Court, Margaret, 176
Cousy, Bob, 46, 50
Cox, Richard H., 165
Cowboys, Dallas, 22
Coyle, Edward F., 270
Csonka, Larry, 15
Cybex equipment, 117, 122, 141–42, 185
Czeisler, Charles, 272–73

Dardik, Irving, 10
Davies, Kelvin J., 61
Davila, Alberto, 87, 91
Davis, Glenn, 108
de Acosta, Jose, 255
Dehydration, 269–70
   effects of, 269
   sports drinks and, 270–71
Dementia pugilistica, 100
deVries, Herbert, 253
Didier, Clint, 13
Diet. *See also* Nutrition.
   athletic performance and, 124–28
   fads, 124–25, 224
   pregame meal and, 127–28
Dillman, Charles J., 81–82, 231
Dintiman, George B., 18
Distance running
   lactic acid production and, 59
   oxygen consumption and, 59
Distributed practice, effects on motor skill acquisition, 202
Diurnal rhythm(s), 274
Dolphins, Miami, 12–14, 28
Donovan, Eddie, 41, 42
do Nascimenti, Edson Arantes, 233–36
Donzis, Byron, 38–40
Dore, Rene, 82
Drag, 148
Drugs, 129–36
   amphetamine(s), 129, 131, 135
   anabolic steroid(s), 130–32, 135
   butazolidin, 129
   caffeine, 130, 223
   cocaine, 129, 135
   cortisone, 129
   human growth hormone, 133
   testing for, 134–36

315

INDEX

INDEX

Musial, Stan, 149, 155
Mutation performance, 281

Nagurski, Bronko, 16
Namath, Joe, 235, 240, 241
Nastase, Ilie, 175–76
National Amateur Athletic Union, 101
National Basketball Association, 41
National Enquirer, 111
National Football League, 15
National Hockey League, 65, 75
Nautilus equipment, 118
Navratilova, Matina, 166–67
Neuromuscular facilitation, 116
Nicklaus, Jack, 193
Niekro, Phil, 146, 248
Nirschl, Robert, 179, 180, 185
Node of vibration, 171
Norman, Robert W., 34, 74, 98
North Stars, Minnesota, 75
Norton, E. F., 257, 258
Nurmi, Paavo, 18
Nutrition, 123–28. *See also* Diet.
  carbohydrate loading and, 7, 125, 220–24
  fad diets and, 124–25, 224
  hypoglycemia and, 128
  pregame meal and, 127–28
  protein requirements of athletes and, 126

Oerter, Al, 248
Oilers, Edmonton, 80
Oilers, Houston, 39
Oldfield, Brian, 16
Olympic Games
  Berlin (1936), 3, 10
  Los Angeles (1932), 57
  Los Angeles (1984), 5, 245
  Mexico City (1968), 256, 281
  Montreal (1976), 4
  Moscow (1980), 248
  Rome (1960), 129
  Seoul (1988), 272
Orioles, Baltimore, 153, 155
Orthoses, 226
Overload principle, 17
Overtraining, 225
Owens, Jesse, 3–4, 9
Oxygen
  blood doping and, 8, 61–62
  blood flow and, 210

  consumption of, 58, 59–63
  hypoxia and, 258, 262
  sideline, 57, 62–64
  transport of, 209, 213
  VO_2max and, 58, 59–63, 208, 250, 252–53, 259, 260–61
Oxygen debt, 57–64

Pacific Select Corporation, 161
Packers, Green Bay, 32
Pain, 107–10
Palmer, Arnold, 187–89, 190, 192, 198
Pastorini, Dan, 39
Patriots, New England, 32, 71
Payton, Walter, 3
Pedoe, Dan T., 213
Pelé. *See* do Nascimento, Edson Arantes.
Pheidippides, 205
Physics
  baseball batting and, 148
  baseball pitching and, 139–44
  basketball shooting and, 42–57
  collisions and, in contact sports, 32–33, 75–77, 93–95
  effective mass of sports equipment, 158
  golf swing and, 188, 191, 193
  tennis racket and, 168, 174, 176–77
Physiology
  aerobic metabolism and, 57–58
  anaerobic metabolism and, 57–58
Pilous, Rudy, 77
Pirates, Pittsburgh, 150
Pitch, baseball, 139–44
  blooper, 138
  curve, 144–46
  fastball, 140
  knuckleball, 146–48
  spitball, 148
  visual tracking of, 148–53
Plante, Jacques, 71–73, 77
Plyometrics, 17
Poikilotherm, 266
Pole vaulting, 4–5
Poupart, Jean, 66
Powerlifting, 112
Power skating, 80–81
Pregame meal, 127
Pressure platforms, 96, 203
Priest, James A., 179, 180
Prince tennis racket, 6, 169
Pronation, 226

319

VO$_2$ max (*continued*)
  genetic component of, 251–52
  marathon runners and, 208, 211

Walker, John, 2
Walsh, Bill, 29
Warriors, Philadelphia, 41
Water polo, 275
Watts, Robert G., 146–47
Weightlifting. *See also* Strength training.
  football and, 16–17
  free weights and, 120–23
  squats and, 121–23
Werblin, Sonny, 240

West, John, 264
White Sox, Chicago, 153, 156
Wicks, Don, 65
Williams, Ted, 138, 148–49
Winslow, Kellen, 29
World Boxing Council, 87
World Cup, 233, 234, 240
Wright, Kenneth, 169

Yanagisawa, Kazuo, 71
Yastrzemski, Carl, 247

Zoff, Dino, 247–48, 249